PROGNOSIS NEGATIVE

Other Health/PAC Books

The American Health Empire

Prognosis Negative

Crisis in the Health Care System

A Health/PAC Book
Edited by David Kotelchuck

VINTAGE BOOKS
A Division of Random House, New York

A Vintage Original, August 1976
First Edition
 Published in the United States by Random House, Inc., New York, and simultaneously in Canada by Random House of Canada Limited, Toronto.

Library of Congress Cataloging in Publication Data

Main entry under title:

Prognosis negative.

"A Health Policy Advisory Center book."
Bibliography: p.
Includes index.
1. Medical care—United States—Addresses, essays, lectures. I. Kotelchuck, David. II. Health Policy Advisory Center. [DNLM: 1. Delivery of health care—U. S.—Collected works. 2. Medical assistance—U. S.—Collected works. 3. Economics, Medical—U. S.—Collected works. W84 AA7 P95]
RA395.A3P76 1976 362.1'0973 75-39078
ISBN 0-394-71757-0

Manufactured in the United States of America

Charts designed by Richard Parsekian and chart typesetting done by Miriam Rodriguez

Grateful acknowledgment is made to the following for permission to reprint previously published material:

"What People Get From Health Insurance" and "Commercial Insurance Companies: Capitalizing on Illness" from "Capitalizing on Illness: The Health Insurance Industry" by Thomas S. Bodenheimer et al., reprinted from *International Journal of Health Services*, Vol. 4, Number 4, pages 583-598, Fall, 1974. Copyright © 1974 by Baywood Publishing Company, Inc. Reprinted by permission of the publisher and the author.

"Blue Cross: What Went Wrong" by Sylvia Law, reprinted from the Introduction and Chap. 2 of the book by the same title. Copyright © 1974 by Yale University. Reprinted by permission of Yale University Press.

"Getting a Fix: The U.S. Drug Monopoly" by Rick Barnhart from *Billions For Bandaids*, edited by Bodenheimer, Harding and Cummings. Copyright © 1972 by the Medical Committee for Human Rights. Reprinted by permission of the editor on behalf of the copyright proprietor.

"Something Must Be Done About Our Nursing Homes" by John Hess, reprinted from *Media and Consumer*, February, 1975. Reprinted by permission of the author.

"Bergman Aides Predicted High Nursing-Home Profit" by John Hess, reprinted from *The New York Times*, February 6, 1975. Copyright © 1975 by The New York Times Company. Reprinted by permission of the publisher.

"Latest Nursing Home Soandal: The Sigety Cover-Up" by Jack Newfield, reprinted from *The Village Voice*, January 13, 1975. Copyright © 1975 by The Village Voice. Reprinted by permission of the publisher.

"Washington Hospital Center Exposé" by Ronald Kessler, reprinted from *The Washington Post*, October 30 and 31, 1972. Copyright © 1972 by The Washington Post. Reprinted by permission of the publisher.

"Hospital Workers: A Case Study in the 'New Working Class'" by John and Barbara Ehrenreich, reprinted from *The Monthly Review*, January 1973. Copyright © 1973 by John and Barbara Ehrenreich. To be included in the forthcoming book, *The Social Functions of Medicine—An Anthology* to be published by Monthly Review Press.

"The Hospital Workers: 'The Best Contract Anywhere'?" by Elinor Langer, reprinted from *New York Review of Books*, June 3, 1971. Copyright © 1971 by Elinor Langer. Reprinted by permission of the author, c/o International Creative Management.

"Origins of the Government Health Insurance Issue" by Theodore R. Marmor, reprinted from the chapter entitled "The Congress: Medicare Politics and Policy" from *American Political Institutions and Public Policy* edited by Allan P. Sindler (Little, Brown and Company). Reprinted by permission of the author.

"The Politics of Health Care: What Is It Costing You?" by Godfrey Hodgson, reprinted from *The Atlantic*, October, 1973. Copyright © 1973 by Godfrey Hodgson. Reprinted by permission of Harold Matson Co., Inc.

"Refused Hospital Bed, Man Held in Robbery" by William L. Clairborne and Alfred E. Lewis, reprinted from *The Washington Post*, March 22, 1972. Copyright © 1972 by The Washington Post. Reprinted by permission of the publisher.

"Hospitals For Sale" by Elinor Blake and Thomas Bodenhemier, reprinted from *Ramparts*, February, 1974. Copyright ©

Preface

This anthology brings together a collection of writings on the U.S. health-care system that have been in demand from the Health Policy Advisory Center (Health/PAC) over the years. The collection examines the industrialization of the health-care system, its impact on patients and health workers, and the forces shaping the system. It then examines the role of the federal government in financing and regulating the health-care system and evaluates proposals for further government intervention in the system, including national health insurance.

These selections have until now been widely dispersed in the literature, throughout the Health/PAC *Bulletin* and in many books, magazines and newspapers. We have tried to provide a consistent intellectual thread throughout by a series of section and chapter introductions that highlight key ideas and point out the relationships between selections.

One significant problem in assembling the selections was the impossibility of covering every major topic of interest about the health-care system. We have chosen a wide range of issues, but particularly regret that we are not able to include an analysis of social relations that characterize the health-care system or of agents for change of the system.

A precursor to this book was developed for a course

on social issues in health care taught at Notre Dame University in the summer of 1974. We thank Paula Woletz, then a student intern at Health/PAC, for helping assemble that earlier version of this book; Peter Robinson of the National Center for Urban Ethnic Affairs and Sister Sharon Stanton of the Catholic Committee on Urban Ministry for their support and encouragement in developing the Notre Dame course; Terry Mizrahi Madison, who helped teach the course; and the many students, faculty and staff whose enthusiastic response encouraged us to refine that curriculum into this anthology.

The staff of the Health Policy Advisory Center helped conceptualize and develop this book. Health/PAC is an independent, nonprofit research and educational organization engaging in analysis on issues of health policy for an audience that includes health-care workers, community groups and students. Since 1968 it has regularly published the Health/PAC *Bulletin*, as well as occasional reports on topics of special interest. Staff members are Barbara Caress, Oliver Fein, David Kotelchuck, Ronda Kotelchuck, Louise Lander, Howard Levy and Steve London in Health/PAC's New York office; and Elinor Blake, Thomas Bodenheimer, Dan Feshbach and David Landau in the San Francisco office. We thank Ken Rosenberg for his help in getting the book to press.

Finally, Health/PAC wishes to thank Mr. Samuel Rubin and the Samuel Rubin Foundation for their generous support over the years.

—October, 1975

Contents

Introduction

To many people the American health-care system appears to be a chaotic conglomeration of health personnel, programs and facilities—thoroughly infested by self-seeking special interests and too disorganized to deal with larger system-wide problems. The problems of the system are manifest: neglect, shoddy care and medical abuse for some; overhospitalization and overreliance on medical technology for most; costly, fragmented, impersonal care for all.

The last decade has seen one proposal for government intervention after another trotted out as panacea for the health-care crisis. On top of the bewildering array of fragmented interests that have comprised the health-care system since World War II have come government-financed programs such as Medicare and Medicaid, with their unfulfilled promise of equal access to health care for all. These have been followed by an alphabet soup of regulatory measures: Health Maintenance Organizations (HMO's), Professional Standards Review Organizations (PSRO's), Comprehensive Health Planning Agencies (CHPA's), Health Systems Agencies (HSA's), plus more than a dozen national health insurance proposals. No wonder observers throw up their hands in dismay at ever making sense out of all these pieces and call this a health-care nonsystem.

In fact there *is* a health-care system—what's more, it is a system in transition. In its first book, *The American Health Empire* (Vintage, 1971), Health/PAC described a system that quite efficiently pursues its own priorities of profits, research and education. Since medical care is often only a by-product of the system, not its foremost priority, the system appears inefficient, a nonsystem, when viewed from the perspective of the patient.

The current American health-care system took shape after World War II, built on advanced medical technology and largely underwritten by Blue Cross financing. It developed from cottage industry based in the physician's office to corporate structure based in the hospital.

No sooner had the system taken on the features of modern industry than, just as in other industries, a period of unparalleled growth and consolidation began. The fuel for this expansion was a vast influx of federal money. During the 1950's and early 1960's government funds were earmarked for research and went primarily to academic medical institutions. Following the enactment of Medicare and Medicaid in 1966, vast sums of money ostensibly for patient care poured virtually without government controls into hospitals and other health-care institutions, ranging from nursing homes and community mental health centers to drug and alcohol treatment centers.

The next five years were a period akin to the heyday of the robber barons during the late 1800's (and the experience of that period largely informed the analysis presented in *The American Health Empire*). Medical empires developed from academic medical centers, swallowing up public and smaller private hospitals through a variety of affiliation agreements. Hospitals grew by leaps and bounds, building new facilities, adding new beds, staff and equipment and expanding outpatient services into the surrounding communities. Health-care costs skyrocketed.

The expansionary visions of health-care providers, not to mention their old-fashioned greed, threatened to kill the goose that laid the golden egg. Annual federal expenditures for health care approached $20 billion by 1970, rising faster than any other major component of the federal budget. Unable to stem the flow of federal health-care dollars, the federal government stepped in, gingerly at first and with more authority later, to regulate the health-care industry. In this effort the government could count on support by the general public, which was complaining bitterly about rising health-care costs, as well as those who were beginning to question the value of the impersonal, technically oriented, crisis care which the system delivered.

If the 1960's were a period of unfettered expansion and corporatization of the health-care system, the 1970's are a period of government intervention to contain and rationalize the system. The central debate today among the powerful interest groups shaping the health-care system is not whether the government will intervene in the system, but the nature and extent of the regulation it will impose in return for its massive investment in the system.

This book attempts to provide an up-to-date overview of the health-care system that sees through the public relations fog enveloping all proposals for federal intervention to the institutional and governmental imperatives that lie behind it. In Section I, we look at internal developments in the health-care system during the 1970's, in particular at the major interest groups that have shaped the system since World War II—medical empires, the health insurance industry and the profiteers within the system. In Section II, we discuss the impact of the industrialization of health care on the health workforce and the response of health workers to that development, both in labor unions and among professional groups. Both of these sections are a necessary prelude to Section III, in which we examine the federal government's increasing intervention in the health-care system and evaluate several recent legislative initiatives, including key national health insurance proposals. In this final section we also include a discussion of the malpractice crisis, a crisis in fee-for-service health care that has already triggered government intervention in the health-care system.

I.
Health Care Institutions

Despite the lingering power of fee-for-service doctors, three forces have been allied since the end of World War II to shape the current U.S. health-care delivery system: academic medical empires, health-care financiers (predominantly Blue Cross) and health-care profiteers (ranging from hospital supply and drug companies to nursing home entrepreneurs). The most striking feature of the system they spawned is how little its priorities have to do with any rational assessment of the health-care needs of the American people and how much they have to do with the particular priorities of each interest group.

Academic medical empires, kingpins of this alliance, contributed to the scientific and technical advances in medicine following World War II—and reaped handsome benefits from them as well. By parlaying federal research grants with a growing prestige that assured plenty of paying patients to fill their beds, academic hospitals have come to dominate health-care delivery in their surrounding areas.

Despite their ability to deliver the world's most advanced hospital care and their vast new powers within the health-care system, the empires' priorities have remained what they had always been: research and education. But the dynamics of scientific research and medical education are different from those of optimal health care. Sometimes the two touch upon and reinforce each other, as in the case of antibiotics, a basic research discovery that turned out to be of enormous human benefit. Sometimes these interests conflict, as in the case of the infamous Willowbrook experiments (where retarded children serving as experimental subjects were injected with live hepatitis virus), in the use of inadequately tested drugs on humans in a headlong rush for experimental results, or in the mundane but equally significant organization by hospitals of dozens of specialty clinics that suit the needs of students and researchers but that may confuse, discourage and sometimes mistreat the patients.

Although there have been incidental relationships between the needs of research and teaching and those of patient care, it is the pursuit of the former that has made the academic medical empires the centers of power that they are today. Thus research stars continue to be the most prestigious members of the medical profession, and new generations of medical students continue to be molded in the image of doctor as medical research scientist.

In the medical empires' pursuit of their particular needs, the financing agencies have been a major ally. Blue Cross, oldest and largest of the private financiers of the health-care system, has for decades been tilting the system toward hospitals by paying only for care delivered in them. This fact is not surprising, since Blue Cross was founded by hospitals during the Depression to help them collect their bills and has been dominated by hospital interests ever since.

But the increasing concentration of health-care delivery in hospitals in many ways conflicts with the requirements of optimal health care. By the very process of concentrating medical resources, hospitals make these resources less accessible to patients. This poses problems both in cases of emergency, when time means life, and in those of marginal medical problems, when people may become discouraged from seeking the treatment their condition requires. In many other cases a person's physical and emotional well-being (which are of course linked) would be better served by treatment at home, at a local physician's office or at a community clinic than in an impersonal hospital setting. This is true in many instances of childbirth, chronic illness or impending death. Sometimes home care just means less bother and expense than hospital care. But whatever these differing circumstances, Blue Cross finances only hospital care and hospital care is what people have to get if they want their medical care to be paid for.

The third major interest group that has shaped the health-care system since World War II are the medical profiteers, especially the hospital supply and drug companies. These corporations have translated technological and medical advances into enormous profits, at the ultimate expense of the patients, and have reinforced the trend toward institutionally based, high-technology medical care.

The first chapter of this section presents background information on public health and health-care financing in the United States, followed by an overview of the role of medical empires, health-care financiers and health-care profiteers in shaping today's health-care system. The next three chapters examine in depth each of these three major forces: medical empires in Chapter 2, the health insurance industry in Chapter 3 and the health-care profiteers in Chapter 4. The readings in each chapter demonstrate the serious deficiencies in health care that are a by-product of the pursuit of narrow private interests. As we examine the development of each of these forces and their impact on health-care delivery, we must remember that patient care is the ultimate measure of the American health-care system—and represents its ultimate failure.

1

The Health-Care Delivery System

THE HEALTH STATUS OF AMERICANS

David Kotelchuck

Health care is now the second largest industry in the United States, larger even than the defense industry. In fiscal 1975, Americans spent $104 billion for health care, compared to $88 billion for military expenditures.[1,2]

Yet everyone who watches television, reads a newspaper or needs a doctor knows that this country faces a health crisis. American health care is expensive—and it's not all that good, either. Some individual patients may receive excellent care, especially if the case is medically interesting or the person wealthy, but for most of us the quality of the health-care delivery system is uneven and woefully inadequate. Public health statistics tell the story of that system—how it reflects and perpetuates differences in health status that in turn stem from social inequalities based on class and race.

INFANT MORTALITY

The infant mortality rate in the United States has been steadily declining since the turn of the century, from 162 infant deaths per thousand live births in 1900 to 17.7 in 1973.[3] But in recent decades the United States has not kept up with the progress in other countries.

In 1955 this country ranked eighth in infant mortality among the twenty leading industrial countries; by 1973 it had dropped to fifteenth (Figure 1). If in 1973 the United States had the same infant mortality rate as Sweden, the lives of 25,000 American children would have been saved. If it had even achieved the rate of Japan, which had the lowest rate among countries of comparable population, size and degree of industrialization, almost 20,000 lives would have been saved.

Three factors highlight infant mortality in the United States. They are the wide variations in infant deaths according to geography, race and class. Mississippi, with a 1973 infant mortality rate of 25.2 deaths per thousand live births, has almost twice the mortality rate of Utah, the state with the lowest rate (12.9 deaths per thousand live births).[4] The infant mortality rate for black children is 65 percent greater than that for white children (26.2 versus 15.8 deaths per thousand live births).[3] Children whose fathers are service workers and laborers show a 50 percent greater mortality rate than those whose fathers are professionals and managers, and this result is true both for black and white fathers separately (Figure 2). There is also a strong association between infant mortality and family income, a rough indicator of class.[5]

The parameters of race and class are linked, of course, and both help explain the mortality differences between states like Utah and Mississippi. Our modern

Rank (1955)	Rate	Rank (1973)	Rate
1 Sweden	17.4	1 Sweden	9.6
2 Netherlands	20.1	2 Finland	10.1
3 Norway	20.6	3 Norway	11.3
4 Australia	22.0	4 Netherlands	11.6
5 New Zealand	24.5	5 Japan	11.7
6 Denmark	25.2	6 Switzerland	12.8
7 United Kingdom	25.9	7 France	12.9
8 United States	26.4	8 Denmark	13.5
9 Switzerland	26.5	9 East Germany	16.0
10 Finland	29.7	10 New Zealand	16.2
11 Canada	31.3	11 Australia	16.7
12 Czechoslovakia	34.1	12 Canada	16.8
13 Ireland	36.8	13 Belgium	17.0
14 France	38.6	14 United Kingdom	17.5
15 Japan	39.8	**15 United States**	17.7
16 Belgium	40.7	16 Ireland	17.8
17 Austria	40.7	17 West Germany	20.4
18 West Germany	41.7	18 Czechoslovakia	21.2
19 East Germany	48.8	19 Austria	23.7
20 U.S.S.R.	—	20 U.S.S.R.	26.3

FIG. 1 INFANT MORTALITY Death Rate Per 1,000 Live Births

Sources: United Nations: *Demographic Yearbook 1957,* 9th Issue (N.Y., 1957) pp. 200-09 and *Demographic Yearbook 1973,* 25th Issue (N.Y., 1974) pp. 256-62

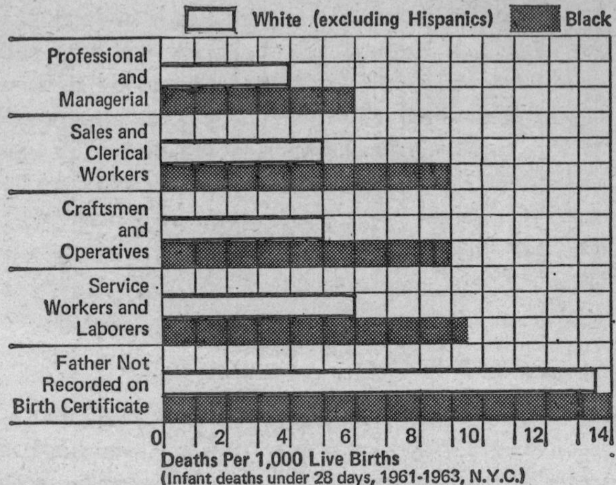

FIG. 2 INFANT DEATHS BY OCCUPATION OF FATHER AND RACE Source: Report in Reference 6, p. 112

health system did not create race and class distinctions, to be sure, but it reflects and reinforces them. For example, a recent study gives striking evidence of the value of maternal health services in reducing infant mortality.[6] The mortality rate of infants whose mothers received inadequate medical care was two and a half times greater than that of infants whose mothers received adequate care. The mortality rate for infants whose mothers received what was considered intermediate care was 50 percent greater than for mothers receiving adequate care. The infant mortality rate in New York City, site of the study, would have dropped by one-third (from 21.9 to 14.7 deaths per thousand live births) if all mothers had had the pregnancy outcome of those receiving adequate care. What's more, the results indicated that improved maternal health services would significantly reduce racial and class differences in infant mortality. Despite such findings, the government is cutting back funds for maternal and child health care. In turn, many hospitals are restricting or eliminating clinics and outpatient centers delivering these services, despite their relatively low cost and hospital protestations of concern about patient care. Thus recent health policies, instead of narrowing class and race differences for infant mortality, appear to be increasing them.

LIFE EXPECTANCY

As a result of improved living standards and recent medical advances, the life expectancy of Americans has increased from 47 years at the turn of the century to 71 years in 1973—an additional 24 years.[7] Most of this dramatic rise, however, had taken place by 1949 when the average life span reached 68 years. In the quarter century since then, life expectancy has increased by only three years. During this period women have fared better than men in extending their life span. By 1973 female life expectancy was 75.3 years compared to 67.6 years for men, the largest difference between the sexes in this century.[7]

For those who have reached age 65, the remaining life expectancy has changed by just three years since the turn of the century, from 12 to 15 years.[8] (Almost all this change in life expectancy at age 65 is due to increased female longevity.) This indicates that improvements in life expectancy during this century reflect improved survival rates for infants and young people, and that organized medicine, despite great expense and effort, has consistently failed to control the chronic, degenerative diseases of old age such as heart disease, cancer and stroke.

As in the case of infant mortality, other countries have advanced more rapidly in life expectancy since the 1950's, while the United States has fallen behind. Between 1955 and 1972 the United States dropped from sixth to sixteenth among the leading industrial nations for male life expectancy, and from third to sixth for female life expectancy (Figure 3).[9,10] Among all United Nations members, the United States ranked a poor thirty-fifth in male life expectancy and an unimpressive sixteenth in female life expectancy.[11]

Within this country the life expectancy of black men is fully 6.5 years shorter than that of white men (61.9 vs. 68.4 years respectively), and the life expectancy of black women is 6 years less than that of white women (70.1 vs. 76.1 years, respectively).[7] The life expectancies of other racial and ethnic groups are not tabulated by the U.S. Census Bureau, but life expectancies are estimated to be 63 to 64 years for native Americans [12] compared to 71 years for all Americans.[7] The life expectancies of Chicanos appear to be intermediate between these two, based on age-adjusted death rates.[13]

ILLNESS AND DISABILITY

In 1972, one out of every eight civilian, noninstitutionalized persons in the United States (12.7 percent) was limited in activity to some degree due to a chronic condition.[14] Of this group, nearly one in four, 3.0 percent of the total population, was totally unable to carry on his or her major activity.

The prevalence of chronic conditions is closely linked to age, income and race. As to age, the 12.7 percent of the population restricted in activity represents 43 percent of those age 65 and over, 21 percent of

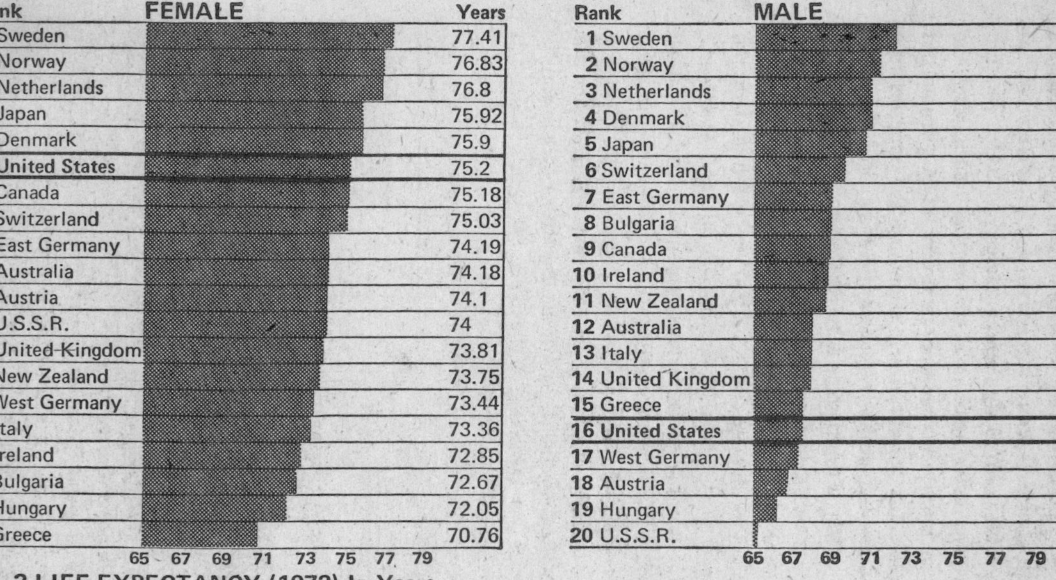

FIG. 3 LIFE EXPECTANCY (1972) In Years

Source: Reference 8

those between 45 and 64 years (who should be at the peak of their earning capacity) and even 8 percent of those between 17 and 44 years.[15]

Even more striking is the inverse relationship between family income and disability. It is a truism, of course, that people with low incomes are poor because they are sick and sick because they are poor. In either case, illness limits their earning capacity, and although they are most in need of health care, they are least able to afford it. Thirty percent of all people whose yearly family income is less than $3,000 are disabled, but only 8 percent with incomes over $10,000 are.[16] The large number of elderly people found in the low-income group contributes to this difference, but even within a particular age group the poor are more frequently disabled than those of higher income. Consider persons 45 to 64 years old. Half of those whose family

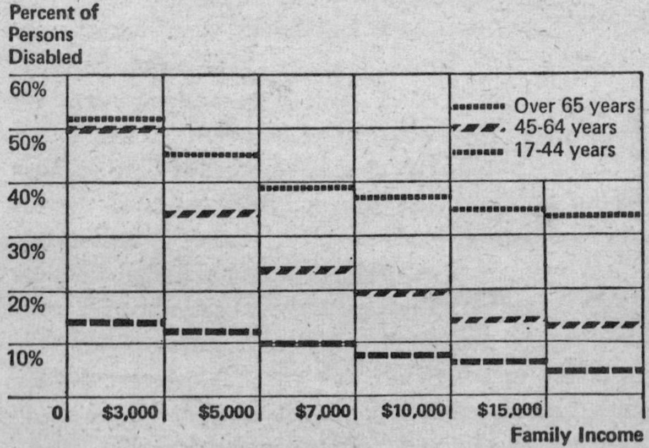

FIG. 4 PERCENT OF POPULATION DISABLED ACCORDING TO AGE AND FAMILY INCOME
Source: Reference 18

income is less than $3,000 are disabled, but only one in eight (13 percent) with incomes of more than $15,-000 are (Figure 4). Similarly, people whose family income is less than $5,000 suffer 60 percent more restricted-activity days each year than the average citizen, 50 percent more days disabled in bed and 60 percent more days in the hospital.[17]

As measured by many different parameters blacks are less healthy than whites. Black adults suffer from activity-limiting chronic conditions about 25 percent more often than whites. What's more, they suffer more severely—blacks are 50 percent more likely than whites to be limited in their ability to move about freely.[18] They experience more days of restricted activity and more days restricted to bed than whites, of course due in part to their lower average income.[19]

HEALTH SERVICES

As we have seen, health problems vary dramatically with race, class, income and geography. But the delivery of health services, instead of compensating for these inequalities, reflects and exaggerates them.

An outstanding feature of the health-care-delivery system is the geographic maldistribution of doctors and other health workers. Alaska has 62.5 doctors per 100,000 people, whereas California has 160 doctors per 100,000 people.[20] Generally, the large industrial states have over 50 percent more physicians per resident than do states in the South and rural Northwest. Within states doctors tend to congregate in metropolitan areas. As shown in Figure 5, counties with fewer than 10,000 people have only 47.5 physicians per 100,000 population, compared to 232.6 for counties with 5,000,000 and over—a factor of five in the doctor-patient ratio.

Population— Non-Metropolitan*	Number of physicians per 100,000 population
Under 10,000	47.5
10,000-25,000	56.6
25,000-50,000	76.1
Over 50,000	103.8
Metropolitan*	
50,000-500,000	140.4
500,000-1 million	161.2
1 million-5 million	194.4
Over 5 million	232.6

*County Census Classification

FIG. 5 PHYSICIAN LOCATION BY COUNTY CENSUS CLASSIFICATION, 1970

Source: *Reference Data on Socio-Economic Issues of Health, 1973 edition,* American Medical Association (Chicago, 1973) p. 120

Similar maldistribution occurs for other health workers. For example, Massachusetts has 649 employed registered nurses per 100,000 population, whereas Arkansas has only 190.[21] As recently as 1969, 134 counties in the United States with a combined population of nearly half a million people did not have even one practicing physician.[20]

Within large cities doctors tend to avoid poverty areas. In Chicago, there are 40 percent fewer general practitioners per 100,000 persons in poverty areas than in other areas, 56 percent fewer specialists of all types and 66 percent fewer board-certified specialists.[22] These trends obviously run counter to patient needs, reflecting instead the social backgrounds and financial aspirations of doctors, as well as their professional interests in being near other doctors and major medical centers. (That this is not simply a matter of doctors pursuing the dollar is evidenced by the many rural communities that cannot get a doctor despite offers of large guaranteed incomes.)

Geographical disparities are also reflected in hospital distribution. The number of hospital beds per 1,000 persons is on the average 60 percent greater in the industrial New England and Middle Atlantic states than in the Rocky Mountain states.[23] Massachusetts, with 11 beds per 1,000 persons, has more than twice as many beds per person as Utah, with 4.7. This reflects too many beds in metropolitan areas, as well as too few in rural areas.

The lack of health personnel and facilities in rural and poverty areas contributes to the traditionally inadequate health care for nonwhite and low-income persons. In 1971, 66 percent of all blacks visited a physician, as compared to 73 percent of all whites; blacks averaged 4.4 doctor visits, as compared to 5.0 for whites.[24] To compensate for the decreasing number of doctors in their neighborhoods, blacks have been making greater use of hospital outpatient clinics in recent years. Thus in 1971 blacks used hospital clinics for 21 percent of their physician encounters, more than twice as often as whites, who used clinics for only 9 percent of their visits.[24] As would be expected, poor people, both white and black, use clinics much more frequently than middle-income and upper-income people.

As a result of this increased reliance on clinics, abetted by federal Medicaid and Medicare financing, the traditional differences of race and class as to frequency of doctor visits is narrowing. It should be remembered, however, that eliminating this gap does not solve the problem of two-class health care. Blacks and poor people suffer from more serious health problems than the average person. An equitable health-care delivery system, with access based strictly on medical need, would thus deliver more care than the average to these population groups, now and for many years to come.

For preventive care and for less acute medical problems, traditional differences in access to health services continue unabated. Half of all white people, but only 30 percent of all black people, visit a dentist at least once a year.[24] Use of dentists by both whites and blacks rises sharply with income. For example, 32 percent of low-income whites, 44 percent of middle-income whites and 61 percent of upper-income whites see a dentist at least once a year.[24] An upper-income person is three and a half times more likely to have a routine physical examination and four and a half times more likely to visit a pediatrician or obstetrician than a person of low income.[25] Generally, physician use for preventive services declines as income declines: in 1964, preventive services accounted for 18 percent of all physician visits by people of high income but only 11 percent for people of low income.[25]

But public health statistics only tell part of the story. Questions about the American health-care system penetrate to the quality of care itself. Studies done in England question the medical value of specialized, coronary care units in hospitals for patients with heart attacks.[26] These studies demonstrate that patients with heart attacks who stay at home do not die any more often than patients who are treated in coronary care units. Women's health activists, for another example, have pointed to the fact that it may be more dangerous to deliver a baby inside a hospital than at home.[27] It has also been demonstrated that some of the procedures routinely used during labor and delivery may adversely affect the baby.[28]

HEALTH COSTS

Whatever or whomever you blame for what's wrong with the American health-care delivery system, you can't say we don't spend enough money for health care. The $104 billion we spent in fiscal 1974 ($485 per person) is larger than all U.S. military expenditures [1,2] and by far exceeds the health-care expenditure of any other country in the world. Indeed, it exceeds the *entire* gross national product (GNP) of Africa for any year and is three-quarters the 1970 GNP of Latin America.[29] This vast sum of money amounts to 7.7 percent of our gross national product.[30] And while it is difficult to compare this percentage among countries (because different expenditures are included in it from country to country), this is clearly one of the largest percentages of GNP spent on health care by any industrial country.[31] For example, Great Britain spends only about 5 percent of its much smaller GNP on health care.

Not only are U.S. health-care costs enormous, they have been growing rapidly in recent years—so rapidly in fact that they are beginning to exceed the capacity of ordinary working people to pay. As shown in Figure 6, between 1960 and 1974 U.S. health expenditures quadrupled and the percentage of GNP spent on health care rose from 5.2 to 7.7 percent.

The medical-care component of the consumer price index is a good indicator for comparing the rise in health-care costs with that of other consumer items. Generally this component has been rising faster than the consumer price index for all consumer items since World War II. But what had been a steady rise during the 1950's and early 1960's took a sharp turn upward after 1966 (Figure 7). It is now generally accepted

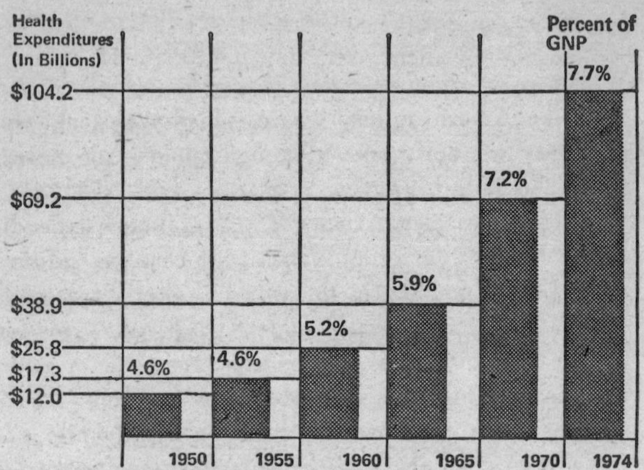

FIG. 6 NATIONAL HEALTH EXPENDITURES AND PERCENT OF GROSS NATIONAL PRODUCT
Selected years 1950-74

Source: Reference 1, p. 5

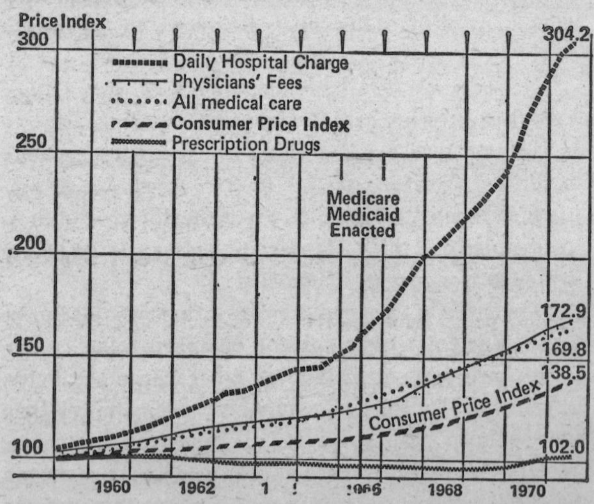

FIG. 7 MEDICAL COMPONENTS OF CONSUMER PRICE INDEX (1960-1970)

Source: Reference 19, p. 17

that the cause of this health-care cost inflation was the implementation of the Medicare and Medicaid legislation in 1966. These programs gave health-care providers access to generous amounts of federal funds with virtually no fiscal controls—and the providers were quick to take advantage. Between 1966 and 1970, while the consumer price index increased by 19.7 percent for all consumer items, hospital daily service charges rose by a whopping 71.3 percent, physicians' fees by 30 percent and overall medical-care costs by 29.1 percent.[32]

Since the implementation of Medicare and Medicaid in 1966, hospital daily service charges have not only led the medical-care component of the consumer price index, they have been the fastest-rising single item in any category on the index.[33] This increase has been largely due to new facilities and equipment and increased staff size at the hospitals, all encouraged by government health spending. (Hospitals put most of the blame on rising workers' wages, especially where workers have become unionized. But payroll expenses have remained an almost constant 60 percent of hospital expenses since World War II.[34] So wages can hardly be the *cause* of the post-1966 inflation, although the increases in wages certainly reflect and reinforce the inflationary trends.)

To protect themselves from financial disaster in the event of serious illness, many Americans have turned to private health insurance plans. According to U.S. government estimates, 78 percent of all civilians under 65 years of age have some insurance coverage for hospital care.[35] But only 35 percent are covered for visits to a doctor's office, and a mere 11 percent are covered for dental care. Private insurance companies, both

Blue Cross–Blue Shield and commercial companies, pay 41 percent of consumer expenditures for health care—75 percent of hospital costs, 49 percent of doctors' fees but only 7 percent of all other health-care costs.[36] For those 65 years of age and over, Medicare covers only 42 percent of health-care costs.[37] Thus, the bulk of health-care costs still falls directly on the consumer.

Left out in the cold entirely are those who have no health insurance of any kind. As would be expected, these are generally the people most in need of health care. For example, while 90 percent of those under 65 with family incomes of $10,000 or more had insurance coverage for hospital care in 1970, only 39 percent of those with incomes under $3,000 had such coverage.[38] Some of those in the lowest income categories were covered by the public Medicaid program. Nevertheless, 25 million Americans have no health insurance at all, private, Medicaid or Medicare.[39]

THE STRUCTURE OF AMERICAN HEALTH CARE

The health-care system seems so chaotic, so unplanned, so uncoordinated, that many people call it a nonsystem. To cure the health-care crisis, they conclude, we must turn it into a system. Specifically, they argue, some form of national health insurance would provide financially shaky hospitals with a stable income. Doctors should be encouraged to form group practices to increase efficiency—the equivalent of corner grocers banding together to open a supermarket. And hospitals and medical schools should be linked together into regional networks that would be able efficiently and rationally to plan for the medical needs of an entire region. More money, more planning, more coordination—that is the standard prescription for the ailing American health system.

But careful examination of the structure of health care indicates that, in fact, there is a health-care system: it is not totally chaotic and unplanned; it seems so only if described in terms of private doctors. Years ago, the doctors did dominate and control health care; however, today health is dominated by institutions—hospitals, medical schools, research laboratories, drug companies, health insurance companies, health planning agencies and many others. Many people don't even have a private doctor any more; the hospital clinic and emergency room have become their doctor. Less than 20 percent of the nation's health expenditures now go for private doctors; most of the rest goes to institutions. And more than nine out of ten health workers these days are not doctors at all, but workers employed by health-care institutions—nurses, dieticians, X-ray technicians, orderlies, laboratory technicians, and so on. The health institutions are big and growing rapidly, and as they grow they are becoming more and more interconnected to form a system.

There are three major components to the existing American health-care system: medical empires, the financing-planning complex and the health-care profiteers, especially the medical-industrial complex.

MEDICAL EMPIRES

Medical empires are the primary units. They are privately controlled medical complexes, usually but not always organized with a medical school at the hub. Radiating out from these centers like spokes on a wheel are a network of affiliations to smaller private hospitals, city hospitals, state mental hospitals, neighborhood health centers and subspecialty programs in areas such as alcoholism, rehabilitation or prison health. To each of these affiliated programs, the medical center provides professional personnel in return for healthy rake-offs of the affiliated programs' resources. In fact, the benefits of such arrangements are often so highly weighted in favor of the medical center that *exploitation* is the only fair description of the relationship—thus the term "empires." These networks of medical centers with their far-reaching affiliations resemble a mother country's relationship to its colonies. This resemblance has been exacerbated by the fact that many of the affiliation relationships are with hospitals, neighborhood centers and special programs in poor communities, most often populated by blacks, Puerto Ricans, Chicanos, Asians or Appalachians.

The empires have their own priorities. Some of these are related to expansion and profit-making, others are related to research and teaching, and still others are concerned with control—influencing policy both locally and nationally. How much any of these priorities relates to patient care is the critical question. The answer is complicated and in many instances not yet fully understood. On balance, however, these priorities are the basis for the exploitative relationship between the medical center and its affiliates.

Take, for example, Einstein College of Medicine (a

medical school) and Montefiore Hospital and Medical Center (a close ally). Together they have come to control most of the medical resources in the Bronx, an entire borough of New York City. Through affiliation contracts, Einstein/Montefiore monopolizes care at three out of the four city hospitals in the Bronx, the only state mental hospital in the borough, several neighborhood health centers, prison health services, several private voluntary hospitals and numerous nursing homes. Of the 6,670 beds in general-care hospitals in the Bronx, 4,500 are controlled by Einstein/Montefiore; most doctors practicing in the Bronx are affiliated with Einstein/Montefiore.

What has this arrangement meant for patients? Perhaps, and this has not been proven, the technical-scientific management of hospitalized patients has improved. But the price for this questionable improvement, questionable both in terms of money and in terms of distorted priorities, is enormous:

- In sheer dollars, the affiliation of the city hospitals to Einstein/Montefiore has increased the money coming into those hospitals by over $37 million a year.
- In the outpatient departments of the affiliated hospitals, subspecialty clinics have proliferated—in some cases to more than a hundred in number. Patients have found their care fragmented, with no single doctor taking responsibility. On the one hand, the patient has no one to see for a common cold; on the other hand, when he or she has a more complicated illness, it takes a visit to three or four separate clinics before a diagnosis can be made, and even then a different doctor may supervise the patient's treatment each visit.
- In the inpatient services (that is, hospitalized patients), all the hospitals were converted through affiliations into teaching institutions. Patients fre-

quently find themselves subjected to unnecessary and occasionally dangerous procedures. Liver biopsies (removal of tissue from the liver), for example, are performed primarily to teach interns how to do the procedure; Caesarean sections and hysterectomies are performed when their medical necessity is questionable at best, so that the residents can gain more experience in performing these operations.

- In research, the affiliations have brought more academic interest to the affiliated hospitals, but not necessarily more patient-oriented controls. In one such hospital, patients admitted for a routine tubal ligation (sterilization) were given medication prior to the operation and then had their ovaries biopsied to determine the effect of the medication on the ovaries. The patients were not asked for their informed consent. Moreover, it turned out that no research proposal had been submitted, as required, to the hospital's research committee.

Besides elevating the medical center's priorities without regard for patients' priorities, medical empires tend to institutionalize the unequal relationship between the mother medical center and the colony-affiliated hospital. This is done in overt ways, with the medical center extracting natural resources from the affiliated hospital. Patients with interesting or rare diseases are taken from the affiliated hospital and brought to the medical center, while patients with mundane medical problems are "dumped" by the medical center onto its affiliates. Likewise, talented medical teachers and researchers located in the affiliated hospitals are asked to spend unpaid teaching time at the medical center. This means that their talents are utilized by the medical center while their salary continues to be paid out of the affiliated hospital's budget. On the other hand, when the affiliated hospital wants the expertise of a researcher at the medical center, it has to pay handsomely for a lecture or consultation.

In addition to such overt discrimination, there are more subtle ways in which inequalities within a medical empire are institutionalized. Patients being referred from the affiliated hospital to the medical center for some specialized procedure, such as cardiac catheterization or cobalt therapy, may end up on waiting lists for months. The scheduling priorities are explicit: private patients come first, clinic patients from the medical center come second and the affiliated hospital's patients come third. Another example is the fact that pension programs and other fringe benefits for the professional personnel on the medical center's staff are significantly more generous than those for the affiliated hospital's staff. The list could go on and on.

Some people may minimize the importance of medical empires. "It hasn't happened here," they will say. "The county medical society is still the strongest force in town." While such an observation may be accurate in many rural and some suburban communities, the nationwide trend is very clear: in Cleveland, Case Western Reserve Medical School controls many of the medical resources; in Baltimore, it's Johns Hopkins Medical School; in Seattle, it's the University of Washington; in North Carolina, its Duke University and the University of North Carolina. And everywhere the results are the same: the structure of health care is organized around the institutional priorities of the medical center and not the health-care needs of the patient. And that disparity of priorities is most accentuated when the individual is not an affluent private patient at the medical center but a poor or uninsured ward or clinic patient at one of its affiliated institutions.

THE FINANCING-PLANNING COMPLEX

The second main part of the health-care system is the financing-planning complex. The most important segment of this complex is the multibillion-dollar Blue Cross operation, whose insurance plans cover 80 million people, four of every ten Americans. Through the publicly funded Medicare and Medicaid programs, Blue Cross administers insurance benefits for an additional 32 million people. Altogether, Blue Cross disburses about half of all hospital revenues.

Because it is by far the nation's largest single health insurer, Blue Cross also plays a very important role in setting health policy: its leaders sit on governmental advisory committees, advise congressional committees and, together with representatives of the big private hospitals, set up and run areawide comprehensive health planning agencies.

Blue Cross is closely allied with the big hospitals. It was set up during the Depression by financially starved hospitals to provide them a guaranteed income, and it continues to be dominated by the major hospitals. Nearly half the members of the boards of directors of local Blue Cross plans (Blue Cross operates in seventy-four localities) are hospital representatives. Needless to say, hospitals and health consumers often have very different interests. Consumers want high-quality, low-cost, relevant health care; hospitals, on the other hand, are often more interested in institutional expansion and the prestige gained through the acquisition of well-known researchers, fancy medical equipment and new and larger buildings. This is why the hospital-dominated Blue Cross has consistently failed to support consumer concerns such as cost and quality control.

THE HEALTH CARE PROFITEERS

The third part of the health system are the health-care profiteers, especially the medical-industrial complex. An alliance exists between the providers of health care (doctors, hospitals, medical schools and the like) and the companies that make money from people's sickness (drug companies, hospital supply companies, hospital construction companies, commercial insurance companies and even companies that provide medical services for profit—profit-making proprietary hospitals, chains of nursing homes for old people, laboratories, and so on). Health care is one of the biggest businesses around, and one of the fastest-growing.

The magnitude of the medical-industrial complex is hard to believe. For example, in 1969 drug companies (Abbott, Upjohn, Merck, and so on) had after-tax profits of about $600 million. The drug industry rated first, second or third in profitability among all U.S. industries during the 1960's, causing *Forbes* magazine, a financial journal, to call it "one of the biggest crap games in U.S. industry."

Hospital supply companies (Becton Dickinson, American Hospital Supply, and so on), which sell hospitals and doctors everything from sheets and towels and bedpans to surgical instruments, X-ray machines and heart-lung machines, had after-tax profits of $400 million in 1969. Proprietary hospitals and nursing homes earned nearly $200 million. (There are even nationwide chains of hospitals and nursing homes run by such businesses as Holiday Inns.)

The commercial insurance companies and the construction firms that build hospitals make additional millions, and, of course, the doctors themselves are still the highest-paid people in the health industry. Even the banks are getting in on the act, with loans to hospitals both for building and for operating expenses. A patient at one of New York's prestigious hospitals, for example, finds that three dollars a day of his or her hospital bill doesn't go for services at all; it goes to the banks for interest payments.

THE SYSTEM IN HEALTH

Not only do all these empires, insurance people, financiers, businesspeople and doctors make a lot of money from people's bad health, they do it with togetherness. Their mutual needs coincide: prestigious medical empires require the manufacture of expensive equipment and the presence of large construction companies; and, of course, only large institutions can afford the expensive products of the medical equipment and drug manufacturers. And all of these groups require the stable, lenient financing of Blue Cross, Medicare and Medicaid and other medical insurers. Their growing interdependence is evident. Increasingly, drug and medical equipment executives, banking and real estate/construction company executives sit on boards of trustees at academic medical centers. Meanwhile, hospital and medical school professionals moonlight as consultants to drug and hospital supply companies and sometimes sit on their boards of directors.

The best thing about the health business is that the profits are sure (as long as you're not a patient or taxpayer, that is). Blue Cross, Medicare and Medicaid hand the doctors and hospitals a virtual blank check. The hospital, in effect, simply tells Blue Cross how much its expenses are, and Blue Cross pays the bill. In the boom years of the 1960's there was no cost control to speak of. The inflation in health-care costs that resulted has led to some belt-tightening more recently, but the accepted definition of a necessary health-care cost remains very generous.

Some costs of course may be necessary for better patient care. But they also may be "necessary" for the purchase of seldom-used and expensive equipment that is available in another hospital across the street; for plush offices and high salaries for doctors and hospital administrators; for expenses incurred in fighting off attempts by unions to organize hospital workers; or for hiring public relations firms to clean up the hospital's poor image in the community. The health industry and the doctors get rich; the consumer and the taxpayer pay the bill.

Even the so-called nonprofit hospitals get in on the fun. All that "nonprofit" means is that such hospitals don't have to pay out their excess income to stockholders. They also don't have to pay it back to their patients in the form of cheaper rates. Instead, they use it to grow; to buy more fancy (even if unnecessary) equipment, more plush offices, more public relations; to pay staff doctors even higher salaries; to buy up real estate, tear down poor people's housing and build new pavilions for private patients.

There is, then, a health care *system*. Its components are, in addition to the doctors, the vast network of health-care resources that make up the medical empires; the financing-planning complex of agencies dominated by Blue Cross; and the medical-industrial complex. But if American health care is provided by such a big, well-organized, interconnected, businesslike system, why is it so poor? The answer is that *health care is not the aim of the health-care system*. The health-care system exists to serve its own ends. The aims of big medical centers are teaching and research.

The hospitals and medical schools seek to expand their real estate and financial holdings. And everyone, from hospitals and doctors to drug companies and insurance companies, want to make profits. Health care for patients is a means to these ends, but is not the sole end in itself. Thus the patients see a system that is expensive, that is fragmented into dozens of specialties, that has no time to treat them in a dignified way, and that doesn't even take care of them very well.

—From "Your Health Care in Crisis," a Health/PAC special report, 4th printing, November, 1972. (adapted and updated)

2

Medical Empires

The downturn of the U.S. economy during the 1970's heralds the end of a period of unrestrained hospital growth. Riding the crest of a whole series of advances in medical science, hospitals received large federal research grants starting in the 1950's and vast sums of Medicare and Medicaid funds starting in the mid-1960's. With this money, plus Blue Cross and other private health insurance reimbursements, hospitals bought more expensive equipment, expanded their physical plants, added many highly trained staff members and offered new specialized medical services to patients. Smaller private hospitals felt compelled to establish affiliations with the academic medical centers so that they could call on these specialized services and avert the risk of losing their patients to the centers altogether. Officials of city and county government, always anxious to rid themselves of the responsibility of running a public hospital, began offering up these hospitals to the academic medical centers. At first the medical centers were happy to get them—to increase their income, acquire additional staff positions for faculty and students and gain access to patients who would provide a large research and teaching population.

All this expansion drove up the cost of health care dramatically, resulting in rising health insurance premiums and contributing to higher government taxes.

By the early 1970's widespread popular opposition to further cost increases developed. In part to manipulate this popular unrest, in part to settle old political scores, but mainly to try to limit government spending, Richard Nixon seriously began to cut back on federal health-care spending at the end of his first term. He slashed medical research and manpower-training funds and in 1971 imposed a wage-price freeze on all industries, including health.

This development has slowed down the expansion of medical empires but it hasn't stopped it. The first two articles in this chapter report on two currently expanding empires—the Boston University and the Duke University medical centers. Besides describing how empires grow, these selections give a glimpse of how empires have traditionally functioned and their detrimental impact on medical care in the surrounding community, especially among low-income people.

The article on the takeover of public Boston City Hospital (BCH) by private Boston University Medical Center shows how the medical services and facilities at BCH were molded to meet the needs of Boston University, in some cases long before the city announced that BCH was up for grabs. Written by a group of health workers at BCH, the article also examines how the cutback in beds at BCH, arranged simultaneously with the Boston University takeover, will force transfer of many BCH patients to other hospitals. Then, highlighting Boston University's fundamental lack of concern for its new patients, the article examines the restrictive admissions policies at Boston University's own University Hospital and its refusal to accept more than a handful of the BCH transfer patients.

The next article, about Duke University in Durham, North Carolina, shows how a local Southern elite with national pretensions has steamrollered ahead with plans to build a new, expanded university hospital that will deliver specialized medical services to a regional and national clientele, while ignoring the health needs of the local community in Durham. Written by two local health activists, the article points out that what Durham needs is not more hospital beds but preventive health programs and accessible primary care, which the Duke facility won't provide.

A particularly complex affiliation relationship is that between public Bellevue Hospital in New York City and its private affiliate, New York University Medical Center, which runs prestigious, private University Hospital. Bellevue and New York University (NYU) have been shaping their relationship for many decades. As a group of staff members from Health/PAC's New York office reports in the fourth selection, the affiliation relationship varies greatly from department to department. In the important medicine and surgery departments, where NYU is strong and especially prizes its independence, there is no formal affiliation contract, and the NYU physicians donate their services to Bellevue. In academically and financially weaker departments, there is a formal contract in which NYU gets paid for staffing the Bellevue departments. In some departments like radiology and pathology, which are particularly expensive to staff and equip, there is also a formal contract totally integrating services at the two institutions. As part of this arrangement NYU does not maintain some specialized pathology services, so that here public funds pay for services to patients in both public and private hospitals. At times this sophisticated ripoff is called, euphemistically, a sharing of services or medicine under one roof.

Most of the articles in this chapter address patient-care problems of poor people in public hospitals. The last selection relates what happened to a middle-class patient who had the misfortune to approach private, prestigious Mt. Sinai Hospital in New York City when she was temporarily without health insurance and had to be admitted through the emergency room rather than under the auspices of a private physician. Her tale of medical horrors is not unique in its general outlines. With minor variations it has been told repeatedly at legislative hearings and before community groups and labor unions. It suggests that problems of quality care are not limited to public hospitals, which are widely acknowledged to be deficient in the care they deliver, but may be found even in those academic hospitals of the medical empires that pride themselves on their superior care.

AS THE NATION GOES, SO GOES BOSTON

Jeff Blum, Jerry Feuer, Kate Mulhern and Joan Tighe

Boston City Hospital (BCH) is the only public acute care hospital in Boston. In 1968 (the last year for which figures are available) it treated a whopping 27.4 percent of all patients treated at Boston hospitals who were Boston residents. The percentage is higher for areas where Boston's Black, Puerto Rican, and working-class white population is concentrated.

BCH is also Boston's major emergency hospital for victims of gunshot and stab wounds and other traumatic injuries. It is the main center for mass hospitalizations arising from serious fires or auto accidents. Any alcoholic who is picked up and in need of medical care will most likely end up there. So will low-income people, no matter what the emergency and no matter where they come from; last year 45 percent of the ambulances arriving at BCH came from outside its official ambulance district.

BCH has been the only hospital in the area where the three major medical schools—Harvard, Tufts, and Boston University (BU)—have co-existed. For most of this century, each of the three has run its own medical and surgical services at BCH while dividing the other services among them. However inefficient, this system has allowed the Hospital to maintain the large staff necessary to care for Boston's poor.

BU TAKES OVER

Like mayors of most cities, Boston's Kevin White has felt himself pressed for funds for a number of years. One of his favorite ways of saving money has been to cut down BCH. In 1971 he froze jobs at the Hospital. In 1972 he unsuccessfully tried to cut the City's contribution to the hospital's budget by almost one-fourth.

In 1973 the ax fell—hard. Within one month the Mayor slashed the BCH budget from $62 to $56 million, eliminated 350 beds (from 850 to 500) and, without prior notice, turned over all medical services at BCH to Boston University Medical Center.

To understand why these changes took place, especially the BU affiliation, we have to look more closely at the interests of Boston's three medical empires. For

Mayor White doesn't make health-care decisions alone; these empires wield tremendous power in determining City health policies.

THE RESEARCH CENTERS DON'T WANT THEM

One result of the existence of the three competing complexes and the numerous hospitals they control is what is commonly referred to as overbedding, a ratio of hospital beds to residents that is far higher than the national average. The gross figures, however, do not speak to the critical question of who has access to those beds. As a medical research center, Boston fills many of its hospital beds with patients from across the country and the world.

"The academic medical centers are referral centers," says Dr. Steven Saltzman, President of the BCH House Officers Association. "They take care of patients with different exotic diseases because enough people come in from all over the world to justify those services. There's no way for [Health and Hosptials] Commissioner Leon White to change that. If he tries to make them into community hospitals, the specialists will leave, but that won't happen because all those people are a lot more powerful than he is. You can't expect a specialist to call a patient from Atlanta who's scheduled for complicated heart surgery and tell him not to come because they have an alcoholic with pneumonia filling his bed."

Poor patients are seen as a burden by private hospitals. Their diseases are boringly similar—complications of years of alcoholism, heart disease, results of inadequate diet, poor housing, unsafe working conditions, and almost no preventive care. They take up beds for longer than the elective surgery patients that hospitals and doctors make money on, because they come in far sicker than a person who has a private physician, who can afford convalescence after illnesses, and who is taken care of in old age.

Unlike BCH, which treats all comers regardless of ability to pay, private hospitals employ a number of devices to restrict access to their facilities. They keep their emergency rooms small and close them at 9 P.M.; charge a fee before letting patients enter a clinic; ask extensive questions about health insurance and ability to pay even before diagnosing the patient's condition; require patients to sign forms—usually illegal—agreeing to have their property and paycheck attached to cover their bills. There is no evidence that these practices are about to be abandoned, especially with the tightening of spending by Medicaid, Medicare, and Blue Cross.

EMPIRES IN THE WINGS

The actual size of these medical empires is always shifting, particularly since the federal government made lavish money available for hospital construction and research in the mid-sixties. Dominant among these three is Harvard, whose medical school controls about ten major teaching hospitals in greater Boston, most inside the city limits. Harvard's primary orientation is to maintain and enlarge its medical complex as an international center of medical specialties—most of the patients in Harvard hospitals don't live in Boston.

Harvard's resources—in money, people, prestige, and power—allow it to outlast or buy off most of its potential critics. This is not to say that Harvard is invulnerable. When it wanted to expand facilities near its major geographical area of concentration, which includes four teaching hospitals and its medical school, pressure from the Mission Hill community stopped it. The medical school, in true Harvard fashion, soon had a solution—an end run. While continuing to exert pressure on its own local community, Harvard took over administrative control of Cambridge City Hospital, a few miles away.

Harvard's move into Cambridge City Hospital may explain its willingness to lose its share of BCH, since both institutions are primarily hospitals for the poor. (Harvard controlled less than 250 beds at BCH and acquired 217 at Cambridge City.) Harvard also had a major research operation going at BCH at the prestigious Thorndike Memorial Laboratories, operated within the Hospital premises but completely controlled by the medical school; it was no problem, however, to move the labs to another part of the empire, namely Beth Israel Hospital, another of Harvard's teaching hospitals.

Boston's other two medical empires are considerably smaller. Tufts controls well under 1,000 beds and does not have the money necessary to attract large numbers of researchers, who contribute to a medical empire's prestige and bring in needed federal money. About four years ago, Tufts faced the prospect either of building up its Department of Medicine at BCH or pulling out entirely, but couldn't make a firm decision one way or the other. As a result of the lack of support from Tufts, the Department was never able to find someone willing to be its chairman. Thus when Tufts got the chance this past winter [1972] finally to rid itself of this albatross, it did so quite willingly, although it went through the motions of submitting a proposal for taking over BCH on its own.

Like Tufts, the Boston University Medical Center is comparatively small. Geographically limited to Boston's South End (although it provides medical staff to several suburban hospitals), BU includes the medical school and the 350-bed University Hospital [UH]. Gaining total control of BCH (where it had formerly controlled about half the beds) meant increasing its bed capacity by a couple of hundred beds with very little added expense.

BU EXPANDS

BU launched an expansion program in 1965. Since then it has built or bought four new buildings, going $14 million into debt in the process. Most of this money has gone for research and teaching space and private physicians' offices. Hence two of its new buildings are the Evans Memorial Research Building and the Doctors' Office Building. Almost no funds have gone to build up outpatient facilities for so-called "clinic patients," a euphemism for the poor.

Recently federal health research cutbacks have forced the BU ship off course. BU has been compelled to change its compass reading and is now coming on as doctor for the surrounding Black and Third World communities.

Spurred on by federal funds for a new residency program and a $5 million seed grant from the Robert Wood Johnson Foundation (as in Johnson & Johnson), BU has proudly announced that Primary Care Delivery (PCD) is now its "central theme." PCD has become the rationale for eliminating specialty services from BCH under BU's auspices and limiting the Hospital to four basic services: medicine, surgery, pediatrics, and obstetrics.

The PCD proposal is carefully couched in terms of commitment to the community, but the community was never consulted in the initial plans for the proposal, nor have concrete guidelines been articulated for the involvement of medical students or the inclusion of patients. The substantive emphasis of the proposal is on the training of physicians, not the delivery of community-oriented health care or the training of community residents to serve primary health-care roles.

Given its emphasis on physician training, the program is caught in a contradiction between its rhetoric of providing "continuity of service" and its projected practice of rotating physicians-in-training through a community. By its character as a pilot research project in health-care delivery, PCD is precluded from providing a general solution for health care delivery problems. Patient care will be provided, but only to those whom BU defines as part of the pilot project.

THE PLOT THICKENS

Both the PCD program and the complementary construction programs of BU and BCH fit in very nicely with BU's assumption of total control at BCH, a fact that suggests something was in the works long before that takeover was officially decided on in February, 1973. BU cites its assumption of responsibility for professional services at BCH as one of the critical developments inspiring it to make the PCD proposal. BU's plans for constructing a new hospital next door to BCH, to replace University Hospital, were publicly discarded in December, 1972. Shortly after the original announcement, a newspaper report quoted an anonymous "highly placed BU official" who hinted at the real reason. He suggested that a new UH might not be needed since "BU Medical School's role at Boston City Hospital might expand if one or even both of the other medical schools that utilize BCH for teaching and research were persuaded to reduce or phase out their participation."

Further evidence of a well-thought-out strategy on the part of BU was its omission of a new outpatient building, despite the fact that the outpatient services at University Hospital are in the oldest and most crowded part of that institution. Interestingly enough, the City is currently constructing a new outpatient building for BCH, a facility that has become a central factor in BU's PCD proposal, which emphasizes "educational settings which focus on the ambulatory instead of the hospitalized patient."

BCH's new outpatient building was originally one part of a plan developed in the late 1960's for a completely new $91-million hospital with 1,000 acute and 300 chronic care beds. Of the rest of the plan, only ancillary facilities have to date been built—a new 28-story, 112-unit apartment complex for doctors (including a swimming pool, gymnasium, and squash courts) and a new nursing school and rooms for 300 student nurses. With the cut in BCH's beds and a concomitant 20 percent cut in its house officers this year, the apartment building is larger than needed by BCH but presumably will come in handy for the house staff at University Hospital.

There are other factors that suggest that the BU takeover at BCH fits in nicely with its own plans and priorities: a few years ago University Hospital closed up its maternity and pediatrics facilities, while BU renovated those services at BCH that it was then operating. Until July, 1973, University Hospital did not even have an emergency room, whereas BCH has one of the largest in the city.

All of this is evidence that the decision to let BU run the medical services at BCH was not made in a week by the Board of Trustees, as they would have us believe. The Trustees' request for proposals to be submitted by all three medical schools was made a week before the decision was announced, and in retrospect was merely a formality. The urgency of winning control for BU is highlighted by the Harvard proposal, which would have closed down those services—pediatrics and maternity—most urgently needed by BU. (Harvard already controls hospitals specializing in those areas.) The City may well have found BU to be the most pliable of these dubious allies precisely because it was the most needy. Or perhaps the prospect of trying to get concessions from Harvard drove the Mayor and his political advisers into the waiting arms of BU. Either way, the decision saves BU millions of dollars in construction money and gives it control of a very large medical complex.

BUT WILL IT WORK?

One critical question is unresolved at this point: can the health needs of Boston's poor communities be met with BCH as a 500-bed institution? The situation looks grim.

During the winter months, BCH normally has a census of over 600 patients. Since the plans call for a 500-bed hospital, this means that about 100 BCH patients willl have to be sent elsewhere. But a majority of BCH admissions are on the danger list and cannot be transferred out. What is more, if other patients are transferred, and the number of danger-list patients at BCH rises, greater burdens will be put on its already overworked staff and the result will be inferior care. (Already the number of staff—but not the number of patients—has been cut in pediatrics and obstetrics.)

The bright young men who set policy for the Department of Health and Hospitals confidently state that there are plenty of empty beds in the private hospitals that can be used to absorb the overflow, and that more efficient management of BCH will work wonders. But their crude numbers games ignore certain realities: on the busy days of the week (Monday to Wednesday) the private hospitals are quite full; in any event, the statistics are all averages, which do not truly describe the health needs of the people of Boston. Their plan to cut down the average length of stay at BCH ignores the fact that BCH patients tend to stay longer because they have nowhere else to go.

The transfer of patients not on the danger list is also problematic. The document spelling out the transfer procedures states that "there is little reason to be concerned that BCH transfers will systematically bump a private hospital's elective patients." This revealing statement, meant to assuage the nerves of money-conscious private hospitals, serves to clarify the real inflexibility in the system: they'll only take our patients if it pleases them.

Evidence from BU's University Hospital reinforces this observation. Under a formal arrangement, UH has agreed to take the first three non-danger-list admissions to BCH every morning. However, since the agreement has gone into effect, UH has often not taken three admissions and has sometimes taken none. After all, as an unnamed UH administrator put it: "As a private, non-profit, voluntary hospital, we cannot just swing open the doors like a drop-in health center, treating anyone who comes in. We already have a deficit of one million dollars." At the same time, UH chief administrator, John Betjeman, was complaining that they couldn't fill their new beds! It seems they are only willing to fill them with certain patients.

If BU-associated hospitals are reacting to BCH transfers this way, one can hardly expect that other private hospitals will come to the rescue. Evidence from the State Senate's Social Welfare Committee suggests that these hospitals have already begun to resist the influx of the poor. "We have documented cases," says a legislative aide, "in which the private hospitals have taken people into their emergency wards and then sent them after the initial work-up to Boston City if they can't pay."

Peter Bent Brigham Hospital (a Harvard institution) came out shortly after the BCH cutback was announced with a new outpatient form by which the patient signed away all rights and agreed to pay the bill by any means necessary. The form, which was probably illegal, was withdrawn after worker and community pressure was exerted. Its introduction, however, is hardly an indication of the willingness to "pick up the slack" that the Mayor's men have imputed to the private sector.

As of late September, 1973, BCH had not yet been fully cut back to 500 beds. At a capacity of 550, the Hospital was full on several occasions during the summer, traditionally its slackest period. Voluntary hospitals have also been full; UH, for example, peaked at a bed census of 110 percent of capacity. BCH will almost certainly overflow in the winter, and the private hospitals will almost certainly not have any beds available or not be willing to use them for BCH's unattractive constituency.

(Jeff Blum, Jerry Feuer, Kate Mulhern and Joan Tighe worked at Boston City Hospital.)

—From the Health/PAC *Bulletin*, October, 1973. (abridged and edited)

SOUTHERN EMPIRE: Cool-Handed Duke

Paul Bermanzohn and Tim McGloin

Durham, North Carolina, has one of the highest venereal disease rates in the country. The fetal death rate is nearly twice the national average. People in Durham are not very healthy, and all indications point to their getting less so.

The health problems of Durham are not due to a lack of doctors or facilities. In fact, health is the leading industry in the city. More than 9,000 people in this city of 135,000 are employed by health institutions. Together the three general hospitals have 1,141 beds. Durham County also has lots of specialized medical services. It has four times the ratio of radiologists to population as the average for the rest of the country, five times that of neurosurgeons, three times the ratio of psychiatrists and six times that of orthopedic surgeons. However, the area has only one-seventh the ratio of general practitioners to population as the country as a whole.

A 1973 study sponsored by the Health Planning Council of Central North Carolina documented Durham's priority health needs as emergency services, preventive health programs and accessible primary care. The study reported that "there appears to be no need to increase the number of beds to serve Durham residents." Undaunted, Durham's powers that be are about to add 250 more beds at two new hospitals, a new medical research center and more specialists per capita. Not surprisingly, these plans coincide with the priorities of Duke University. And according to Terry Sanford, Duke's President, "Our University can only be great with a great Medical Center." The crown jewel of this complex is to be a brand-new, sparkling $91-million hospital.

Duke University was created by the family of Washington Duke, founder of the American Tobacco Company. Mr. Duke's descendants and their various financial interests are intertwined with the expansion of Duke's medical center. Just as American Tobacco grew into one of the largest and richest corporations in the country (41st in net profits), so Duke grew into a major university.

In order to be a great medical center, Duke needs access to a community hospital from which to draw its teaching material and an academic hospital in which to do its research and make its money. The power structure of Durham has been obliging in both respects. A new community hospital is now under construction, and work is about to begin on the new university hospital.

HEALTH IN THE LAND OF WEALTH

Lincoln and Watts Hospitals, the old, traditionally segregated community hospitals used by the people of Durham, are both deteriorating. It has been clear for some time that new facilities are needed. A new community hospital that will combine the two old ones into one unit is now under construction. But this $21-million, 500-bed hospital is not being designed to meet the health needs of Durham's people.

They are not getting the accessible primary care that the Health Planning Council (HPC) study documented as their number one health need. Durham County Hospital is being built miles away from the center of the city. Although promised when the new hospital opens, there is not now a bus line which travels out to it. The site is in a section of Durham County owned by a leading real estate developer and the city's biggest banker. Together they are promoting nearby suburban residential development. To enhance the attractiveness of the area to the upper and middle classes and maximize the developers' profits, a "medical park" for private practitioners is being built adjacent to the new hospital.

But Duke Medical School couldn't care less about the hospital's inaccessibility, as long as its needs are being met. Its medical students will rotate through the hospital; the Medical School will run the department of surgery; and the family medicine training program, which Duke now operates at Watts, will be transferred to the new hospital. And finally, the County Hospital's 30 percent "service" beds will function as the receiving end of Duke's policy of refusing admission to persons "when other facilities are available . . . more appropriate to the patient's financial circumstances."

FROM DUKEDOM TO KINGDOM

Long content to be just a quiet monument to J. B. Duke's memory, in the past ten years Duke University has decided to "go national." This decision represents not only the desire to create an institutional name (the Harvard of the South), but also reflects the ambitions of the men in power at Duke. A growing and powerful institution is an important base for their own personal advancement.

The University as a whole is in an excellent position to grow. Its trustees come from deep within America's ruling elite. Native North Carolina industry is well represented by such giants as Burlington Mills (in the person of Henry Rauch, retired board chairman), R. J. Reynolds Tobacco Company (Charles Wade, Senior Vice President), Hanes Corporation (Clifford Perry, Treasurer) and the state's largest bank, the Wachovia (pronounced "walk over ya") Bank (three leading officials). A major financial resource is the Duke Endowment Fund, the world's third largest foundation.

The University's national connections are no less prestigious and wealthy. Representatives of the Ford Motor Company, Mobil Oil, the Shell Oil Foundation and the Chicago Board of Trade sit on its board, along with two ambassadors from the Rockefeller empire—John Knowles, formerly of Massachusetts General Hospital, now president of the Rockefeller Foundation, and Nancy Hanks, a former Nelson Rockefeller assistant and executive secretary of the Rockefeller Brothers Fund.

A major asset in Duke's climb to national power was the recent acquisition of Terry Sanford as its president. A liberal ex-governor of North Carolina, Sanford ran for president in 1972, posing as a Southern Jack Kennedy. In addition to his political credentials, Sanford is an agile fund raiser. In 1973 he announced an "Epoch Campaign" to raise $162 million for the University's endowment; as of May, 1974, over $40 million had been received.

The power behind the throne at Duke is J. Alexander McMahon, Chairman of Duke's Board of Trustees. After several years as President and chief operating officer of North Carolina Blue Cross/Blue Shield, he was named President of the American Hospital Association. McMahon served on the Health Services Committee of the Cost of Living Council, which administered President Nixon's Phase II wage-price freeze.

McMahon's presence on the Duke Board of Trustees provides the major link between the Duke group, with its national connections and aspirations, and Durham's local power structure. McMahon became the first President of a unified Blue Cross/Blue Shield in North Carolina. Before him, the Blues had been a collection of insurance agencies with loose ties to each other. McMahon presided over their merger and coordinated the construction of a $9-million glass and steel structure in Durham to serve as headquarters for the merged organization. In 1971, as the new building opened, the Blues reported a net loss of $5.4 million and announced a 32 percent rate increase, all the time insisting that the building and the rate increase were not related. For the past two years the Blues have finished in the black, a record marred only slightly by a lawsuit lodged by the Internal Revenue Service for overcharging 40 percent of their subscribers. They were charged with violating 15 pricing guidelines, a "mistake" affecting 650,000 North Carolinians. It seems that McMahon as head of the Blues was violating the pricing guidelines he was helping to make in Washington, as a member of the Cost of Living Council's Health Services Committee.

THE CROWN JEWEL— DUKE'S NEW HOSPITAL

No medical empire is complete without its imperial headquarters. All of Duke's power, with its national and local connections, has coalesced around its proposal for a new Duke Hospital. Deciding that 200 of the beds in its existing 800-bed hospital are obsolete, Duke commissioned a major accounting firm to establish the financial feasibility of a new hospital. It conveniently concluded that the resources were available for the construction of a $91-million, 1,000-bed facility. All 1,000 units will be single-bed rooms, thus further emphasizing Duke's highly specialized inpatient priorities.

To provide the operating costs of the new hospital, Duke projects a 73 percent increase in average gross costs a day—from $151 to $263. This increase, of course, will be reflected in the Blue Cross premiums paid by local people and in the amounts of public money turned over to the Hospital from Medicaid and Medicare.

Sixty million dollars of the cost of the new hospital is to be raised through long-term debt floated at the local banks. The remaining $30 million or so is to be obtained from hospital operating funds and private sources. Duke Hospital is freeing up this money in predictable ways. Those services that are most profitable are expanded, and the rest are either constricted or the fee scale is raised. For example, visits to Duke's profitable private diagnostic clinic have increased 73 percent since 1967, while the public clinics have seen only a 4 percent increase in the same period. Since 1971 the private clinics have continued to grow while public clinics have remained at the 1971 level.

In the double-think language of Wallace Jarboe, Director of the University's Office of Project Management, "We are not cutting back on outpatient services. That is the terminology of the auditing firm. . . . What we are doing is *freezing our losses.*"

Another method employed by Duke for generating funds for the new building is through lowering personnel costs at the existing institution. A hiring freeze has been in effect for many months. A recent memo from the director of employment at the hospital, Robert A. Duncan, instructed the deans, department heads and division chiefs that "No one is to be hired for the biweekly payroll at a rate above the minimum for the position unless approved by me" and that "new employees may be hired below the minimum" up to 10 percent. Jobs requiring skilled technical people are going to untrained workers to save money. One repercussion of this policy has been three job actions by various categories of employees. The dietetic workers, the microbiology technicians and the data terminal workers have walked out because of low pay and understaffing.

The microbiologists' job action was the most recent and also the most dramatic of the three walkouts. Immediately after they walked off their jobs in late May [of 1974], Duke Hospital suspended them for 30 days. Although there were only six workers in this job category, they appealed to their fellow hospital employees and were successful in gaining support at rallies and meetings. Because of the extensive coverage in the press, the unsanitary, overcrowded and understaffed Duke labs became a local scandal. Because of the support of other hospital workers, the press coverage and the indispensable nature of their work, Duke had to capitulate to the technicians' demands. Three weeks after the walkout began, the microbiologists were reinstated at a higher salary, four more technicians are being recruited and the lab space is being cleaned up and expanded. As Duke increasingly squeezes its employees to raise the necessary money for the new hospital, job actions may become more frequent and more militant.

HEAVY-HANDED DUKE

As Duke Medical School has expanded, so has the opposition of people in Durham to Duke's imperial plans. When the new hospital proposal was first announced, a coalition of community people and health workers formed in opposition to it. Since all new capital construction that is either publicly financed or underwritten must be approved by the local comprehensive planning agency, this coalition was able to voice its disapproval at a public hearing. This effort made a real impact at the local level, and obtaining local agency approval of Duke's plan required heavy-handed intervention by George Watts Hill, Sr., Durham's leading businessperson and for 38 years chairman of the Blue Cross board. At higher levels in government, however, Duke's influence has been more pervasive and approval easier to get.

The Duke experience had been a result of that convergence of factors that make for the growth of a medical empire. An impressive array of nationally connected figures has been drawn to Duke to abet and encourage its expansion. There is a local power structure both unified and determined to back up with its money and influence the wide-ranging plans of the University—plans that not only put feathers in their caps but also money in their banks. Despite the opposition of community people and health workers, this mixed chorus sings a familiar song—the people be damned.

(Paul Bermanzohn and Tim McGloin have been active in community health struggles in Durham, the former as a member of the Durham Health Collective of the New American Movement (NAM) and the latter as a member of Citizens Concerned About Durham Health Care.)

—From the Health/PAC *Bulletin*, July/August, 1974. (abridged and edited)

BELLEVUE HOSPITAL: Growing Up Absurd

Louise Lander, Constance Bloomfield and Jonathan Morley

On November 15, 1973, the City of New York proudly dedicated the new Bellevue Hospital. The speeches at the dedication ceremony predictably dwelt on Bellevue's glorious past and projected an even more glorious future in its magnificent new facility. What the speechmakers predictably failed to acknowledge was the role of private health institutions, at Bellevue as much as elsewhere, in shaping public hospitals to fit their own needs. In other cities this phenomenon has led to the closing, leasing or contracting of public hospitals; in New York a more sophisticated accommodation of the public sector to the private is being shaped. Here a new public hospital has been designed to serve essentially as an annex to an elite private medical center, serving its needs primarily and the public need only coincidentally.

SETTING THE STAGE

Around the world, people know about Bellevue, even if they mistakenly think it's only a psychiatric hospital. It's historic—dating back to 1736 and probably the nation's first public hospital. It's big—with 1,550 beds, it's the fourth largest hospital in the country. Its emergency services are frantic—their 102,000 annual patient visits include the most critical of emergencies and form the basis of the legend that "If you sit in Bellevue emergency for a few nights you will see everything there is to see in this world." It's where people come who have nowhere else to go.

INTRODUCING THE NEW YORK UNIVERSITY MEDICAL CENTER

Bellevue exists in the shadow, literal and figurative, of its neighbor to the immediate north, the New York University Medical Center, which includes NYU Medical School, University Hospital, and assorted institutes of research. For over a century NYU Medical School has based its teaching program on the large and varied supply of clinical material available at Bellevue. University Hospital patients don't qualify as material for a medically "balanced" teaching program; that institution prides itself on being a superspecialized referral hospital for the private patients of the Medical School faculty—no ordinary illness need apply. Nor, might we add, need Medicaid patients apply, UH being the only voluntary hospital in the City that declines to participate in the Medicaid program. Patients looking for a clinic won't find any, and emergency cases will probably end up at Bellevue before they find UH's well-concealed, unstaffed emergency room.

The presence of Bellevue, in other words, has conveniently saved NYU from the annoyance of having to respond to the medical needs of the poor while at the same time supplying NYU with the bodies of the poor in a setting, namely teaching, where it finds them useful. NYU's own facilities then serve to consolidate its ties to its faculty by giving them a place to hospitalize their patients and, to the extent that space permits, to conduct their office practice.

At the concrete level of physicians—teachers, researchers, and clinicians—Bellevue and NYU virtually merge. NYU is the entry point for physicians who work at Bellevue. With minor exceptions, every attending physician at Bellevue is a faculty member of the Medical School and an attending at UH. Conversely, acquiring those NYU credentials requires undertaking an obligation to do "service" at Bellevue. In most cases, the chairmen of the Medical School's academic departments, in addition to becoming chiefs of the corresponding service at UH, also become the corresponding chiefs of service at Bellevue. It is frequently, and proudly, said that the medical staff is the "connecting tissue" that binds the two institutions together.

THE POLITICS OF AFFILIATION

Into this long-existing milieu came during the 1960's the drive of the City's then Department of Hospitals to place the municipal hospitals under an affiliation system, whereby various voluntary hospitals and medical schools contractually agreed to provide medical staff to municipal hospitals in exchange for a lump-sum payment. NYU was offered an affiliation contract around 1966, at a time when Columbia's and Cornell's medical schools, which had had relatively small pieces of the action at Bellevue, were being asked to devote their efforts to other City hospitals. Many of the prima donnas of the NYU medical hierarchy—the chairmen, for example, of such key departments as medicine and surgery—declined to rise to the bait. Freedom, it seems, is still in some circles more important than cash—freedom, that is, from any semblance of public accountability, such as an affiliation contract might impose. There was also for these department chairmen the critical question of control; the affiliation contract requires that the affiliate designate a full-time chief of service for each department of the affiliated municipal hospital. The Chairman of the Medical School's Department of Medicine, for example, who also, of course, is chief of the medicine service at University Hospital, obviously wouldn't qualify and just as obviously would have to give up his power to run the show at Bellevue.

These considerations persuaded many department chairmen that NYU should decline the City's kind offer of payment for what, after all, they had an academic incentive to do for free. Other department chairmen felt the need for an infusion of funds to be sufficiently pressing to outweigh the attendant disadvantages. The upshot was a compromise in the form of a partial affiliation contract covering only certain specified services.

AFFILIATION: TO BE OR NOT TO BE?

In some departments affiliation means a formal affiliation contract between the NYU Medical Center and New York City's Health and Hospitals Corporation (HHC), the agency that now operates the municipal hospitals; in other departments the term implies a gentlemen's agreement of many decades' standing whereby NYU provides medical staff without either the payment or the nominal public control that a formal contract involves.

The Department of Medicine, for example, is not covered by the partial affiliation contract because Dr. Saul Farber, the department chairman, has always been unwilling to accept money and the possibility of control from anyone but NYU. Similarly with surgery —"We need the money," Dr. Frank Spencer, its chairman, admits; the problem with a contract is that the "superb physicians" on the NYU staff have preferred to donate a portion of their valuable time to Bellevue rather than get paid and have to put up with such harassments as signing in and out. The point seems to be that if labor is charity, the recipient can't complain if it's provided at the convenience and for purposes that serve the benefactor.

Some of the departments that the affiliation contract covers—namely, intermediate care, home care, and the chest service—are also services that rank low on the hierarchy of academic importance. (The intermediate care service, for one, has no internship or residency program.) The official explanation is that the City's contract offer was accepted for these services because running them represented an additional burden that NYU assumed with the departure from Bellevue of Columbia and Cornell, a burden it wasn't prepared to take on without financial support. One suspects that the lack of academic interest in such programs also has something to do with NYU's willingness here to submit to a formal affiliation arrangement.

Pathology and radiology, on the other hand, are both covered by the affiliation contract and are both academically important. Apparently these service chiefs decided it was simply impossible to equip and staff what they considered a modern, adequate department without an infusion of funds, whatever its source. This has not, however, meant that Bellevue physicians in these services must sever all ties with NYU. In radiology, for example, NYU guarantees to Bellevue the full-time equivalent of 11 physicians; the department, however, is perceived as one department for both Bellevue and NYU's University Hospital, with physicians shuttling back and forth as the need arises. (The physicians receive a full-time salary in the form of an NYU check, partly representing affiliation funds, partly NYU funds.) The theory is that this arrangement gives Bellevue the advantage of a super-specialist whose specialized talents aren't needed on a full-time basis. The relationship between bookkeeping and reality under such an arrangement, however, remains an open question.

In pathology, the affiliation gives NYU a double advantage. The pathology service at UH doesn't include neuropathology, pediatric pathology, or obstetrical-gynecological pathology: these are "unified services" that are located at Bellevue. These pathology procedures, in other words, are done for UH patients as well as Bellevue patients by pathologists whose salaries are paid by the HHC through the affiliation contract. If there's a flow of money from NYU to Bellevue to pay for the procedures done for UH patients, no one —including NYU's affiliation administrator, who says it's "not an affiliation matter"—seem to know about it.

Pediatrics by a stroke of luck found a way to be both prosperous and unaffiliated, at least for a while. The service used to suffer from a lack of staff and facilities sufficient to do more than run a disjointed, emergency-type program. When Congress legislated the Children and Youth (C&Y) program in 1966, NYU was quick to jump at the opportunity to obtain relatively unfettered federal money. With a million and a half annual federal dollars coming directly to NYU, Dr. Saul Krugman, the department chairman, developed a showpiece comprehensive-care department, with its own labs, its own pharmacy, and UH's only computerized medical records system. Regrettably, federal money got tight a few years ago and the amount of the C&Y grant was no longer sufficient to cover the department's needs; to make up the deficit, Krugman took his physicians off the C&Y budget and negotiated an affiliation agreement to cover their salaries. As in radiology, most of the doctors are on full-time salary but spend part of their time at NYU, mostly doing research. Krugman doesn't agonize over whether their time actually spent at Bellevue corresponds to that part of their salary paid by the HHC; after all, he reasons, Bellevue "is where the action is" and consequently where doctors prefer to be anyway. He is proud to point out that his own office as department chairman is not at NYU but at Bellevue—where it immediately impresses the observer as a lushly carpeted, walnut-paneled, air-conditioned oasis in a desert of bleakness.

The same considerations that made many NYU figures wary of the affiliation mechanism also made them uneasy about the legislation enacted in 1969 creating the Health and Hospitals Corporation. If the HHC lived up to its press releases, it might get actively involved in the running of what NYU faculty saw as their operation at Bellevue. The legislation also had a provision mandating the creation of a community advisory board to each municipal hospital, something that NYU feared might get in its hair. Having failed to ward off the HHC's creation, many at NYU now bemoan the fact that a feature of the legislation permitting the creation of subsidiary corporations to the HHC, one for each City hospital, has never been implemented. Their line is couched in terms of the benefits of decentralization, but one suspects their motivation relates to the possibility of a subsidiary corporation, if controlled by NYU, becoming a mechanism for diluting the HHC's control over the goings-on at Bellevue.

OUR LABS, YOUR ELECTRIC BILLS

Some of the goings-on at Bellevue, which neither Bellevue administration nor the HHC has very much to say about, relate to research. (NYU's research operation is not trivial. Its 1972 research budget was in the neighborhood of $60 million, mostly representing lab research.) Bellevue's buildings include about 48,000 square feet of research lab space, used by NYU researchers paid by research grants coming to NYU, on research that Bellevue's administration knows little or nothing about. The maintenance costs of these labs—including electricity for the air-conditioning that is present in the labs but absent in the wards—are paid for by Bellevue, since the HHC has never gotten around to figuring out what a square foot of such space costs to heat, light, and electrify.

INNOVATING WITH OUTPATIENTS

Before extricating ourselves from the intricacies of the Bellevue-NYU relationship, we should pass by the Outpatient Department, where we find the beginnings of an arrangement that may have interesting implications for the future of that relationship. The traditional, and still predominant, setup in the clinics is direct payment by the HHC of clinic attendings, assigned by NYU to fulfill their service obligation there. Their rate of pay—$13.30 an hour for two-hour sessions—is viewed around NYU as extortionately low and only possible as the price of a faculty appointment and admitting privileges at University Hospital. Reportedly the session physicians typically come late and leave early, with the bulk of medical care being provided by the house staff.

A departure from this arrangement was established two years ago with the creation within the Outpatient Department of a medical group practice, known as the Comprehensive Care Unit. The unit is staffed by 18 physicians representing different subspecialties of internal medicine, who are salaried at the rate of $10,000 a year for 10 hours of work per week, six at scheduled clinics and four reserved for unscheduled patient visits. For a small number of clinic patients—2,200 out of a total Outpatient Department census of about 40,000—this means being assigned a primary physician who will see the patient at every visit and who is even accessible, via telephone answering service, any time of the day or night.

Organizationally, the Comprehensive Care Unit brings the clinics into a middle-class pattern of providing ambulatory care that may set the stage for bringing the middle class into the clinics. Fiscally, the unit is innovative in creating salaried positions for ambulatory-care physicians. (Their checks are signed by the HHC, although their selection remains the responsibility of NYU.) Most of these doctors spend the other three-fourths of their time on NYU salary, teaching and/or doing research, their comprehensive care salaries in effect permitting NYU to pay them less than it would otherwise have to.

ENTER THE NEW BELLEVUE

Bellevue's administration is advertising the newness of its new hospital in terms that go beyond its air-conditioned rooms and high-speed elevators. According to Bellevue's 1972 *Annual Report:* "This building will represent a radical departure from both the philosophy and logistics of care in the existing plant. Its opening presents a unique opportunity to change the concept of Bellevue as only a hospital for the sick poor to Bellevue as a true community hospital with a primary dedication, still, to those without sufficient funds to carry the expenses of their medical care." Given the demographic changes that have made Bellevue's immediate community into a middle-class neighborhood, that reference to "a true community hospital" sounds like its means a middle-class hospital—something, perhaps, like an annex of University Hospital.

The first step in the annexation would be through

the further development of the group practice arrangement now established at Bellevue's Comprehensive Care Unit. The *Bellevue Comprehensive Plan*, an elegantly produced document prepared by the consulting firm of Westermann-Miller Associates (after extensive consultation with the folks at NYU), cites the possibility of using outpatient space at the new hospital to expand the group practice method of organization "to make complete patient care services available to the mixed income population within Bellevue environs. . . . It would permit private physician services to those who both wished and could afford them, but the program itself would not be economically discriminatory."

As to NYU's reaction to the question of moving the middle class into the new Bellevue, Dr. Frank Spencer, the chairman of surgery, notes University Hospital's long waiting lists for elective surgery and goes on to observe that what motivates middle-class elective surgery patients to wait several weeks for a bed at UH rather than use a Bellevue bed is the wretchedness of Bellevue's physical facilities rather than the mystique of the private doctor-patient relationship. "Our main concern at the new Bellevue is that it be fully utilized. With its superb facilities and the shortage of hospital beds in Manhattan, it should be fully used. If normal Bellevue patients do not fill the beds, other members of the public will need education to use the beds effectively."

It might be noted in this connection that the operating room capacity of the new Bellevue is sufficient to double the number of surgical procedures currently performed at the old Bellevue, assuming a low average of three procedures per room per day. Spencer is an open-heart surgery specialist and projects an increase in the number of coronary bypass operations that will be done at Bellevue in its new facility. "Economically, we'd love to use the new Bellevue for open-heart surgery," says Dr. Ivan Bennett, Jr., NYU's Dean and Director. The procedure is inordinately expensive and involves a loss of several thousand dollars per operation. Obligingly enough, Bellevue included in its discretionary budget for the 1973–74 fiscal year a $1.1 million item for an expanded cardiac surgery program. Some observers note that the capacity of the new Bellevue for open-heart surgery far exceeds the needs of Bellevue's traditional clientele.

The objective conditions that make the new Bellevue an attractive object from NYU's perspective are summarized in the Westermann-Miller plan: "The opening of the new Hospital will generate new opportunities for the Bellevue-NYU relationship to develop. The new Hospital, with its image radically improved from what has historically been associated with Bellevue, represents a potential expansion of private practice beds for NYU faculty, a powerful inducement to continued NYU participation, especially in the light of NYU's limited bed capacity. The new Hospital will also provide more and better facilities for clinical training programs."

SHARING OF SERVICES

As a companion concept to the new Bellevue as community hospital, Bellevue's administration sometimes bandies about the concept of sharing of services, more grandly known as "medicine under one roof." The trial balloon for the idea was floated by Manhattan Borough President Percy Sutton in an address at NYU Medical School's 1972 commencement. Heralding "a magnificent opportunity . . . to establish the pilot project of a huge ultra-high quality medical complex where equal medical services could be provided to rich, middle class, and poor alike in the same, well-equipped facility," Sutton put forth a vision of "the University Hospital, the Veterans Administration Hospital (VA), and Bellevue Hospital all operated as a single institution within a unified health concept."

In a sense, sharing of services is nothing new. We have already noted the sharing of pathology services—Bellevue does it free of charge for University Hospital's patients, Bellevue's ophthalmology service also does testing for University, and Bellevue's pediatric intensive care unit is sophisticated enough for University to send over an occasional premature infant in distress. The VA Hospital sometimes gets into the act; it does a sophisticated gastroenterologic procedure that isn't done at the other two hospitals.

As far as anyone on the outside can tell, what's going on by way of planning to expand such arrangements bears little relationship to the grandness of the "medicine-under-one-roof" concept but is bogged down in such particulars as how to administer radiation therapy to the combined clientele of Bellevue and University Hospitals. NYU has beefed up its radiation therapy capacity with a new linear accelerator—it is, after all, vying for designation as a national cancer center—while Bellevue has canceled its orders for equipment for the radiation therapy suite in the new building. The two parties have initiated negotiations over the logistics and cost of getting radiation therapy to Bellevue's patients at University Hospital, which reportedly have reached an impasse over what Bellevue regards as an exorbitant price. Note that sharing of services seems to mean that a service done at Bellevue for University Hospital patients is free, but not the reverse.

In any event, the tentative plan is for Bellevue to maintain one cobalt unit (as opposed to its original plan for two of them plus a linear accelerator) to treat patients who can't safely be transported between the two hospitals. This raises the interesting question of why these patients couldn't be admitted directly to University Hospital. After all, NYU seems to plan to admit elective surgery patients who might otherwise wait for a UH bed directly to Bellevue. It may be that Bellevue is reluctant to give up radiation therapy altogether, or it may be that NYU is more willing to share the City's hospital with its patients than to share its hospital with the City's patients.

THE MANAGERS VS. THE MEDICAL PATRIARCHS

Despite the interdependence of Bellevue and NYU, the long-range outlook for collaboration between the municipal hospital and the elite private medical center is that the going may, more than occasionally, get rough. NYU clearly needs Bellevue for teaching material, lab space, income, and for the possibility it offers for an expansion of NYU's brand of medicine to NYU's brand of patients. On the other hand, NYU is clearly unhappy about the fact that dealing with Bellevue brings it into contact, and conflict, with the Health and Hospitals Corporation. NYU's physicians are clearly unhappy at the prospect of any outside entity calling them to account.

"The Corporation doesn't understand physicians," says Dean Bennett. "No one trusts the HHC, and no one would say anything that suggests a dependency relationship on the HHC," says Dr. Albert Keegan, director of radiology at Bellevue. (That last remark may explain the fact that NYU has drawn up a contingency plan for use in the event it loses Bellevue as its teaching hospital.) More positively, NYU spokesmen are quick to attack the Corporation as an aloof, overcentralized bureaucracy, preoccupied with balancing its budget and failing to account for the uniqueness of particular institutions.

However strongly one may criticize the HHC for its bureaucratic bumblings, it is clear that NYU would find fault with any public agency that attempted to exercise an overview of its operation—thus its oft-repeated complaint that the affiliation contract doesn't provide enough flexibility for it to run things as it thinks best. It is also clear that whatever the extent of its interest in ensuring that public funds aren't squandered, the HHC has virtually no interest in programmatic planning for the benefit of its clientele. There is no evidence, for example, that the HHC has taken any part in planning for the new Bellevue other than rubber-stamping deals made by NYU and Bellevue's administration. There is no reason to believe, in other words, that there is any real danger to NYU of the HHC imposing a re-ordering of its priorities, heavily weighted as they are in favor of teaching and research.

At the level of NYU's physicians, however, there is irritation bordering on bitterness at the HHC's attempts to keep track of time actually spent at Bellevue; the cursed timesheet seems to symbolize a refusal by those blasted bureaucrats properly to acknowledge the privileged status of the medical profession. (A study of physicians' perceptions of New York's municipal hospital system, commissioned by the Society of

Urban Physicians, a group of attendings and service chiefs at the City's municipal hospitals, noted a common resentment by physicians created by the feeling that they were "being converted into employees who do not have a role in making decisions in areas in which their professional judgments are necessary.") Working for NYU then becomes preferable to working for Bellevue-HHC, not because the latter is a municipal bureaucracy but because it demands accountability and exercises control in ways that the physicians would resent coming from any source.

(Louise Lander, as well as being a Health/PAC staff member, was a member of the Bellevue Community Board. Constance Bloomfield was a Health/PAC staff member. Jon Morley was a Health/PAC summer intern and a student at NYU Medical School.)

—From the Health/PAC *Bulletin*, October, 1973. (abridged)

DEAR DR. POMRINSE: Next Time I'll Go to Bellevue

What follows is the somewhat abbreviated text of a letter from a patient to Dr. S. David Pomrinse, Director of New York City's Mt. Sinai Hospital, an 1,150-bed voluntary teaching hospital that joins with the Mt. Sinai School of Medicine to form the Mt. Sinai Medi-

cal Center. A "Consumer Guide to New York City Hospitals" published by New York *magazine includes this description of Mt. Sinai: "One of New York's great teaching hospitals, Mt. Sinai has the distinction of being both a specialty referral center and a primary hospital for its community. Its large number of superspecialists attracts a highly qualified house staff. . . . Emergency department is highly recommended." The letter, whose author is especially well trained to evaluate the adequacy of hospital care, throws a somewhat less glowing light on what it concretely means to be a patient in such a distinguished institution.*

Dear Dr. Pomrinse:

From Thursday evening, November 15, 1973 to Monday, November 19, I was an inpatient at Mt. Sinai Hospital. I am writing to you about my stay because of your position and the fact that I am a graduate of the Mt. Sinai Hospital School of Nursing and devoted close to five years of working experience to Mt. Sinai after my graduation in Adult and Child Psychiatry.

On Wednesday, November 14, I went to see my own physician because of a leg infection which had become quite severe. On Wednesday evening I had cold, shaking chills and a temperature of 103.6 degrees. On Thursday afternoon, I phoned my doctor and he urged me to go to the Emergency Room of Mt. Sinai and be admitted. He notified the Emergency Room and the chief medical resident there.

I went into the ER, informed them who I was and that I was to see the chief resident. They stated that they had no knowledge of this matter, became quite belligerent and hostile to me and told me I had to go to the admitting office. I stood there with my friend (also a former staff member) at a loss. After some minutes, a volunteer agreed to call the chief resident. She returned in a few moments to inform me that he had stated that he didn't know anything about it. At that point the doctor walked by, heard the conversation and ignored it. Some minutes later, my friend went to the door of the staff area and asked what was to be done, and at that point the chief resident acknowledged having spoken to my doctor and took me into the treatment area. He informed me that he did not think I should be admitted. He said he could either admit me or we could wait until he spoke with my doctor on the phone to discuss it.

THE AGONY OF ADMISSION

At this point, I should say that I was very ambivalent about admission. I felt physically ill and had a great deal of leg pain, making it almost impossible to walk; however, I was in great financial difficulties and knew a hospitalization would be a great added burden at this point.

Five months ago I completed my graduate degree in Psychological Counseling. While a student I worked part-time in nursing and other capacities to support myself. From last June until about two weeks before hospitalization, I had been unemployed, working only part-time as a nurse-counselor in an abortion facility, and had no health or hospital coverage. I had incurred many debts, including government loans necessary to see me through graduate school. Two and a half weeks before hospitalization, I had begun working as an individual and family therapist at a facility for adolescents. Hospital coverage in this position would not begin until February 1974, and of course I was concerned as well with whether I would be allowed to keep my position or get sick time benefits since I had just begun working. For these reasons, I told the resident I would wait until he conferred with my doctor. The resident then disappeared for over and hour and I sat and waited. On his return, the resident got in touch with my doctor, who had been trying to return his call for some time.

After consultation, it was decided that I should have an incision and drainage and if most of the difficulty was due to an abscess, I should be sent home; if, however, most of the problem was from the cellulitis in my leg, I should be admitted. The resident took me to a surgical intern. I had blood cultures drawn and an incision and drainage. Up to this point, the only person who had spoken to me as a human being was the surgical intern. It was obvious that the emotional as well as physical trauma I was experiencing was of no consequence to any member of the Emergency Room staff.

The surgical intern felt, after doing the incision and drainage, that I should be admitted. The majority of the inflammation was cellulitis. He looked for and paged the medical resident, who never appeared and could not be found. The intern told me the surgical resident (who had walked into the treatment room for approximately 60 seconds, looked at the incision and drainage and left) had stated that I should not be admitted but would have to return daily to the ER to have my leg taken care of, packing changed, etc. I informed the intern that this was not feasible for two reasons: I refused to be put through such a dehumanizing and degrading experience daily and I live alone on the fifth floor of a walkup apartment, and going up and down those stairs was not possible in my condition. The resident said that was my problem, there was nothing he could do about it if I wanted treatment. The surgical intern suggested that I go home; he could not find the medical resident and saw that I was obviously in pain, feverish and distraught. I accept my mistake in having left at this point.

On returning home, I called my doctor and told him of my experiences. He called the resident, and I was told to return to the emergency room for admission. I refused, feeling physically and emotionally drained and having no desire to see that staff again. I was told to go directly to 4 North. When I arrived there, I was told to go to admissions. This was approximately 10 or 10:30 P.M. I could hardly walk, I had not eaten for some time and I was quite weak and upset. I asked if someone from admissions could come over there and without investigation was told no.

I went to admissions and was informed that unless I was prepared to pay $1,400, I could not be admitted. I explained my financial situation and informed them that I was a graduate of the School of Nursing. After again conferring with my doctor, I returned to the Emergency Room on foot. I was at this point put in a wheelchair, to be brought to 4 North. Up to that point the only thing I had been given was a $10 ER bill. I arrived on 4 North at 1:30 A.M. Friday.

THE INPATIENT AS OUTCAST

I was given the usual physical and a case history was taken. I also informed the doctors of my history of reactions to medications. I was given no medication, although I had been put on Oxacillin by my doctor. Finally, at 11 A.M., after inquiring of both nursing and medical personnel, I was given my first dose of Oxacillin since arriving.

I had met several of the house staff but had no idea who was in charge of my case and soon found out that there was a complete lack of communication between any of the staff. If I asked about the medication or anything else, I was put off or told that "the doctor" would be told. He (whoever he was) never was informed. For the three days I was hospitalized, it was only by hitting the right person by luck that anything was communicated. Even then frequently nothing was done.

By Friday afternoon I had severe, explosive diarrhea and severe nausea. I had not eaten anything for some time and never did eat during the entire hospitalization. I asked to see the doctor about these symptoms, and many hours later kaopectate was ordered. The doctor never acknowledged what I had told him about the nausea and retching except to say that my symptoms weren't dramatic enough for him to do anything about, it was just the infection. I have had this type of reaction with other antibiotics, but he would not believe it was from the medication. When I told him I had eaten nothing (he had not been told by the nursing staff, although they had removed my trays and commented about it during these three days), he laughed and said, "You haven't eaten?" He told me he would give me nothing. His manner was always flippant, arrogant, patronizing and egotistical. This seemed to be the attitude of several of your medical house staff from my observation of their behavior toward myself and my roommates.

I discovered also that the nursing staff, especially on evenings, were totally uninvolved and uncaring of the patients. I received remarks to the effect that I could change my own dressing. Although at home I kept my leg elevated, fixed a cradle to keep the blankets off my bed, fixed a doughnut to keep my heel from being irritated, kept myself on bedrest and made some clear fluids, in the hospital I was for the most part ignored and none of these things were done or even offered. Even my temperature and blood pressure, which were ordered four times a day, frequently were not checked more than twice a day. Twice during my stay, in the evenings, I put on my light to ask for something for nausea. The bell was turned off at the nurses' station, and no one ever acknowledged it. My roommates had to help me back to bed from the bathroom several times.

Friday evening I went to the nurses' station to ask the chief resident what was happening. I stood there, talking to the resident; another resident came by and interrupted our discussion. They then proceeded to go off together. The chief yelled back over his shoulder, "Oh, I'll be back in a while." I was dumbfounded. I was angry and stated that I wasn't finished talking. He was not being called away for an emergency, he just seemed totally uninvolved in talking to a patient.

Saturday morning, when a few doctors made rounds, I again asked for something for the nausea. They looked at me and said, "Nausea, since when are you nauseated?" They didn't know. I don't know if there was anything written in my chart by either nursing or medicine, whether they hadn't read it or whether they just weren't concerned. They left with, "We'll order something," and that was the last time I heard anything about it.

At this point I should say that I was very emotionally upset about this whole experience. When I was in nursing school we learned that sick people, especially patients in a hospital, are more vulnerable and need help not only physically but also emotionally, socially, religiously and sometimes economically. We were taught to see and respect the whole person. What I was seeing was a lack of concern about any of these areas, including the physical. I know I wasn't the sickest patient at Mt. Sinai, but there is no excuse for the lack of concern and caring on the part of all disciplines of the supposed team.

Saturday afternoon I did by chance meet a very nice resident, whom I begged to help me. Having been a patient at Mt. Sinai himself on previous occasions, he seemed to understand and spent a few moments talking with me and did order something for my symptoms. Finally Saturday evening the antibiotic was discontinued. This was done only because my own doctor had come up to the unit and I informed him of my symptoms. The house staff had told him nothing, despite the fact that he was the attending on the unit. . . .

ENTER THE BILL COLLECTOR

On Monday I asked to see the social worker. I told her of my financial difficulties, and she told me to go to Patients' Accounts. I was still not well and still shaky on my feet. I walked to Patients' Accounts, was kept waiting for some time, was passed from one person to another. I told the man who finally spoke to me about my financial situation and asked about Medicaid. He excused himself, saying he was going for a pad of paper; he returned 20 minutes later to inform me not only that I could not receive Medicaid, but also that he had spoken to my place of employment and stated that I was employed there. (I had not denied that I had started working there two and a half weeks before.) He then informed me in a very nasty tone that I owed Mt. Sinai $200 per month until my bill was paid.

I told him this was impossible, asked if the payments could be less per month and again explained my financial difficulties. He refused to compromise in any way and would not let me go until I signed a paper stating that I owe Mt. Sinai $200 per month. . . .

This experience was a nightmare for me; it angers me, it dehumanized me. I know it was worse for me because I am a nurse with medical knowledge of what can be done for patients; because psychology is my field and I'm aware of feelings and attitudes more in myself and others; because I'm a woman who felt surrounded by men who haven't begun to understand people; because I spent three years being educated at Mt. Sinai, learning and believing everything in the opposite way from the way I was treated; and because I speak up for what I believe in and this, I am sure, was a threat to a lot of the staff.

I am left with three things after my hospitalization. The first is an eight-pound weight loss (which I appreciate), the second is information I am utilizing in writing an article and the third is the sad knowledge that one does not enter a hospital to get better, one enters to not get worse—hopefully!

Yours with concern,
Nancy Shamban, R.N., M.A.

—From the Health/PAC *Bulletin*, September/October, 1974 (abridged).

3

The Health Insurance Industry

As the most important institution in the health-care financing-planning complex, Blue Cross has played a key role in the development of the health-care delivery system. Through its reimbursement policies and its representatives on state and local health-planning boards, Blue Cross has favored hospitals and helped make them the dominant institution in this country for the delivery of health care. Following a brief introduction on what people get from health insurance—how much it costs, which health services it does and does not cover and what types of insurance most people have—this chapter will then concentrate on an examination of Blue Cross.

The major selection of this chapter is an excerpt from the book *Blue Cross: What Went Wrong?* by Sylvia Law. It demonstrates that Blue Cross is most accurately seen as the financing arm of the hospital system and is thus more responsive to the interests of the hospitals that control it than to those of the subscribers whose premiums support it.

In the hermetically sealed environment of local Blue Cross plans, many instances of outright corruption have developed, a fact that is documented in the Law selection. But the most serious objection to Blue

Cross is its failure to restrain hospital cost inflation and its policy of paying hospitals only. This has skewed care toward hospitals when experience has shown that many services currently delivered in hospitals can be better delivered in a home or community setting.

The final selection in this chapter, by Thomas Bodenheimer, Steven Cummings and Elizabeth Harding, discusses commercial health insurance companies. It demonstrates that commercial health insurance is no more nor less than a financial venture by major insurance empires that, unlike Blue Cross, have no interest in health care itself. Their interests are most closely aligned with those of the profit-making corporations comprising the medical-industrial complex.

WHAT PEOPLE GET FROM HEALTH INSURANCE

Thomas Bodenheimer, Steven Cummings and Elizabeth Harding

For an insurance company, illness is not a frightening and uncomfortable experience, it is a golden opportunity. And today, when people are willing to spend a great deal of money to avoid possible financial ruin through illness, payment for health care at the time of illness is gradually being replaced by the mass financing of private health insurance: regular collection of small amounts of money from everyone to pay for the care of people who are sick. The questions then remain: How much money is collected and from whom? What types of institutions receive and pay out the money? How much is paid out and to whom?

We contend that private health insurance institutions have taken the progressive concept of mass financing and have used it for their own benefit and that of the health care providers. They are indeed capitalizing on people's illness.

About 160 million Americans presently hold private health insurance policies. Many buy the insurance as part of a group such as a company, union, or professional organization, with their premiums often being deducted automatically from their paychecks. About 40 million have the far more expensive individual health insurance, and these people tend to be employees without access to a group, the unemployed, the self-employed and sporadically employed, and the elderly or sick.

Many insurance policies will not insure or will only partially insure the ill. Blue Cross states in one policy, "If at the time your application is reviewed a condition is found which excludes you from enrollment, you may be given an opportunity to join with a waiver for that condition." In other words, if you are sick, you can buy our policy and your medical expenses will be covered, but only if you get a different illness.

The elderly, under experience rating, pay more for health insurance. A Prudential policy offering hospital coverage costs $318.36 per year for a 26-year-old female and $482.36 for a 58-year-old female. Women are generally charged more than men for the same coverage because they use medical care more frequently. And people with chronic illness such as high blood pressure or diabetes must pay more for insurance, if they can obtain insurance at all.

All types of health insurance have deductibles and uncovered or partially covered care. Deductibles refer to the amount the consumer must pay for services before the insurance company will pay. A major medical plan offered by Connecticut General begins paying for covered services after the consumer has paid a $750 deductible. A similar plan by Prudential has a $400 deductible, and Equitable offers major medical plans with from $500 to $2000 deductibles.

Insurance companies generally make patients pay part of the costs of services. Partially covered care is expressed in two ways: the first is called co-insurance —we pay 80 per cent and you pay 20 per cent; the second is limited coverage—we pay for 60 days of care, you pay the rest. Insurance salesmen call this "sharing the risk with us." A group Blue Cross plan requires the policyholder to pay 20 per cent for almost all services received outside the hospital, and 20 per cent of the hospital bill after 70 days; the plan pays only $100 for outpatient psychiatric care. Innumerable additional examples could be listed.

Every insurance policy leaves many medical services uncovered. The best examples of such services are dental care, outpatient psychiatric care, preventive care, and outpatient drugs. A Connecticut General major medical insurance policy pays for no outpatient care at all. A group basic benefit plan offered by Equitable pays for no visits to doctors' offices, no psychiatric care, no dental care, and no outpatient drugs.

About 20 per cent of the population has no private surgical and hospital insurance, 28 per cent has no in-the-hospital physician insurance, 55 per cent has no insurance for physician visits, 48 per cent has no insurance for prescribed drugs, and 93 per cent has no dental insurance.[1]

An average family of four has the following medical needs: yearly physical examinations by a doctor for all members, four visits to the doctor for illness, a yearly dental checkup and needed dental work, prescription drugs for three members, and an eye examination and glasses for one member. The standard insurance policy will pay for none of these services and costs the family about $350 per year.

Private insurance advocates claim that deductibles, uncovered, and partially covered care prevent the consumer from "overusing" health facilities. In reality, however, two studies show that out-of-pocket payments mainly prevent lower-income people from using needed services.[2] With the average person covered for only 42 per cent of health costs,[1] and with these costs rising each year, out-of-pocket expenses even for insured middle-class people can be financially disastrous, as the following examples show:[3]

- In 1969 the daughter of two federal government employees had a sudden attack of intestinal disease with complications in the liver and lungs. She was hospitalized for 44 days, with a bill of $7571. Even with her parents' comparatively good insurance, the family had to pay $1550 out-of-pocket.
- In 1965 an engineer was stricken with kidney disease. In three months he ran up medical bills of $24,000. His Blue Cross and Blue Shield policies left $9000 unpaid. The patient lost his $3000 in savings, sold his car and some furniture, moved to a small apartment, and went on welfare.

—From "Capitalizing on Illness: The Health Industry," by Thomas Bodenheimer, Steven Cummings and Elizabeth Harding, *International Journal of Health Services*, 4, 583 (1974). (abridged)

BLUE CROSS: What Went Wrong?

Sylvia Law

It is widely acknowledged that the American health care crisis is primarily one of organization, administration, and accountability. Blue Cross is at the heart of the administration of the present medical care delivery system.[1] Over $22 billion a year, about one-third of the national health care dollar, are spent in hospitals.[2] Blue Cross provides about half of hospital revenues, administering over $11 billion in 1970. Public funds comprised over half of Blue Cross payments to hospitals—$4.9 billion under Medicare, $1.2 billion under Medicaid, and $545 million under other federally financed programs.[3]

Blue Cross is a complex animal, impossible to characterize in a few words. For example, it may be seen as the financing arm of American hospitals, with a primary obligation to provide them, on an equitable basis, with a stable source of income to be utilized as they judge necessary. If this is regarded as its primary role, then Blue Cross's responsibilities to subscribers and to the public are to offer hospital insurance benefits at competitive rates, to maintain a financially sound rate structure, and to pay hospitals promptly for services provided to subscribers. Alternatively, Blue Cross may be seen as a quasi-public agency with primary responsibility to the public and to its subscribers. If this is its primary role, then its obligations are to offer benefits that will enable subscribers to obtain quality health care services economically, to monitor the quality of care provided subscribers in participating hospitals, to utilize the collective power of its payments to encourage hospitals to establish programs that will best meet subscribers' health needs, and to refuse to reimburse hospitals for charges that are excessive or do not meet subscribers' needs. Finally, with respect to the public funds it administers, Blue Cross may legitimately be viewed as an agent of the government, with an obligation to carry out the policies of Congress and of the administrative agencies responsible for publicly financed medical programs. Confusion as to the proper role of Blue Cross is common and pervades the organization itself, the state regulatory agencies, Congress, and the Department of Health, Education and Welfare.

In a nutshell, this book [*Blue Cross: What Went Wrong?* by Sylvia Law, Yale University Press, 1974] finds that Blue Cross is most accurately characterized today as the financing arm of American hospitals. It argues that money for hospital care, and health care generally, should be administered by an agency—whether Blue Cross or some other—which is primarily responsive and accountable to the public interest, and particularly the interests of the individuals who use and pay for health care services.

A UNIQUE AMERICAN INSTITUTION

Blue Cross is the child of the Depression and the American Hospital Association. The period from 1875 to 1915 was one of major development of medical institutions in this country, and by 1920 the now familiar pattern of community voluntary hospitals and local autonomy in health matters was established.[4] During the 1920s there was growing recognition of the need for some mechanism by which middle income people could finance extraordinary costs of hospitalization. Hospital insurance was virtually nonexistent.[5] In October 1927, the president of the American Hospital Association described the organization's "ultimate objective" as

> providing hospitalization for the great bulk of people of moderate means . . . [who are] confronted with the necessity of amassing a debt or the alternative of casting aside all pride and accepting the provisions that are intended for the poor . . . Let us keep in mind the *raison d'être* of our existence, vis.: the provision of hospitalization for the patient of moderate means, consisting of 80 per cent of the entire population. The wise solution of this great problem will inscribe the name of the American Hospital Association in the hearts of the people for all time.[6]

The solution most often proposed then was public education; people should be taught to save for large medical expenses.[7] The Depression, however, provided the impetus for a movement away from public education toward the development of the comprehensive Blue Cross network. Hospitals were hard hit by the Depression. In one year, from 1929 to 1930, the average hospital receipts per patient fell from $236.12 to $59.26. Average per cent of occupancy fell from 71.28 per cent to 64.12 per cent. Average deficits as a percentage of disbursements rose from 15.2 per cent to 20.6 per cent.[8] The hospitals had an immediate interest in developing a stable source of payment for services and also had the technical and financial resources to create such a program. Of 39 Blue Cross plans established in the early 1930's, 22 obtained all of their initial funds from hospitals, and five were partially financed by hospitals.[9]

There was by that time a variety of small, voluntary plans for the prepayment of medical expenses, particularly the predictable expenses incident to childbirth.[10] The largest of these plans, and the one generally credited as the progenitor of Blue Cross, was initiated in 1929 by Dr. Justin Ford Kimball in Dallas, Texas. As executive vice president of Baylor University, Dr. Kimball found the unpaid bills of many local schoolteachers among the accounts receivable of the university's medical facilities. In order to assure payment to the university, he enrolled 1,250 teachers in a program to prepay fifty cents a month for 21 days of semi-private hospitalization at the Baylor University Hospital.[11]

From the 1930s on, the American Hospital Association sought to promote and control the development of monopolistic Blue Cross organizations. Preferred corporate status and tax treatment were important in the growth of Blue Cross, and these publicly conferred advantages were intensified by the private policy and control of the AHA. The [state] enabling acts do not refer to Blue Cross by name but rather allow the establishment of "hospital service corporations." Although theoretically there could be several competing hospital service corporations in any one area, the enabling acts typically require that the corporation establish cooperative agreements with the majority of hospitals in the area served. Furthermore, AHA policy has required that, in order to use the Blue Cross emblem, a hospital service corporation must establish agreements with 75 per cent of the area hospitals,[12] and the AHA generally authorized use of the emblem by only one hospital service corporation in any given area.[13] Thus, historically, the combination of public enabling legislation and the private power of the AHA has assured that there is only one Blue Cross organization in any given area and that it is, to some degree, controlled by the hospitals.

By 1938, 1.4 million people in the United States had enrolled in 38 Blue Cross plans. Private insurance companies provided hospital insurance to only 0.1 million people. During the forties Blue Cross expanded at a rapid pace; the private health insurance industry also grew, but more slowly. Several factors contributed to the rapid growth of Blue Cross: it began writing contracts with employers and contracts having nationwide coverage; health insurance increasingly became a matter for collective bargaining, with labor supporting Blue Cross; and employment and wages mushroomed during World War II.[14] In 1945 Blue Cross claimed 61 per cent of the hospital insurance market, compared with the insurance companies' 33 per cent. But in 1951, for the first time, the number of people with private commercial hospital insurance (40.0 million) surpassed the number enrolled in Blue Cross plans (37.4 million),[15] and throughout the fifties and sixties Blue Cross was unsuccessful in competing with the commercial companies. At the end of 1969 Blue Cross had an enrollment of 70.6 million, or 35 per cent of the civilian population under 65, while the commercial insurance companies provided hospital coverage to 100 million people, or 57 per cent of the civilian population under 65.[16] The passage of Medicare and Medicaid legislation in 1965, however, gave Blue Cross a boost that reestablished its dominance in terms of hospital payments as a whole.

BLUE CROSS VS. COMMERCIAL INSURANCE COMPANIES

Two major characteristics have distinguished Blue Cross from most commercial insurance companies: payment of service benefits to hospitals rather than cash benefits to the individual insured; and community rating, that is, the provision of benefits to all members of the community at the same rate, rather than higher rates to high risk groups.

The Blue Cross commitment to the payment of service benefits to hospitals means, simply, that while commercial insurers generally pay the individual a fixed dollar amount per day or period of hospitalization, and the individual bears primary responsibility for the payment of the hospital bill, Blue Cross gives the subscriber the assurance it will settle his bill with the hospital, with the subscriber bearing responsibility only for the coinsurance, or deductible, specified in the policy. The original American Hospital Association standards for the approval of hospital service plans required that, "Benefits in member hospitals should be expressed in 'service contracts,' which describe specifically the types and amounts of hospital services to which the subscribers are entitled."[17] Over the years, however, as a result of competitive pressures, an increasing number of Blue Cross plans have offered subscribers indemnity rather than service contracts.[18]

The second major distinction between Blue Cross and commercial insurers was the Blue Cross promise of service to the community. Initially all Blue Cross plans offered hospital insurance to all members of the community at uniform rates,[19] one rate for individuals and one rate for families, while commercial companies offered more favorable rates to those groups and individuals who were actuarially less likely to make claims.[20] Since low income families and the aged tend to utilize hospital services more than the general population, these groups are helped by community rating.[21] During World War II, as organized labor began to press for more adequate health benefits and other insurance companies began to compete for this growing business, Blue Cross, after a decade of internal struggle, abandoned its commitment to community rating.[22] Today most Blue Cross plans offer group experience-rated contracts, particularly for larger group policies, as well as community-rated policies for those individuals who are not able to obtain a group policy through their work or otherwise.[23]

LOCAL PLANS, THE BLUE CROSS ASSOCIATION, AND THE AMERICAN HOSPITAL ASSOCIATION

Membership in the national Blue Cross organization is critical to a local Blue Cross plan. The advantages of membership include: use of the official Blue Cross emblem and seal; the right to exclusive provision of Blue Cross benefits within a territorial area; national advertising, public relations, and lobbying; the use of information gathering, processing, and dissemination apparatus; and mechanisms for coordination of national accounts and for the transfer and acceptance of subscribers who move from one plan's territory to another's. With the advent of Medicare, membership in the national organization became even more valuable. The national Blue Cross Association (BCA) contracted with the Social Security Administration for the administration of the Medicare program, and the

BCA now serves as protector and interpreter for local plans vis-à-vis the federal government.

The name "Blue Cross" and the Blue Cross insignia were owned by the American Hospital Association until 1972.[24] The relationship between the AHA and Blue Cross plans has been close throughout Blue Cross history, as we have seen. In 1936, as part of its effort to promote the establishment of prepaid hospitalization plans, the AHA created a Committee on Hospital Services, which in 1946 became the Blue Cross Commission of the AHA.[25] Until 1960, the commission performed the national coordinating function among Blue Cross plans. In 1960, most of the commission's functions were transferred to the Blue Cross Association, a nonprofit Illinois corporation. The BCA and AHA maintained close coordination through interlocking directorates, with the AHA designating three members on the BCA board and BCA designating two members on the AHA board. Other functions, including the administration of the approval program for use of the Blue Cross insignia, were retained by the AHA. In 1971, the AHA and Blue Cross agreed in principle that the ownership of the Blue Cross name and insignia should be transferred to the BCA,[26] and this transfer became effective on June 30, 1972.[27] The two groups also agreed to eliminate their interlocking directorates and substitute a joint committee to facilitate communication between them.[28] AHA officials stated that the change was made as "a response to changing public attitudes" and emphasized that it did not represent a "cooling off" in the close relationships between Blue Cross and the AHA.[29]

CORRUPTION UNCHECKED

In 1971, the Subcommittee on Antitrust and Monopoly of the Senate Committee on the Judiciary heard extensive testimony on the operation of BCA review of local plan performance, with particular reference to the Richmond, Virginia, plan. The hearings revealed that BCA's claim of national review of local plans is predominantly public relations puffing. Testimony showed that throughout the late sixties the administrative costs of the Virginia plan were among the highest of any Blue Cross plan in the nation.[30] Subsequent investigations prompted by public and congressional concern revealed gross mismanagement. For example, the plan had 119 rented automobiles and could not account for their use.[31] It paid for staff memberships in various country clubs and owned stock in a country club.[32] Two years after Medicare began, the plan moved into an $8 million office building. One million dollars was spent to decorate and furnish the building, and most of the purchases were made, without competitive bidding, from a firm whose sales manager was chairman of the Building Committee of the Blue Cross board.[33] The plan paid $198,000 to a profit-making data processing organization but received no identifiable service. The assistant general manager of the plan was also a member of the board of the data processing organization, but he never revealed this relationship, because he believed that there was no conflict of interest.[34]

In October 1968, while these policies were in effect, the Richmond plan was given a "Total Plan Review" by the BCA. The final report, while noting low productivity and high cost per claim, was laudatory.

> The team was particularly impressed with the overall corporate structure and organization of the plan. . . . The executive management group of the Richmond plan displays a progressive and confident attitude. . . . There is an atmosphere which is conducive to innovation and change aimed at improvement. . . .
>
> It was favorably noted that a good start has been made toward greater refinement of the budget, cost accounting, etc. in the financial area. The Richmond plan has made great strides towards attracting and retaining qualified personnel. This is true with respect to physical surroundings, progressive atmosphere, etc.

Despite this clean bill of health, by early 1970 public attention prompted the BCA to reexamine the plan. Internal BCA memos subpoenaed by the Senate committee revealed that the 1970 investigation was primarily concerned with public appearances. One national official recommended that a BCA team be sent in "in the interest of preserving the National reputation as opposed to assisting the Plan." Another BCA official visiting Richmond concluded that BCA should

> refrain from moving in since we know the bad news that might erupt. . . . Richmond could blow up. It is a real "can of worms." But we know enough bad things without necessarily sending in a team to get more information. However, I also recognize that the National Associations must preserve their dignity and be prepared to answer questions. . . . Nevertheless, this is another case of "locking the barn door after the horse has departed."[36]

It seems that local malfeasance is a subject for national concern only when it approaches the level of scandal or illegality. Even then BCA efforts are directed first toward preventing adverse publicity, then toward correcting the problems.

While corporate waste through high administrative costs is significant, it is not the central issue in evaluating Blue Cross performance. In Richmond, administrative costs represented only 5.4 per cent of the earned subscriber income, the balance being payments to hospitals.[37] The key issue of public concern should be what Blue Cross does to ensure that hospital costs are reasonable. Not surprisingly, the evidence was that the Richmond plan did not pursue any form of hospital cost control. The executive director of the plan was asked, "What if your audit [of hospital books] indicated clearly wasteful practices? What do you do?" He responded, "Well, Mr. Chairman, I am not aware of our audits ever uncovering wasteful charges, and I really wouldn't know what we would do if we ran into them." [38]

Because of the difficulty in obtaining information about the internal operations of Blue Cross, it is not possible to know whether the Richmond operation is typical. Probably it is not.[39] However, such mismanagement is not unique. For example, the General Accounting Office and a subcommittee of the House Committee on Government Operations found that during 1966–67, Washington, D.C. Blue Cross kept an average of more than $10 million in federal funds in noninterest-bearing accounts in Washington banks. Larger amounts, estimated in excess of $15 million, were kept in noninterest-bearing accounts from 1961 to 1965.[40] Several members of the Blue Cross board, including the treasurer, were officers and board members of the banks in which the monies were deposited.[41] From 1963 until 1971 Illinois Blue Cross had between $7 and $15 million deposited in noninterest-bearing accounts in a bank at which the chairman of the board served as senior vice president and an additional $2 million in noninterest-bearing accounts in a second bank, one of the officers of which was also on the Blue Cross board.[42]

Periodic investigations by congressional committees are obviously an ineffective means to discover whether plans operate efficiently or to encourage such operation. As the facts concerning the mismanagement of the Richmond plan unfolded, the Subcommittee on Antitrust and Monopoly grappled to find some mechanism of public accountability—some means by which the interests of the public and of subscribers could be protected. Senator Hart asked, "There isn't any outside discipline, either the Virginia Corporation Commission or legislative body or the National Blue Cross, that could do other than sort of wonder. Nobody could correct, is that right, absent the internal discipline?" The chief executive officer responded, "Mr. Chairman, I would say you are absolutely right, but that responsibility rests purely on the shoulders of the boards of directors. . . . The moment they found the level of spending which they couldn't quite stand, they acted immediately." [43]

BLUE CROSS BOARDS OF DIRECTORS

The local Blue Cross board has the primary—and often the sole—responsibility for determining policy and assuring accountability within the plan. In the 1960's, the assertion that Blue Cross boards were publicly responsive was a major selling point in persuading Congress to give Blue Cross a key role in the Medicare program.[44] Although citizen control of local Blue Cross policy has always been emphasized in Blue

Cross rhetoric, it is only within the past few years that there has been serious scrutiny of the actual composition of Blue Cross boards.

Hospital representatives currently dominate Blue Cross boards. The AHA Standards for Approval, now taken over by the BCA, require that at least one-third of the board members represent the contracting hospitals, and some enabling acts require hospital representatives on the board.[45] In 1970, according to BCA figures, 56 percent of the members of local boards were health care providers, 42 percent representing hospitals and 14 percent representing the medical profession.[46]

A case can be made that hospital representatives have no proper role on Blue Cross boards. Because the federal and state governments have delegated to Blue Cross the public functions of: (1) paying for publicly financed hospital care; (2) determining the reasonableness of hospital costs; and (3) using payment processes to encourage rational planning and utilization patterns, the place of provider representatives on Blue Cross boards can certainly be questioned. For example, the chairman of the Massachusetts Rate Setting Commission and special counsel for health affairs commented:

> If we regard Blue Cross as having a responsibility to "regulate" hospital costs—and I most certainly do—then we can look upon this arrangement as those who are regulated actually being the regulators of themselves. The counterbalancing and resolution of discrete interests which should be the heart of any regulatory process is lacking.[47]

The criticism of provider members on Blue Cross boards is not primarily that they are self-dealing or necessarily incapable of avoiding conflicts of interest.[48] Rather, the problem is that provider representatives are primarily responsible to hospitals rather than to subscribers or the public. It is unrealistic to expect that, as Blue Cross board members, hospital representatives will challenge hospital policies on cost control, area planning, or reorientation of services, when these are policies they have developed. Hospital representatives will seek to maintain the autonomy of the hospital.[49]

As presently constituted, even the public board members often do not protect or reflect subscriber interests. Although in 1970 44 per cent of the members of local plan boards were "public" representatives, examination reveals that under present structures public representatives are an elite group with little resemblance to subscribers. In most Blue Cross plans public representatives are selected by the incumbent board.[50] In twenty-one plans they are selected by the hospital representatives.[51] In Washington, D.C., the public representatives are appointed by the commissioner of the district. Subscribers elect public representatives in only eight plans, including the Philadelphia plan.[52]

Compared to other plans the Philadelphia board has democratic selection procedures. However, it is not in fact open to subscriber control or participation. In 1971 the plan bylaws were amended to allow subscribers to vote for board members, with nominations made by the incumbent board or by petition with 300 subscriber signatures. In 1971 and 1972 subscribers nominated candidates to run against the nominees of the board. Through advertisements in local newspapers and through contacts with large organizations holding group contracts, the plan management solicited proxy votes for the board's candidates. In both years the plan refused subscriber requests to publish a ballot that would allow subscribers to cast votes for the insurgent candidates and to publish information about the position of various candidates on questions of plan policy. In 1971, the subscriber candidates received over 1,000 votes, but the management slate won with about 3,000 votes. In 1972, the subscriber candidates received over 4,000 votes, but management had increased its effort and obtained 16,000 proxy votes.[53] During the intervening year there had been substantial adverse publicity about Blue Cross, as Insurance Commissioner Herbert Denenberg criticized the plan for failure to hold down hospital costs. It is difficult to believe that the fivefold jump in votes for the incumbent board reflected a vote of confidence or popularity. The number of votes obtained by the management appears to reflect the amount of management resources devoted to the collection of proxies rather than subscriber endorsement of management policy and competence. The subscriber candidates had no financial support but depended on volunteer efforts of those concerned about Blue Cross policy. There are no limitations on the resources which the plan can devote to insuring the election of a board that will support current policies and management.[54]

The Philadelphia plan directors are not representative of the plan's subscribers. Twelve of the 32 directors are directors of banking and financial institutions. Two sit on the boards of major real estate companies, one is the president of a company with major interests in hospital supply, and others are business executives.[55] Two directors represent organized labor. The typical board member is white, male, over 40, and wealthy; departures from this norm are few. The Philadelphia board does not even reflect the broad range of the city's hospitals; in 1970 five of the city's most influential hospitals had more than one representative on the board.[56]

The pattern in Philadelphia is typical of the rest of the country. Blue Cross Association data show that the 824 members of local plan boards designated as public and consumer representatives include: 311 business executives, 116 physicians and surgeons, 90 retired people, 73 bankers, 54 lawyers, 39 labor leaders, 34 university and school officials, 23 investment advisers, 17 religious leaders, 8 real estate men, and 59 people in a variety of other positions.[57] Of these public representatives, only 18 are women.

Labor representatives on Blue Cross boards are often cited as the representatives of ordinary subscribers. There is no evidence that they have played such a role.[58] Further examination of labor members of Blue Cross boards is needed. One hypothesis is that labor representatives have been content to obtain relatively favorable rate treatment for their own members.[59] Blue Cross critics charge that community-rated subscribers, who pay substantially higher rates, subsidize the organized experience-rated subscribers.[60] No one would be the wiser if a plan were to offer favorable group rates based not on experience but on political influence, representation on the plan board, or other extraneous factors. Only Blue Cross has the information needed to determine whether such discriminatory rate setting exists. Insurance commissioners do not obtain sufficient information to know whether experience rates are justified on the basis of actual experience and administrative savings resulting from the group contract; certainly community-rated subscribers do not have access to such information.[61] Aggressive scrutiny of Blue Cross policies and pursuit of institutional reform would require enormous effort and tenacity and could quickly put labor representatives into direct conflict with plan administration and board members from the hospitals. Given that labor representatives constitute such a small minority on a Blue Cross board and given that they are accountable to a constituency that is probably not demanding reforms in the Blue Cross structure, it would not be surprising to find labor members playing a quiet role in Blue Cross governance.[62]

Within the present Blue Cross board structures, there are some reforms that can and should be instituted. Although neither the BCA nor the insurance departments presently scrutinize board members for direct conflicts of interests, such a probe could be conducted. It would be a fairly simple matter for the BCA, state insurance departments, or the federal government as administrator of Medicare to gather and publicize information on the affiliations of Blue Cross directors and on the major organizations with which the plan contracts and banks. Simply gathering such information and making it public would do much to curb the more flagrant abuses of Blue Cross power.

The more fundamental question of who governs Blue Cross, and to whom it should be accountable, requires a more comprehensive solution. It is an illusion to believe that effective public control of an institution as complex and influential as Blue Cross could be achieved easily or with minor reforms.

—Excerpts from Introduction and Chapter II of *Blue Cross: What Went Wrong?* by Sylvia Law (New Haven: Yale University Press, 1974).

COMMERCIAL INSURANCE COMPANIES: Capitalizing on Illness

Thomas Bodenheimer, Steven Cummings and Elizabeth Harding

Commercial insurance companies did not become important in the health field until after World War II, when the Blues were already well established. Labor unions, as part of their negotiations with management over wages, began to demand health benefits for workers and as these benefits were fought for and won, employers started to pay part of employees' wages into health and welfare funds, which were used to buy private health insurance at group rates. Commercial companies grew rapidly during the 1950's. They captured much of the labor union market by experience-rating relatively young, healthy worker groups, while Blue Cross continued to offer them more expensive community rates.

Unlike the Blues, which were put together to assure the payment of bills to the hospitals and doctors, commercial insurance companies sell health insurance purely for the purpose of making a profit. About 1000 companies offer health insurance, with about 115 million people holding some type of commercial policy. In 1972, the commercials took in $14.3 billion in premium income.[1] Thus the total volume of commercial insurance is somewhat greater than that of the Blues, though no one commercial company comes close to Blue Cross in size.

The ten largest commercial health insurers are Aetna, Travelers, Metropolitan Life, Prudential, CNA, Equitable, Mutual of Omaha, Connecticut General, John Hancock, and Provident. In 1970, Aetna took in over a billion dollars in health premiums.[2]

Most of the top health insurance companies are also the biggest life insurers. These giants represent an enormous concentration of wealth and political power in America. Prudential and Metropolitan Life, the two largest, each have $30 billion in assets, making them far bigger than General Motors, Standard Oil of New Jersey, and ITT, and the equals of Bank of America and Chase Manhattan Bank. In 1970, supposedly a bad year for health insurance, the life insurance business boomed. In that year Prudential and Metropolitan Life received premium income (life, accident, health, and other policies) of almost $4 billion each and net income from investments of $1.4 billion each.[2]

The major insurance companies are closely tied to the largest U.S. banks and manufacturing corporations through enormous financial empires. The Rockefeller family interests control or heavily influence the Metropolitan Life and Equitable insurance companies, Chase Manhattan Bank, Standard Oil, Mobil Oil, IBM, and numerous other corporations. The Morgan empire (the legacy of J. P. Morgan) includes the Prudential Insurance Company, the Bankers Trust and Morgan Guarantee Trust banks, General Electric, and U.S. Steel. Of 28 directors of Metropolitan Life, 23 sit on the boards of banking institutions, particularly Chase Manhattan. Eighteen of Prudential's 29 directors sit on bank boards. Half of Equitable's directors are on bank boards with an especially close relation with Chase Manhattan.[3]

These facts are given in order to make the point that commercial health insurance policy is ultimately set by very rich and influential people in U.S. society. The money that comes into the hands of these companies, constituting one-half of the net savings of individuals in America,[4] is used in several ways: (a) to make huge loans ($185 million daily) to corporations, thus supplying much of the money needed for corporate expansion; (b) to buy large blocks of stock in corporations so that the insurance company can effectively control the corporations; (c) to finance real estate developments and urban high-rise buildings; and (d) to influence politicians through campaign contributions and other favors (for example, W. Clement Stone, chairman of Combined Insurance, the thirteenth largest health insurer, gave $1 million to Richard Nixon's 1968 campaign, another million to the 1972 campaign, and received a preferential ruling from the Price Commission in 1971 to raise insurance rates).[5]

Commercial insurance companies have a different relationship with doctors and hospitals than do the Blues. Whereas the Blues make contracts with hospitals and doctors regarding how much they will pay, a commercial company contracts with the patient and does not deal with the providers directly. Thus patients often have to fight to collect the money from their insurance company.

Commercial companies formerly paid the patient only a stipulated sum of money for each service, for example, $50 per hospital day despite the fact that the daily charge might be $80. Many individual policies are still written this way. One plan advertised in a San Francisco newspaper pays $100 per week ($14.28 per day) for hospital care while hospital rates are around $100 per day. The advertisement contained the sentence: "When hospital emergency strikes, you can say 'Thank Heaven, we didn't have to borrow a cent.' "

However, commercial group plans have generally changed due to competition among themselves and with the Blues. Many of these plans now pay the full daily hospital rate, though with the usual deductibles, co-insurance, and limitations. Commercials thus have become concerned with the rapid rise in hospital charges since they too must pay out more when the rates go up.

In 1972, commercial companies collected $14.3 billion in insurance premiums and paid out $10.6 billion in benefit payments.[1] On the average, group policies pay out in benefits 96 percent of the premiums collected, whereas individual policies pay out only 51 percent. Clearly, individual plans pay far fewer benefits and thus are of less value to the buyer than are group plans.[6] Different companies pay out higher or lower percentages of their premium income depending on whether they have more or less group coverage. In 1970, Aetna and Travelers paid out 90 percent of their premium income; these companies overwhelmingly sell group insurance. Metropolitan Life and Prudential paid out around 85 percent of premiums, whereas Mutual of Omaha paid only 73 percent and Combined Insurance (run by former President Nixon's friend W. Clement Stone) paid out only 43 percent of its largely individual premiums.[2]

In light of the profit orientation of insurance companies, it may come as a surprise that in 1970, the commercial insurance industry spent $600 million more in benefits and administrative costs than it collected in premiums. Aetna, the largest commercial insurer, collected $1 billion in 1970 premiums, paid out $984 million in benefits, spent millions more in administration, and consequently had what is called an underwriting loss of $13 million on its health insurance. In 1969 Aetna similarly lost $28 million on health insurance; in 1968, $16 million; and in 1967 it "gained" $6 million. In 1970 Travelers "lost" $41 million in health insurance; Metropolitan Life "lost" $18 million; Connecticut General "lost" $37 million; and Combined Insurance "gained" $16 million.[2] By 1972, however, the companies as a whole were doing better, as we will describe later.

Are health insurance companies really losing money? The answer is no. First, commercial health insurance is closely linked to life and other forms of insurance. A large amount of group commercial insurance (perhaps $2–3 billion a year) is bought by companies who pay for workmen's compensation, disability, life, accident, and health insurance for their employees. These companies generally study the policies of several insurers and buy all the insurance in a package from one insurance company. Thus, an insurance company that makes a good offer on health insurance will sell more of the highly profitable life insurance, and the apparent health insurance losses are actually bringing in greater profits in other types of insurance.

Secondly, the health insurance losses do not take investment income into account. When Aetna collects $1 billion in health insurance premiums, it does not pay this money out in benefits right away. The money is available for investment, which produces a profitable return. Aetna's total investment income in 1970 was $344 million.[2] Since 55 percent of Aetna's premiums are from health insurance, one can assume that Aetna earned $190 million in investments from its health business. Thus the $13 million in "losses" is erased, and Aetna actually profited immensely from its health insurance.

Private health insurance institutions have no reason to exist in the health care system. They are presently in the health business to make money—for themselves, for doctors, and for hospitals.

The only reasonable thing to do with the health insurance industry is to abolish it. Health care can be financed by government collection of taxes and payment directly to health centers and hospitals, without profit.

But it is not enough to abolish insurance companies. The entire notion of insurance is unfair. With insurance, people get what they pay for. Sicker people pay more than healthier people; the elderly pay more than the young; and lower-income people pay the same premiums as wealthy people, thus taking a larger percentage of their earnings.

The entire philosophy of insurance is in sharp conflict with the concept of health care as a right. If health care is a right, money should not be a consideration in receiving it. Health care should be free to everybody at the point of delivery and should be paid for by a progressive tax based on ability to pay. The insurance concept—that people receive only what they pay for—should be thrown out along with the insurance industry.

—From *International Journal of Health Services*, 4, 583 (1974). (abridged and edited)

4

Profiteering in Health Care

There is no question that enterprises such as drug companies, hospital supply and equipment companies and commercial insurance companies are involved in health care for the explicit purpose of making a profit. Their proponents insist, however, that there is no conflict between making a profit and serving the health needs of the American people.

The selections in this chapter demonstrate the fallacy of that proposition. The opening selection, by Rick Barnhart, shows that patients have had to pay a high price, both literally and figuratively, for the profits of drug companies. These companies are expert in using the patent laws as a means of avoiding free-enterprise competition and keeping their prices at enormously inflated levels. Even worse, from the patient's point of view, are the drug industry's expensive advertising and promotion campaigns, which are aimed at expanding the range of symptoms for which its products are prescribed beyond all reasonable medical need, and covering up its products' negative side effects.

The search for profits by the nursing-home industry has created an even uglier scene than that by the drug industry. The venality of nursing-home entrepreneurs in New York City and the high-level political connections that protected them are outlined in three short articles by reporters from *The New York Times* and *The Village Voice.*

The nursing-home scandals, reflecting as they do the conflict between profit-making and decent patient care, have spurred proposals for the abolition of profit-making institutions, at least in the nursing-home field. The difficulty with that approach is that it ignores the problem of the profit-making that goes on within nonprofit institutions. This problem has long been apparent in the case of hospitals, most of which in this country are organized as private, nonprofit institutions, so-called voluntary hospitals. Profiteering within hospitals, whether voluntary hospitals or proprietary (profit-making) hospitals, is the next concern of this chapter.

Three groups within hospitals, including nonprofit hospitals, have traditionally been in a position to use the hospital as an arena for profiteering—namely, trustees, administrators and doctors. Such profiteering is nowhere better illustrated than in the remarkable series of reports on Washington Hospital Center, a voluntary hospital, by Ron Kessler of the Washington *Post.* Kessler exposes many instances of corruption, both petty and grand, by trustees and administrators, as well as price-gouging by the physician who directs the hospital's pathology laboratory.

Another arena for profit-making in hospitals, again including nonprofit ones, is hospital construction, which in many areas has far outstripped the need for hospital beds. In the next selection, Bob Nichols and associates at the Oklahoma Consumer Protection Agency discuss overbedding in Oklahoma City, showing how profitable hospital construction is for banks and construction companies and how costly it will be for the people of Oklahoma City.

GETTING A FIX: The U.S. Drug Monopoly

Rick Barnhart

There are in America some 2,000 companies dealing in pharmaceuticals for human use. One hundred and thirty-six comprise the Pharmaceutical Manufacturers Association (PMA), which accounts for 95 percent of prescription drugs sold on the domestic market.

The drug industry itself is largely a noncompetitive enterprise. Despite the fact that no company controls more than 7 percent of U.S. prescription drug sales (a fact that PMA has cited to prove the competitive nature of the drug industry), we must remember that drug markets are separate and noncompeting. That is, the sale of tranquilizers does not cut into the market for antibiotics; and the sale of neither cuts into the market for anti-inflammatory agents. There is no price competition between drug companies in general, but between companies producing a particular chemical entity. Therefore, we must examine individual drugs and determine how many companies control their markets. Senator Kefauver found that of 51 chemical entities comprising at least ⅔ of prescription drug sales, 27 had only one producer, 8 had two producers, 10 had three, and none had more than seven. For better than half the entities considered the producer company had no competition at all, and for the remaining drugs competing companies were few.

PATENTS AND PRICES

The number of firms producing and selling a new drug is limited primarily by patents and licensing practices. A company developing a new drug receives a patent that prohibits other companies from producing the same drug for 17 years. The patent leaves the producer "free to charge what the traffic will bear." Thus, a patent ensures a virtual monopoly over the drug, a monopoly that can be extended by "judicious spacing of improvement patents, or by making slight changes in the drug's molecular structure, allegedly increasing its potency, efficacy, or safety." [1] The combination drug is another mechanism by which drug companies extend their patents and their price monopolies, as Dr. Calvin Kunin testified before the Nelson Committee:

> If I were in industry, and I were in danger of losing my patent with which I have reaped my fortune over many years and I wanted to retain that patent, then I would combine that drug with something else so that I have a new proprietary agent. This is the way of keeping this within one's own pocket.[2]

In short,

> the production of nonpatented drugs will give only moderate profits while the production of patented drugs will give abnormally high profits. Drug manufacturers have attempted, therefore, by every conceivable means to divert the market into the sale of high-profit patented drugs. Let us note at this point that

an estimated two thirds of sales of the larger manufacturers are for patentable drugs.[3]

How far the industry is willing to go to get patents and profits is illustrated in the case of tetracycline. The Trade Commission concluded:

> . . . that Pfizer was directly and culpably responsible for the procurement by misrepresentation (of the results of their own research) of a monopoly over a product which had cost the American public millions of dollars . . . that Cyanimid withdrew its own application for the tetracycline patent after a deal was made with Pfizer to divide up the American market for the product . . . that the procurement of these patents had enabled Cyanimid and Pfizer to establish noncompetitive and fixed prices . . . from 1949 through 1953 to the great damage of millions of Americans.[4]

The profits realized through this strategy are tremendous; the average net income/sales equals 9.0 percent, twice the industrial median of 4.8 percent. This ratio ranges as high as 15.0 percent (SK&F) [Smith, Kline and French], 15.9 percent (Merck) and 18.5 percent (Searle). Net income/invested capital equals 17.9 percent, almost twice the industrial median of 11.7 percent. This ratio goes as high as 24.3 percent (Merck), 24.9 percent (SK&F) and 27.9 percent (Searle).[5]

When a company introduces a new drug, the drug is given two names, a generic name and a brand name. The generic name is generally long and hard to remember while the brand name is often catchy and popular. For example, Roche's tranquilizer with the well-known brand name Librium has as its generic name chlordiazepoxide hydrochloride. When Librium's 17 years of patent protection are over, any company could make chlordiazepoxide hydrochloride and can either call it chlordiazepoxide hydrochloride or can give it another brand name. Roche, of course, will continue to have a competitive advantage because doctors and patients know the name Librium.

Among the most significant components of high pharmaceutical profit is the abnormally high price of brand-name drugs. The price of brand-name drugs has virtually nothing to do with production costs and other industrial expenses, but rather is based upon the maximum the public in its medical need can be induced to pay. From among numerous examples consider prednisone. Schering's name brand, Meticorten, sells for $102.57/1000 while Wolins (a large respected wholesaler of generic drugs) sells prednisone for $4.40/1000.

The companies usually defend their business strategy, including patent monopolies and high prices, with the following arguments: (1) there is strong competition and high risk within the industry; (2) the high cost of quality control added to other production costs causes prices to be high; (3) brand-name drugs are superior to generic drugs; (4) vital research and development costs are high. All these arguments can be easily refuted.

Competition and risk: There are two types of competition: price competition and competition by advertising. Price competition means that a company lowers its prices in order to get more buyers. As already suggested there is virtually no price competition in the drug industry, since either one company has a monopoly on a particular drug, or two or three companies fix the prices of a drug. There is, however, intense competition for a greater share of the market through advertising. This competition does not reduce the price for consumers; in fact, it raises prices with high advertising costs.

Nor is the drug industry so risky an enterprise as its spokesmen would have the public believe. H.E.W.'s *Task Force on Prescription Drugs* concluded that "the exceptionally high rate of profit which generally marks the drug industry is not accompanied by any particular degree of risk or by any unique difficulties in obtaining growth capital." [6]

Cost of quality control and production: The *Task Force* also found that "any company large or small, brand-name or generic name producer can institute and maintain an effective quality control program, and most companies have apparently done so. The cost of such a program has been estimated to be about 2.4 percent of sales." [7] Economic analysis before the Nelson Committee has indicated that the cost of quality control is really a very small component of the total costs, and that the cost difference between a minimally satisfactory program and an extremely scrupulous program would not begin to account for the price differences observed between a generic drug and its name-brand equivalent.[8] We must conclude, therefore, that the high price of drugs is not a function of quality control costs at all.

Superiority of name-brand quality and efficacy: In 1966 a U.S. Food and Drug Administration (FDA) study of drug potency covering 4573 drug samples from 236 manufacturers—though by no means absolutely conclusive—indicated "that, although 7.8 percent of generic samples were found violative, the figure was 8.8 percent for trade names." [9] The industry's claim that generics do not perform with the therapeutic efficacy of the trade-name drug is a flimsy one at best. Dr.

Robert H. Ebert, Dean of the Harvard Medical School, recently sent a memo to the Faculty of Medicine stating:

> Almost all studies show that generic drugs and name-brand drugs are indistinguishable in therapeutic effectiveness, purity, or accuracy of labeling.
>
> The exaggerated and probably false distinction between brand-name and generic drugs claimed in advertising by drug firms is regrettable.
>
> The Faculty of Medicine should maintain its awareness of such questionable practices in the marketing of drugs and counteract this practice through their own habits of prescription writing and those they teach to their students.

Generally the only difference between generic and name-brand drugs lies in the physical state of the active ingredient (particle and crystal size) and the nature of inert substances (bases, disintegrants, and binders). The drug industry claims that these differences create significant variations in therapeutic effect and therapeutic reliability. To prove the superior quality and reliability of their name-brand drugs, drug companies and the PMA parade testimonials from doctors and pharmacists before both the public and the rest of the medical profession. But they do not cite controlled clinical studies from objective sources because in the realm of scientific investigation the conclusions have gone heavily against their argument.

Research and development: The drug industry notes that numerous new chemical entities of great therapeutic significance have been introduced in a remarkably short time; to this end the industry spends three times as much of its own money on research than any other major industry; and, therefore, its high prices are necessary to ensure these vital medical advances. The PMA claims that of 823 "single new chemical entities" introduced between 1940 and 1966 the U.S. industry invented 502. Senator Nelson found, however, that the definition of "single new chemical entity" included the class of drugs known as molecular manipulations (minor changes in the molecular structure of drugs without necessarily changing the drugs' effects).[10] The *Task Force* concluded:

> Since important new chemical entities represent only a fraction, perhaps 10 to 20 percent of all new products introduced per year, and the remainder consists merely of minor modifications of combination products, then much of the industry's research and development activities would appear to provide only minor contributions to medical progress.[6]

Of the 502 drugs introduced by the U.S. industry perhaps as few as 40 were of any real medical significance. Recall that the reason for molecular manipulations and combinations is to extend the duration of patent monopoly and to introduce drugs onto the market at higher prices. Since up to 90 percent of drug industry research and development is devoted to this maneuver, the money invested by the drug companies is not a reflection of concern for medical progress as much as a reflection of concern for maximum profits.

Thus, we have exhausted the drug industry's strongest arguments in defense of its prices and business strategy. None is substantial. The price of these monopolistically controlled name-brand drugs is unjustifiably high, and the profit to which these prices contribute is correspondingly exorbitant.

FOREIGN EXPANSION

Another factor in the industry's business strategy that contributes heavily to high profits is its expansion into foreign markets. "Since the patent system applies throughout the western world . . . the ease with which U.S. patents may be registered almost anywhere abroad, ensures that a U.S. patent holder will not be bothered by foreign competition."[4] With no significant competition, U.S. drug companies set up factories in other countries, use the cheaper labor, lower tax rates and lower overhead costs of these countries, and send the profit back to the United States. Since most of these factories are highly automated and therefore employ relatively few people, they do not help the unemployment problems of underdeveloped countries. With factories set up all over the world, the companies are in a fine position to corner the market in each country with the same business strategy to which the American public is subjected. Moreover, when the FDA belatedly regulates a dangerous drug within the U.S., the company can and does continue to sell that drug overseas (see the case of chloramphenicol below).

ADVERTISING AND PROMOTION

There is another component of drug profit, one of growing concern to the public, medical profession, and government alike: the expansion of domestic markets beyond actual medical need by means of promotion and advertising. The demand that creates the market for a drug is relatively fixed. That is, barring epidemic fluctuations in a disease, the need for appropriate drugs remains roughly the same and, therefore, the demand for such drugs should be relatively fixed. This poses a real limitation to market growth; the only way to influence the relationship and increase the demand for a given drug is to maximize the medical needs for which it is recognized as indicated. For example, if I produce an antibiotic specific for a given class of organism, and the incidence of disease these microbes cause is relatively fixed, then the demand and market for my antibiotic are also fixed. This relationship would, of course, tend to limit my profits. If, however, I can convince the prescriber that the drug is effective against an additional class of organisms, then my market and profits will expand. The drug industry has used this strategy with uncommon and often disastrous success. Thus, marketing practices are aimed primarily to influence the physician to prescribe (a) only a given brand-name drug, (b) for as many conditions as possible, often regardless of contraindications (potential dangerous situations).

The backbone of the drug marketing system is the brand (trade) name. "Once the trade-name product has won wide acceptance by physicians, it is difficult to supplant. Thus it may stubbornly hold its market share despite subsequent development of more advanced competitive products or increased competition following expiration of the patent."[11] The overwhelming proportion of drugs sold today are brand-name, and laws are such that even a prescription for generic drugs stands a 50–50 chance of being filled with name-brand products. Forty-four of the 50 states have anti-substitution laws making it illegal to fill a prescription for a particular brand with any other. Generic prescriptions, however, may be filled with any brand, so although 6.5 percent of new prescriptions are for generics, roughly half of them are filled with expensive name-brands.

The industry's campaign for its name-brand begins early. With medical students "the strategy of names takes on great importance. For it is during his training that the student begins to associate useful drugs with the trade-names as well as, and often in place of, their generic names." [12] The campaign of indoctrination to brand-names is carried out on a massive scale and on many fronts. Marketing expenses absorb anywhere from 15 to 35 percent of the industry's sales.[6] The magnitude of this expenditure is roughly three times that used by U.S. manufacturing in general.

Companies invest marketing funds in various ways to gain the medical profession's acceptance of its name-brands. To the tune of $3000 per physician per year the industry can treat each M.D. to: (1) brochures and journal advertisements, (2) free product samples, (3) displays and hospitality at conventions, (4) grants for research, professors' salaries, and academic courses, (5) detail men, and (6) "gifts" to medical students and doctors.

Probably the most significant of these promotional activities is the detail man. In one AMA survey, "65% of physicians listed these company representatives as the 'most effective' source of the doctor's information on new drugs." [13] Apparently the industry is well aware of this fact since the force of detail men often accounts for ⅙ to ⅕ of all employees. In fact, for twenty large firms, salesmen's and detail men's compensation amounts to $200 million or ⅖ of total marketing costs.[13] Dr. Dale Console, Medical Director for E.R. Squibb for many years, speaks of the purpose of detail men:

> The primary purpose of the detail man is to make a sale even if it involves irrational prescribing and irrational combinations.
>
> During my time in the drug industry I had a close ongoing relationship with detail men. It was from them that I learned the simple maxim, "If you can't convince them, confuse them." [14]

Since the enormous cost of the detail men can be counted as a tax-deductible business expense, the public winds up paying for a large portion of the industry's detailing in addition to paying brand-name drug prices. Paraphrasing Oliver Wendell Holmes: if all the detail men were dumped into the sea it would result in the betterment of mankind and detriment to the fishes.[14]

The next most significant marketing activity is advertising. "In composing advertising . . . drug companies are . . . open to a strong temptation to imply a wider range of uses than the FDA has explicity approved, to underplay the harmful side effects . . . and to neglect contraindications." [13]

Herein the strategy of increasing demand beyond actual medical need becomes reality, for experience has proven that the drug companies are not only tempted; they all too often give in to their temptation, sometimes with medically disastrous results. The Drug Act was amended in 1962 to stem advertising abuses, but "with only ten men to handle the job, the agency [FDA] could not hope to cover the field in a comprehensive way." [13] So even with the strengthened law "advertising failures" persist. During one recent period, January, 1967, to April, 1968, the FDA required 21 remedial letters for advertising abuses to be issued by 20 different companies including Roche, Abbott, Pfizer, Geigy, Squibb, Upjohn, Searle, and Parke-

Davis.[15] One can only wonder how many letters would have been required had the FDA a more adequate staff.

There are many specific examples of misrepresentation in promotion and advertising. We will consider two such examples in some detail, examining the role of these most important aspects of drug marketing, ads and detail men.

"Indocin, the Merck brand of indomethacin (a drug similar to aspirin) was recognized from the first as a drug with significant capacity for adverse effects . . . its promotion over the first year of its approved marketing improperly presented the drug to the medical profession—both as to range of effectiveness and as to the margin of its safety." [16] The advertising (1) claimed that the drug "extended the margin of long term safety without any evidence to support the claim," (2) offered the drug for "arthritis disorders" though it has not been approved for such conditions, and (3) "In the 'brief summary' of information on side effects and contraindications some of the major warning information was left out—such as the fact that indomethacin itself had caused ulcers, and that the drug should not be administered to children." [16]

A series of bulletins entitled "Profit Improvement Promotional Program—Indocin" distributed to all of Merck's sales associates gives an indication of the role of their detail men in backing up the distorted advertisements. One bulletin contains a blatant confession that the company was "making claims over and above those approved by the FDA. The detail men were being told to influence physicians to use Indocin for unapproved uses." [17] The text of another bulletin indicated what Senator Nelson's Committee characterized as "disquieting attitudes of the firms' employees toward the medical profession and the patient:" [18]

> "Tell 'em again, and again.
>
> "Tell 'em until they are sold and stay sold.
>
> "You've told this story now, probably 130 times. The physician, however, has heard it only once. So go back and tell it again, and again until it's indelibly impressed in his mind and he starts—and continues to prescribe 'Indocin.' Let's go.
>
> "Now every bottle of 1000 'Indocin' that you sell is worth an extra $2.80 in incentive payments. Go get it. Pile it in!!!"

Chloromycetin, the Parke-Davis brand of chloramphenicol, is an extremely dangerous drug with a high risk of inducing serious and even fatal anemia. Its indicated range of use for rational prescribing is extremely narrow. The company was aware of these facts in 1960 when it marketed the drug and both promoted and advertised the drug without a statement warning of the potential hazards.[19] Physicians were encouraged to use chloramphenicol for a multitude of conditions that did not reflect the risk taken with the drug. People on therapy began to sicken and die, and a warning was finally required. But promotion had been so effective that even by 1967 four million people were being treated with the drug even though "90 to 99% of these patients received it for non-indicated cases."[20] The effects of the indiscriminate use of chloramphenicol have been international, and in countries without legal requirements for warnings, chloramphenicol is still advertised without an appropriate statement of risk.[21] In order to shore up the Parke-Davis' declining chloramphenicol profits the Defense Department bought 10 million capsules for the South Vietnamese army and civilians, to be used in the usual indiscriminate manner.[22]

Referring to the entire chloramphenicol story, Senator Nelson commented:

> No other example . . . more dramatically demonstrates the ineffectiveness of the medical leadership of the nation on drug education when measured directly against the power and persuasiveness of drug company promotion and advertising . . . against the combined authoritative voice of the whole medical profession, drug company promotion has carried the day without drawing a deep breath.

The total impact of the drug industry's business strategy upon the health of the American people (and as foreign expansion grows, upon the health of people in other countries) is staggering. The confusing proliferation of name-brand drugs, the promotional distortions that lead to misprescribing and overprescribing, all contribute to the "1,500,000 hospital admissions annually attributed to adverse reactions to drugs." [23] We should not assume that this is the full extent of the damage either, for due to inadequate reporting and the tendency of doctors to underplay clinical results that might reflect poorly upon their professional judgment, this figure is almost certainly a gross understatement. The situation has become so serious that it is now estimated that one hospitalized patient in three (33%) is affected by adverse drug reactions.[24]

CONCLUSION

The PMA has characterized their industry as "an outstanding system for the discovery, production and distribution of drug products . . . the most dynamic and the most innovative of any country in the world."

But we have probed deeper and have asked: Outstanding for the discovery, production, and distribution of what sort of drug products, and for what purpose? Dynamic and innovative to what principal end and for whose primary benefit?

The answer to these questions does not appear to be improved human health and welfare, but rather increased profit and power for the drug industry. Numerous therapeutic advances have been developed and marketed, it is true. But evidence is strong that often these advances are secondary benefits of a primary strategy to maximize profit. Monopolies that cost the drug consumer billions in high prices are hardly therapeutic, neither is fraudulent price fixing that costs the public millions. The thousands of duplicative, confusing, useless drugs marketed over the years do not represent medical progress nearly so much as extended patents and increased profits. And none of us is any healthier for misleading promotion and advertising that costs millions in taxes and causes immeasurable damage in confused physicians, medically irrational therapy and adverse drug reactions.

We all need the production of high-quality drugs as well as the research and development of pharmacological advances, and the primary purpose of the drug industry should be to provide society with these vital commodities at maximum quality and with minimum expense. But the drug industry of this country is an unjustifiable, monopolistic profiteer of international proportions. Its primary purpose today is the exploitation of society for private financial gain. The cost of the drug industry to the consumer goes far beyond high prices. And that cost is much too high!!

—Excerpts from Chapter V of *Billions for Bandaids*, Thomas Bodenheimer, Elizabeth Harding and Steven Cummings (eds.), San Francisco Chapter, Medical Committee for Human Rights (1972).

SOMETHING MUST BE DONE ABOUT OUR NURSING HOMES

John L. Hess

In 1965, Congress created yet another machine to manufacture money. It was called Medicaid, and its express purpose was to solve the crisis of the rising cost of medical care for the aged poor. But Congress in its wisdom offered this welfare job to private enterprise, and left it to each state to run its own programs.

The wolves came running. A new federal program now hitting $10-billion a year was an invitation to steal, on a big scale. Operators with no skill whatsoever became millionaires overnight. The biggest killings were made in nursing homes.

While each of the 50 states has its own way of fouling up, the basic principle of Medicaid is that the less an operator does for the patient, the more he puts in his pocket. Many of the states use a per-diem rate. Wherever reporters have investigated, they found that patients were being starved and neglected to maximize returns.

One not uncommon cause of death in America not listed in medical statistics is this: An old person seeking help in the night to go to the toilet can find none. So the patient must either pass the night in cold filth or try to manage unattended. Many fail. Death is eventually listed as pneumonia, or natural causes.

The New York Legislature decided nothing was too

good for our senior citizens and enacted a cost-plus system. Since the same persons who had been ripping off welfare agencies long before Medicaid came along were involved, the situation was essentially the same, except that the take was far bigger than in per-diem states. At an average of $15,000 a year per patient, New York has the costliest program in the country. It is bleeding patients and taxpayers alike.

In four months of investigation for *The New York Times*, I found:

> The private nursing-home industry in New York City is largely controlled by an interlocking syndicate headed by one man. This group is linked to scores of other nursing homes around the country.
>
> Conditions in the nursing homes were in flagrant and massive violation of city, state and federal standards, and these violations had been recorded by inspectors year after year for at least two decades.
>
> Civil servants who sought to correct these conditions were repeatedly overruled by their politically-appointed superiors.
>
> No Medicaid facility had been audited before 1971—that is, the government accepted the nursing homes' word about what they spent—and only one in 10 had had a single spot-check of its books since then.
>
> The spot-checks revealed, as might be expected, widespread padding of bills, kickbacks, no-show jobs and various other types of criminal behavior. But the politicians refused to order thorough audits.
>
> No nursing-home operator in the state had ever been prosecuted or even asked to pay an administrative fine, although the files showed hundreds of allegations of misconduct.
>
> The "punishment" for being caught cheating is that the operator eventually may have to pay back the money—after exhausting all appeals. The crook gets interest-free use of taxpayer funds for up to 10 years, and his legal and lobbying expenses are fully paid by Medicaid.

> Many legislators doubled as lobbyists for nursing-home operators, some of them collecting law fees, insurance business and campaign contributions in return. No major public official was altogether untainted by some contact with the mob.

At this date, there are half a dozen investigations under way, all stemming from the *Times'* disclosure. But I must say that I am not overly optimistic about their outcomes.

An old Tammany Hall statesman once said, "Reform is a morning glory." This goes for muckraking, too. We rake up a little muck, and move on; the money boys stay. Unless the independent prosecutor who has been appointed picks up this story and runs away with it, the present clean-up will only be temporary and conditions will eventually return to what they were.

—From *Media and Consumer*, February, 1975.

BERGMAN AIDES PREDICTED HIGH NURSING-HOME PROFIT

John L. Hess

When Bernard Bergman bought the Park Crescent Hotel in the nineteen-sixties and prepared to turn it into a nursing home, his associates advised Wall Street analysts that it should be clearing a net profit of

$833,500 a year by 1973, according to a document in the hands of investigators.

That would come to $1,600 a year for each of the 520 beds and to an annual return of 57.5 per cent on the $1.45-million that the promoter told the State Health Department he had originally invested in the project.

Actually, auditors of the department maintain that this sum was soon withdrawn to be invested in other Bergman projects, and that the nursing home was built entirely with borrowed funds.

The Park Crescent, on Riverside Drive at 87th Street, reported to the department that it cleared $193,000 in 1972 but lost $149,000 in 1973. The report for 1974, on which Medicaid reimbursement will be based, is not yet available.

$78,000 IN SALARIES

Despite the 1973 loss, Park Crescent paid Mr. Bergman and his two sons, Stanley and Meyer, $78,000 in salaries, for unspecified services.

Congressional auditors have told the Senate Subcommittee on Long-Term Care that "no show" jobs for operators and relatives were a common phenomenon among the 41 nursing homes and venders whose documents it subpoenaed January 21.

Other dominant patterns, a committee aide said, were inability to account for patients' personal funds, and "an apparent identity between venders and operators, accompanied by inflated costs."

Thus far, the committee has been slowed in its efforts to determine what the real profits of nursing-home operations are, especially since many homes report that their debts exceed their assets, and that they lose money on Medicaid. However, the State Welfare Inspector General's office computed last year that one home was clearing 40 per cent on investment.

Mr. Bergman told the Senate Subcommittee on January 21 that his career in nursing homes had been "very little profitable, when you consider what we had been working under." In an interview read into the record on Tuesday, he said he was not a millionaire.

DIFFERENT DATA GIVEN

Documents filed by Mr. Bergman's accountant, Samuel A. Dachowitz, for credit purposes give a somewhat different picture. One set, previously reported, put his net worth at nearly $24-million, most of it in nursing homes, and showed a rise of $4.3-million in a single year.

Another Dachowitz report, made available to *The New York Times*, said Mr. Bergman had a "net cash flow income" of $748,120 from 13 of his nursing homes in the 12 months ended February 28, 1971.

Cash flow is a term commonly used to show how much money is left in a business at the end of the year after all cash expenses, including interest and amortization, have been paid. It is not the same as net income for tax purposes, which comes after depreciation. Indeed a landlord or other businessman may well have a substantial cash flow but no taxable income.

The Bergman list did not include the Park Crescent, but it did show a cash flow of $99,600 for "Towers Nursing Home and Liberty House." Towers was losing money, according to its report to the State Health Department. Liberty House was a subsidiary of Medic-Home Enterprises, Inc., a publicly owned company controlled by Mr. Bergman, which leased the building to Towers. The amount of the rent, billed to Medicaid, has been challenged by the State Welfare Inspector General's office.

Witnesses at a hearing of the Temporary State Commission on Living Costs last week testified that the White Plains Nursing Home had a $600,000-a-year contract for food and dietary services with a company based in a hardware store, and owned by the home's purchasing agent.

—From *The New York Times*, February 6, 1975. (abridged)

LATEST NURSING HOME SCANDAL: The Sigety Cover-up

Jack Newfield

At last, after 20 years, Bernard Bergman seems to be on the run. The Justice Department, the Attorney General of New Jersey, several New York DAs, the United States Senate, and the Stein Commission, are peeling away the layers of ghoulish greed.

But Bergman is not the only *gonif* [*crook*, freely translated—ed.] in the nursing home racket. The whole industry is the red light district of health care, where real estate operators and political influence peddlers play monopoly with old bodies.

Look at Charles Sigety.

Sigety began as a Republican bureaucrat; in 1958

he was the first assistant to Attorney General Louis Lefkowitz. Later, in 1962, he became executive director of the state housing and financing agency under Nelson Rockefeller.

By 1972, Sigety owned the Florence Nightingale Nursing Home at 175 East 96 Street, and was trying to build a second home two blocks away. To open his second home, landlord Sigety evicted dozens of families, mostly the poor and the elderly living on welfare. Sigety's harassment tactics were so brutal that he was fined $10,000 by the city's Office of Rent Control.

As the landlord for 129 East 97 Street; 114, 116, and 128 East 98th Street; and 1506, 1508, 1514, and 1516 Lexington Avenue, Sigety deprived his tenants of heat, hot water, a super, and locks on the front door; he also hired a managing agent named Bennett Cohen, who, according to testimony by tenants, threatened them with a loaded gun. In addition, Sigety sent the tenants false telegrams saying they had lost their case.

Despite his fine for harassment, and despite report after report on miserable conditions in his first nursing home, Sigety received a license to open his second home from the necessary city and state agencies.

On October 4 of 1974, the office of State Welfare Inspector General William Meyers completed a field audit of the finances of the Florence Nightingale home. The audit only covered one year—1972.

Nevertheless, the accountants found $40,571.26 worth of Medicaid cheating—billing the taxpayers for nonhealth related expenses, and improperly charging them to Medicaid.

Among the personal luxuries Sigety was reimbursed for by Medicaid were:

Parking fines—$105
A hotel room in Germany—$279

The Harvard Club—$621
G & G Wines and Liquors—$382
Szechuan Gardens—$135
K & D Liquors—$617
D. Sokolin (wine)—$318
Sherry Lehman (wine)—$385
Stevens Public Relations—$1,250
Yale Club—$190
Metropolitan opera subscription—$841
Icelandic Airlines—$554
Telephone bill for Sigety's home in Pennsylvania—$1,309
Renee Moss Antiques—$2,355
Lord & Taylor (rugs)—$496
International Persian Rug—$1,000
Percy Sutton [Manhattan Borough President—ed.] Testimonial dinner—$100
Real estate taxes on a boarded-up building—$2,742

As a result of all this padding, the monthly Medicaid rate per bed in Sigety's nursing home was an incredible $1,444 as of January 1974. This is among the highest in the state.

In 1973, the total Medicaid reimbursement to the Florence Nightingale home was $4,395,782.

Three months after this audit was completed, its findings have still not been released to the public, or forwarded to any law enforcement agency.

One reason for this apparent cover-up is that Sigety and Inspector General Meyers are close personal friends, and have been comrades in Republican party politics for more than 15 years.

On December 10, 1974, an acquaintance of mine noticed Meyers and Sigety having a cozy lunch together at the Auto Pub on Fifth Avenue. So this week I called Meyers and asked him about it.

"Yes, I did have lunch with Charley last month," he acknowledged.

I asked Meyers if he could recall ever having a private, social lunch with any other person he was supposed to be investigating.

"No, I never did," Meyers said. "Sigety is the only one."

What is so special about Sigety?

"Charley and I are good old friends. I worked with Charley years ago in the state division of housing."

Did he asked you about the Florence Nightingale audit?

"Yes. He asked if he could see it when it is released. I told him we had no policy on that."

(Meyers got his housing job after working for the Rockefeller campaign in 1958. Sigety also worked for Rocky in 1958. Meyers was named Inspector General by [then Governor—ed.] Malcolm Wilson last year.)

It seems clear to me that Meyers is now severely compromised. It also strains credulity to believe that Attorney General Louis Lefkowitz, another close friend —and former employer—of Sigety's, will aggressively investigate the Medicaid fraud at Florence Nightingale.

Luckily, the incorruptible Robert Morgenthau is now the district attorney of Manhattan. He can be trusted to convene a grand jury to find out why Sigety has billed the public for liquor, parking fines, tickets to politicans' dinners, public relations, and hotel rooms in Germany, while his elderly patients were being neglected and mistreated.

A city health department report on Sigety's Florence Nightingale home, dated February 16, 1972, detailed dozens of violations uncorrected since the department's previous visit. The report concluded: "The management of this home continues to show indifference to the requirements and recommendations of this department." Previous inspections of the Sigety home had shown filth in the kitchen, no recreation for the patients, fire hazards, inadequate nursing staff.

—From *The Village Voice*, January 13, 1975.

WASHINGTON HOSPITAL CENTER EXPOSÉ

Ronald Kessler

CONFLICT OF INTEREST MARKS HOSPITAL CENTER MANAGEMENT

"You'll get a better deal with friends than with strangers."

This is the philosophy that has guided Thomas H. Reynolds while managing Washington Hospital Center's financial affairs for most of the center's 15-year existence.

One of the friends that Reynolds did business with was American Security & Trust Co., Washington's second-largest bank. But while the bank got a good deal by doing business with the hospital, it is clear the hospital, and its patients, got a bad deal by doing business with the bank.

Until two years ago, the hospital's balances in an American Security checking account typically hovered at around $1 million and ranged as high as $1.8 million. The account paid no interest—so the bank had the use of the money at no cost.

Using the most conservative assumptions, the hospital lost at least $50,000 a year in interest it otherwise would have received. Indeed, after the banking arrangement was changed and the balances were lowered, the hospital took in annual interest of $82,000 that it hadn't previously received. Jose A. Blanco Jr., former controller of the hospital, attributes that largely to the elimination of the interest-free policy at American Security.

An annual $50,000 loss of interest amounts to an extra $1.50 on the average patient bill at the center.

Reynolds concedes he was the one who placed the account at American Security and set the policy that sent the hospital's balances there soaring above $1 million. He says he feels the policy was "prudent."

Reynolds is hardly a disinterested party. Until he retired last year, he was a vice president and the second man in charge of the trust department at American Security.

The interest-free policy was changed when several non-banker trustees of the hospital warned of the possibility of civil suits against the trustees if the information ever got out. However, there is evidence that the new arrangement with American Security continues to favor the bank at the expense of the hospital.

Asked about relations between the bank and the hospital, Joseph W. Barr, president of American Security, referred all questions to the current treasurer of the hospital, John E. Sumter Jr.

"I don't want to comment," Sumter said. "All I know is the hospital is running well, and utilizing its money well, and it stands on its record." As for the interest-free money, Sumter said, "I don't know anything about a $50,000 loss."

Sumter is senior vice president for commercial loans at American Security.

To many critics inside and outside the hospital industry, such conflicts of interest—and the detrimental effect they can have on a hospital—illustrate the lack of public accountability of hospitals and explain in large part why hospital costs have skyrocketed.

"What the hospitals don't realize is that they're supposed to be run for the public," says Herbert S. Denenberg, the Pennsylvania insurance commissioner who has investigated hospital trustees' conflicts of interest in his state. "The bankers on the boards think they're run for themselves," he says.

At various times, 10 of the 38 trustees of the hospital center and four former trustees have been involved in conflicts of interest when they or their companies did business with the hospital, a Washington *Post* investigation has found. Often the business was given to the trustees at their own direction.

A conflict of interest, according to Nathan Hershey, coauthor of the *Hospital Law Manual*, a standard reference work used by the hospital center's own attorneys, is when a hospital trustee does business with the hospital, automatically giving him conflicting interest on both sides of the transaction.

The hospital center's conflict-of-interest dealings, the *Post* has found, have ranged from catering contracts to malpractice insurance to purchase of stock of local banks by a trustee committee composed primarily of officers and directors of those banks, who also generally have personal holdings in the banks.

D.C. law specifically prohibits any trustee of a charitable institution that receives any federal money from doing business with the institution. The hospital center is incorporated in D.C. as a charitable institution, and it gets about a third of its operating funds from the federal government through Medicare, Medicaid and other programs. The D.C. law requires that trustees in conflict resign.

At the hospital center, competitive bidding was sought for only one of the transactions involving conflicts of interest by trustees. In the one exception, the bidding was limited to those banks—American Security, Riggs National Bank, and Union Trust Co.—whose officers are trustees of the hospital.

There is no evidence that any of the trustees involved in the conflicts abstained from voting or participating in the decisions, and in several instances there is evidence that the trustees involved in the conflicts themselves made the decision to give themselves the hospital's business.

There is also no evidence of any public disclosure of the conflicts. Indeed, many of the conflicts have been carried on in such secrecy that other trustees say they were unaware of them, and some of the trustees involved in the conflicts refused to discuss them when asked to do so by this reporter.

One such trustee is George M. Ferris, Jr., president of Ferris & Co., a local stock brokerage firm. One of the firm's Virginia brokers, Michael G. Miller, Sr., is the broker who buys and sells the stock held by the hospital's $4.5 million pension fund.

Why was Miller, a Virginia broker relatively new to the business, chosen by the center to receive commissions for buying and selling its stock? Sumter, of American Security, which administers the pension fund, concedes Miller was picked by Reynolds, who is Miller's father-in-law.

HOSPITAL CENTER OFFICIALS USED CONNECTION TO REAP PROFITS

It was the old American success story. A Cuban immigrant, penniless after fleeing the Castro regime, turns an idea into a $2-million-a-year company that plans to sell stock to the public.

But in this story, the immigrant, Jose A. Blanco, Jr., had more than an idea. He also had a large first customer for the services his company would offer. The customer showed no signs of wanting to haggle over the price for the services. Indeed, the customer was convinced that only Blanco could do the job.

The reason is understandable. The customer was Blanco.

It was 1970, and Blanco was controller and an assistant administrator of Washington Hospital Center, the Washington area's largest private, nonprofit hospital.

Blanco, who was in charge of data processing, decided the existing facilities at the hospital for billing, keeping track of patient records, and accounting through the hospital's computer were less than adequate. He decided the best solution was to hire a private, outside company to provide these services. And he decided he would start the company he needed.

While making $39,000 a year as a full-time employee of the hospital center, Blanco formed Space Age Computer Systems, Inc., to provide data processing services to hospitals. The firm's first customer was the hospital center, and other customers quickly followed.

If there was ever any question whether or not the center would go along with the idea, it was quickly dispelled when Blanco's boss, Richard M. Loughery, administrator of the hospital, accepted stock free of charge in the new company, and became one of its directors. Blanco concedes that five other administrative officials of the hospital, including the assistant controller and the internal auditor, bought stock in Space Age at $1 a share.

To further help the new company along, it was given $50,000 by the hospital. The payment was described as a "deposit."

Blanco and Loughery say they see no conflict of interest in their dual roles and say they did nothing wrong.

After *The Washington Post* began investigating Space Age and its relationship to the hospital center, the hospital's board of trustees ordered Loughery and the other assistant administrators to give up their stock in Space Age. Blanco was dismissed as controller of the hospital and was made a consultant to the center for a year. Samuel Scrivener, Jr., the center's president, says competitive bidding will now be sought on the data processing contract.

How Blanco and Loughery were able to start a private company using hospital center funds, and the effect that this had on the center's operations, provide an example of the lack of public accountability of hospitals and give insight into why hospital costs have risen since 1965 at four times the rate of other consumer prices.

Before Blanco became controller of the hospital center, he had taught business courses and raised cattle in Cuba, and later participated as a part of the landing force in the abortive Bay of Pigs invasion in April, 1961. A certified public accountant with a quick mind and professorial approach, Blanco became controller of Methodist Evangelical Hospital in Louisville in 1961. He was a consultant to the hospital center before he became its controller in July, 1967.

In that same month, Blanco, his brother, and another Cuban expatriate started their first commercial venture—a business billing company. At the time, Blanco was a full-time employee of the hospital center.

Three years later, Blanco found the center's existing computer system lacking and decided he would supply the services he thought were needed.

Normally, hospital controllers are responsible for running a data processing department as part of their duties, but Blanco saw his duties as controller differently.

"What I know in my brains is mine. I am paid to be controller of Washington Hospital Center—that's it," he said, indicating the job doesn't entail supervising data processing.

There was little doubt the center's key officers would approve the plan. Loughery, the hospital administrator, accepted free stock in the new company and became one of its directors.

The president of the hospital at the time, Thomas H. Reynolds, said he felt the center could get a better deal on a contract if it was with an employee of the hospital.

"Their jobs are on the line," said Reynolds, who retired last year as an American Security & Trust Co. vice president and second man in charge of its trust department.

Finally, the man who was then treasurer of the hospital, and to whom Blanco reported on financial matters, also raised no objections. The former treasurer, Samuel T. Castleman, then also an American Security senior vice president, was made a director of Space Age and given an option to buy 10,000 shares of its stock at $1 a share.

Castleman and Reynolds were two of the four trustees who gave formal approval to the Space Age contract and agreed to give Space Age $50,000 as a "deposit." Reynolds described the four as the members of the center's executive committee minus its doctor members. He said doctors are "totally lost" in dealing with financial matters.

Other trustees who later found out about the approval said it was given by a "rump" session of the executive committee. All but one of the four were themselves doing business with the hospital center.

The $50,000 was to represent the payment for the last month of the Space Age contract, if the contract was ever terminated. Blanco last year returned the money to the center, without paying interest on it, because he said he had been advised he would have to pay taxes on it. He said he still wants the money, but in a nontaxable form.

If Blanco had paid 8 per cent interest on the money, it would have yielded the Hospital Center $4,000.

Blanco claimed such a deposit is common in the hospital data processing business. Other companies, asked about this, said they had never heard of a deposit.

One company, McDonnell-Douglas Automation Co. in St. Louis, said it makes an installation charge when new equipment is needed or employees must be trained.

Blanco did not have these problems. The employees in the hospital center's data processing department were simply switched to the Space Age payroll. The leased International Business Machines computer already at the center was taken over by Space Age, although the lease continued to be in the center's name.

This way, Space Age could take advantage of the average 20 per cent discount IBM gives the hospital center as a nonprofit institution. Space Age, which must pay for the computer rental, thus cut 20 per cent from its most important cost of doing business. Blanco says IBM is aware of this arrangement.

Blanco's two hats, as controller of the hospital and president of Space Age, presented other difficulties. Blanco the controller had the responsibility of insuring that Blanco the Space Age president paid his rent for use of office space in the center's Physicians Office Building, did not overcharge the hospital, and got paid the correct amount.

Blanco, the Space Age president, and other Space Age employees under him, decided when the hospital's requests for special computer analyses went beyond what was provided in the Space Age contract and what the extra charge for these analyses would be. Sometimes the request for these special analyses was made by Blanco the controller.

"It used to crack me up that a controller could essentially write his own check (to himself)," said one former employee of Blanco the controller.

Other former employees say Blanco spent the majority of his time on Space Age business, ignoring hospital problems for weeks or altogether because he was too busy flying around the country looking for new Space Age customers.

"The hospital became a base of operations for Blanco. The guy was almost never there. Sometimes it was comical," a former employee said.

PATHOLOGIST PAID A PERCENTAGE OF THE PROFIT IN DEPARTMENT

In the basement of Washington Hospital Center is the relatively modest office of a man who makes approximately $200,000 a year.

He is not the head of the hospital center, whose administrators get about a quarter of Martens' pay. He is not the head of one of the center's major medical departments, whose chiefs also get about a quarter of Martens' compensation.

Martens runs the hospital center's laboratory, which performs chemical tests and analyzes patient tissues. He is a medical doctor in the field of pathology, the study of human diseases and tissues.

As hospital pathologists go, Dr. Martens is not particularly well paid. Congressional testimony and interviews with hospital administrators and accountants indicate many make $300,000 a year and at least one in the Washington area makes $500,000 a year.

Nor are pathologists the only ones so favored. Hospital radiologists, who interpret x-ray photographs, and anesthesiologists, who administer anesthesia during surgery, are similarly well compensated.

The reason they are is one of many illustrations of why it costs $170 a day to be hospitalized at an institution like Washington Hospital Center and why hospital costs have risen at about four times the rate of other consumer prices since 1965.

Testimony before the Senate Antitrust and Monopoly Subcommittee, a 1967 Justice Department suit against the pathologists, and interviews with hospital administrators and accountants and pathologists indicate a simple explanation for the high compensation.

The pathologists and other hospital medical specialists have a monopoly on the services they offer, and they use it to force hospitals to give them an unusual form of compensation.

This is how the practice works:

Pathologists are given what many experts call a monopoly on hospital laboratories under a principle laid down by the Joint Commission on Hospital Accreditation, which gives hospitals their coveted accreditation. The principle: hospital laboratories should be run by pathologists.

Whether this is justified is questioned by many experts who say a hospital laboratory is much like a manufacturing plant: most of its work is concerned with testing blood, urine, and other patient samples with automated machinery, and this process should be administered by a technician skilled in efficient management methods and quality control.

Doctors in private practice generally send patient samples to independent, commercial laboratories that often are run by technicians or biochemists. These labs hire pathologists on salary to perform the work that only they can do—analyze tissues and give interpretations of test results to doctors when requested.

A 1969 Northeastern University study supported by the U.S. Public Health Service concluded that costs to patients in hospitals are raised by "inefficient management" and "often backward methods" of laboratories run by pathologists who lack management skills and have no desire to learn them.

Pathologists counter that a laboratory not run by a pathologist does poor work. However, several pathologists, including Dr. Martens, conceded that they have no evidence to support this contention.

Whatever the justification, hospitals are bound by the accrediting group to put pathologists in charge of their laboratories. Pathologists, in turn, refuse to work in the laboratories unless they are given a percentage of the profits.

Until 1969, according to a Justice Department suit against the College of American Pathologists, the specialty's professional group, accepting a salaried position with a hospital was cause for possible expulsion from the group.

The college's canon of ethics included this rule: "I shall not accept a position with a fixed stipend in any hospital . . ."

An exception was made for those hospitals run by the local, state, or federal governments, presumably because laws would prohibit government institutions from giving profits to individuals.

In practice, there was, and is, another exception. Pathologists will work on salary for a university hospital. The result, says Dr. Gillespie, is that pathologists of equal qualifications work for $28,000 to $40,000 for university hospitals but receive $200,000 and more from general hospitals.

The College of Pathologists agreed in 1969 to omit the antisalary canon and other rules from its ethics as part of a settlement of the Justice Department suit.

The suit charged that pathologists had illegally forced patients to pay "excessively high prices" for lab tests by agreeing, often in writing, to a series of monopolistic practices.

Dr. Martens' compensation last year cost each patient entering the hospital center an average of 79 cents a day, or $6 on the average total bill.

Last year, he was given $429,595. This represented 23 per cent of the net profit of the lab after salaries, supplies, bad debts, and discounts to third party insurers had been deducted from the lab's gross income from patients of $4.8 million.

Out of his payment, Dr. Martens says, he paid about $24,000 for additional salaries of residents or interns, and he paid the salaries of the five other pathologists working for him at the time.

Talks with these doctors indicate their salaries fit the pattern of hospital lab compensation throughout the country: a relatively high salary of $65,000 for the second man in charge and salaries of $25,000 to $35,000 for the less senior pathologists.

The sum left over for Dr. Martens: a minimum of $200,000.

Despite the $6 that the average hospital center patient pays for Dr. Martens' services, Dr. Martens concedes he has little to do with the bulk of the work of the lab. Most of this work consists of chemical testing, a task performed by technicians who stamp the name of Dr. Martens or another pathologist on the test report given to the physician requesting the test.

Nor is Dr. Martens always at the lab. Despite the $200,000 he earns there, he works at the hospital center job only part time; he has a similar position at Hadley Memorial Hospital, where he is paid a percentage of the gross income of that hospital's laboratory. (Hadley refused to say how much Dr. Martens is paid there.) He also operates farms in Virginia.

The hospital lab is "strictly a monopolistic, moneymaking proposition," Dr. Edward R. Pinckney, a Beverly Hills, Calif., pathologist, has testified before the Senate Antitrust and Monopoly Subcommittee. He says prices to patients could be considerably reduced if hospitals hired independent laboratories to perform tests.

A comparison of prices charged for the same tests by Washington Hospital Center and two local, independent labs bears this out:

Test	Hospital Center	Lab A	Lab B	Av. Difference
Routine urinalysis	$ 5	$2.50	$ 1.00	186%
Complete blood count	7	3.75	2.00	143%
Pregnancy test	11	3.75	3.50	204%
Mono test	6	3.50	5.50	33%
Routine tissue	18	10.00	15.00	44%
12 channel (SMA 12)	25	5.00	5.00	400%

The average difference shows the additional price that hospital center patients pay when compared with the average price of the two independent labs for the same test.

The independent lab prices are those charged to doctors, who generally draw samples themselves. National Health Labs estimates it could perform all the functions of a hospital lab for no more than an additional 25 per cent on its regular prices.

Why don't hospitals use independent labs to cut charges to patients?

Dr. Jacques M. Kelly, head of National Health Laboratories, Inc., says that despite the 1969 Justice Department consent decree, pathologists continue to have a "lock" on hospital labs and an "ex officio" agreement that they won't do business with an independent lab, unless they own it.

One reason independent labs are able to charge lower prices is that they are largely automated. The 12-channel test—which measures 12 ingredients ranging from glucose to protein in blood—is performed by a $75,000 machine that does at least 60 blood samples an hour.

Dr. Martens says he hasn't bought such a machine for his lab because there still are problems with "balancing" it.

The Northeastern study suggested another reason. It says that the machine saves so much labor that it would pay for itself in a week if run eight hours a day. But the study says hospital labs often don't buy the machine because the expenditure would come out of the pathologist's compensation. The salaries of technicians who perform the same test by hand, the study says, are paid for by Blue Cross and other third-party insurers.

"Thus there is little incentive for a hopital to invest in automation," the study says.

But if the hospital center's lab became more automated, there is little reason to believe prices to patients would go down. This is because under his agreement with the center, Dr. Martens sets his own prices. He, in turn, gets a percentage of the profit the prices produce.

—From *The Washington Post*, October 30 and 31, and November 1, 1972. (abridged)

OKLAHOMA CRUDE: Everything's Gushing Up Hospitals

Bob Nichols with the assistance of Eric Johnson and Deborah Roher

During the past two decades hospitals have sprung up throughout the United States like MacDonald hamburger stands. Now there are too many hospital beds to fill with sick people and the beds stand idle.

In Dade County, Florida, about 7,500 beds are needed but within two years the County will have 12,000 beds. This is not an isolated instance; the pattern is being repeated across the country. St. Louis has 714 beds too many, San Francisco 1,130 excess and Honolulu 1,000 empty beds.

Since overbedding is a national problem (though a few cities like New York are exceptions), one has to conclude that either hospital officials are monumentally inept planners or else that hospital construction serves some purpose other than providing sufficient beds for the infirm. Oklahoma City is a good place to look for some answers because perhaps in no other city are the politics of overbedding more transparent.

For a city of 700,000 people, Oklahoma City has a lot of hospitals—18 nonfederal hospitals to be exact. Of these, however, only five account for most of the patient admissions. All except the University of Oklahoma-related University Hospital (UH) are private voluntary hospitals: 195-bed Presbyterian, 595-bed Baptist Memorial Hospital, and two Catholic institutions, 181-bed Mercy and 800-bed St. Anthony's Hospital.

Unlike many cities, Oklahoma City has no municipal or county hospital. However, like other cities, Oklahoma City has many medically indigent patients, perhaps more than ten percent of the city's census. Up until recently (see below), patients without hospital insurance of any kind were admitted to UH, a state facility related to the state medical school. Indeed, UH served as the "dumping" ground for the other hospitals in the city. Unlike most other cities, UH served more or less the role of a public hospital—it was the hospital of last resort.

PRESERVING THE LAST FRONTIER

Oklahoma City suffers (or thrives) from an untamed frontier mentality or ethos. Mr. E. K. Gaylord, the town's 100-year-old patriarch and power broker, was one of the illustrious gentlemen who invaded Indian Territory prior to statehood in 1907. At age 100 he is a bit more sedate but no less powerful. He or his minions have membership on almost every key public agency and private board (more later about how those relate to hospitals) and he and his son publish the state's two leading statewide newspapers, *The Daily Oklahoman* and the *Sunday Oklahoman*, as well as Oklahoma City's evening *Oklahoma City Times*. The empire also controls WKY Radio-Television. Thus the family molds public opinion for at least one million readers and listeners.

Hospitals are important for the image of men like the Gaylords. They proclaim the idea that the "West has been won" and are a convenient display of the City's refinement. The truth is, however, that building new hospital pavilions is also good for business.

The hospital building boom started about 20 years ago, just about the time that Oklahoma City hospitals changed their corporate status from profit-making, tax-paying to nonprofit, tax-exempt voluntary hospitals. Two events convinced Oklahoma City businessmen, who then as now controlled the hospitals, that it was better to switch than fight. In 1947 Congress passed the Hill-Burton Act designating many millions of dollars of federal money for hospital construction. The money had to go, however, only to nonprofit hospitals. Then in 1954 the Internal Revenue Service revised its regulations to grant special tax exemptions to voluntary hospitals. For Oklahoma County these rulings save the hospitals some $20 million a year.

While it was said to have been the intent of Congress and the Internal Revenue Service that this money be used for care of the medically indigent, this isn't how it worked out in Oklahoma City (or, for that matter, anywhere else). Instead the money has been spent building unneeded, in fact, empty hospital beds. A quick look at how hospital bed need is calculated will prove the point.

BUILD WE MUST

A good way to determine about how many short-term acute beds the community should have is to use the locally accepted ratio of four beds per thousand resident population (4/1000), which assumes an 85 percent occupancy rate. The primary patient origin area of the Oklahoma County area hospitals is the Oklahoma, Canadian, and Cleveland County area. The population of this area is about 674,000 people. This produces a bed need of 2,696 short-term beds at 85 percent occupancy.

The expected increase in the population is going to produce a three-county population of 700,000 people in 1975. This creates a need for 2,800 short-term hospital beds.

However, the three-county area will have a projected 4,746 short-term beds in 1975 for a surplus of 1,946 beds. Each one of those excess beds is costing about $50,000 apiece to build and about $20,000 apiece to maintain each year. The surplus will be at least 1,000 beds for 30 years, for a total cost to the community for unneeded facilities of over $650 million.

The local Oklahoma City hospitals that are building the excess beds are borrowing the money to do it, expecting to raise patient fees for the next 30 years in order to recover the cost of construction and of maintaining the empty (non-income-producing) beds. When construction is completed the maintenance costs are figured into the overhead costs of the hospital and tacked onto the bills of the patients occupying some of the beds. One hospital which has completed its construction and is already doing this is St. Anthony's Hospital.

St. Anthony's Hospital
1968 to 1972 percent change

Average Daily Census up 1.6%
Number of Beds up 46%
Operating Expenses up 51%
Total Revenue up to 62%
Net Income up 190%

In 1968 the hospital averaged 438 patients a day. By 1972 while the number of beds had increased 46 percent (by 259 beds) the number of patients had increased only 1.6 percent (seven) per day.

Some of the 51 percent increase in operating costs was passed on to patients in the form of higher per-patient-day charges. The hospital determines per-patient-day charges by dividing the number of patient days for the whole year into the cost of operating the facility for a year. The increased cost is then passed on to the government and to private insurance plans and from there on to taxpayers and subscribers. From this perspective it is obvious that everyone, except the hospitals responsible for the costs, pays through the ear. Indeed, overconstruction of hospitals and related facilities is the greatest single factor causing national hospital cost inflation (217 percent over the last ten years).

But inflation is only one of the costs which result. In order to keep ahead of the game and maintain their "surplus funds," hospitals must begin eliminating "unprofitable" services. Some hospital services, such as medicine and surgery, always make money and are used to subsidize money-losing services such as emergency rooms and outpatient departments. To save money Oklahoma City hospitals are cutting back on the number of patients being seen in their emergency rooms and outpatient departments and the number of no-pay and part-pay patients. This has been the major source of care for many of the city's medically indigent, which the hospitals obligated themselves to serve by acquiring tax exemption. Patients are now charged a preadmission deposit so that if a family can't pay the deposit, the patient is refused admittance or service. This allows the hospital to divert the money from patient care to paying construction and operating costs of empty beds. This is underscored by further data from St. Anthony's Hospital:

St. Anthony's Hospital
Operating Data
1968 to 1972 percent change

Average Daily Census up 1.6%
Number of Beds up 46%
Occupancy Rate down 31%
Emergency Room Visits down 32%
Outpatient Visits down 54%

As the number of emergency room visits and outpatient visits has decreased from 1968 to 1972 the same services at University Hospital have until recently shown a dramatic increase. As working people have been refused at St. Anthony's Hospital, they have gone to University Hospital in search of medical care for their families.

In Oklahoma City overexpansion is not limited to St. Anthony's Hospital. Presbyterian Hospital's capacity will increase from 195 to 412 beds when its new facility, now under construction, opens. Mercy Hospital will go from 181 to 400 beds and Baptist Hospital projects an expansion to 800 beds from its present 595.

By 1975 the Oklahoma County area hospitals will have an average occupancy rate of 55 percent because of the added bed-days. But this is not enough to pay the operating costs and mortgages. A minimum of an additional 87,000 income-producing patient days will have to be found somewhere to help the hospitals meet expenses. They are nowhere to be found.

CHOICE, NOT CHANCE

Miscalculations such as these just don't happen by accident. The fact is that long after it was known that Oklahoma City was fast heading for an excess number of beds, the most powerful business leaders kept relentlessly pushing for further hospital expansion. In 1969 the Community Council of Central Oklahoma, whose members are the wealthiest and most influential business leaders in the community, passed a resolution changing the name of their own Health and Hospital Planning Council to the Areawide Health Planning Organization (AHPO) of Central Oklahoma. The Department of Health, Education and Welfare then cooperated by designating the organization the local comprehensive health planning agency.

By 1970 the AHPO's staff was pitted in opposition to their own Policy Board over the issue of hospital expansion. The Board, composed of hospital administrators and trustees, doctors, government representatives and wealthy "consumers," was pushing full steam ahead for more hospital construction. The staff, and anyone else who cared, knew that no more beds were needed. Oklahoma City was being inundated with hospital beds. An independent consultant to the AHPO Board confirmed the staff's judgment. The consultant reported that, ". . . the community will have 916 excess beds by 1975." A subsequent report concluded that there would be:

> $35 to $50 million in capital expenses wasted.
>
> $20,000 per bed per year in operating expenses with no off-setting income.
>
> Extreme pressure on hospitals to make use of the beds to increase income, resulting in unnecessary hospitalization.

A severe limitation in the hospitals' ability to explore new forms of health care due to heavy debt burdens incurred for unused beds.

Increased costs of hospital care, passed on to the patient.

Increased difficulty in maintaining medical staff rules and regulations due to relative ease of shifting practices from one hospital to another.

Increased pressure on hospital administration to meet physician demands for duplicative expensive equipment, for fear of losing the medical staff necessary for maintaining the highest occupancy possible.

Naturally, the Policy Board was not persuaded and further hospital expansion was mandated. Since that time the boards of various hospitals with representation on the Policy Board have proposed that an additional 695 short-term hospital beds be built by 1977. This would simply waste another $34 million.

WHO PROFITS?

"Profit" is a dirty word in the hospital industry. Yet profit is as important to nonprofit hospitals as it is to General Motors.

Some profits in hospitals are obvious—for example, the $100,000 a year salaries garnered by radiologists, anesthesiologists and pathologists. Chances are, however, that the hidden "profit makers" will prove to be of greater importance. Doctors may not profit from overexpansion but other people sure do. Aside from construction companies, which profit directly, lawyers, architects, surveyors, appraisers, management consultants and money lenders—banks and insurance companies—profit handsomely. After all, no hospital can self-finance major construction, so the hospital must borrow money for expansion. The money must, of course, be paid back over a period of 20 to 30 years with interest, which is where the money lenders make their profit.

In Oklahoma City this amounts to big money. The tax-exempt bonds issued by the Oklahoma Industries Authority (OIA) to expand Baptist Memorial, Presbyterian and St. Anthony's hospitals total $89.4 million. The OIA is a public-trust State agency established by statute to ensure the economic and industrial growth of Oklahoma. After the OIA funding of the three nonprofit hospitals, the hospitals' anticipated 1973 to 1978 surplus (profit) zoomed to a total of over $56 million (this figure derives from the hospitals' own bond feasibility reports).

OIA's chairman is Edward L. Gaylord, son of the 100-year-old Indian raider and Oklahoma City's leading media baron. OIA does business with Oklahoma City's First National Bank and Trust Company, whose Chairman of the Board sits as a trustee of OIA. The Bank actually profits in at least three ways: on the interest it receives on loans to the hospitals; on investments it makes on the lump-sum money OIA deposits for hospital construction in the first place; and on the expected investment of the projected $56 million "surplus" of OIA-funded hospitals.

In the last analysis, after including only the money paid on the principal and interest, Oklahoma City health-care consumers will have to foot an astronomical $180 million for the hospital overexpansion now in the works. Of course, the consumers' loss is the banks' gain.

UNIVERSITY HOSPITAL

Until 1973 patients refused admittance to Oklahoma City voluntary hospitals were at least assured of getting into UH. As many as 50 percent of UH patients were medically indigent. This arrangement was agreeable to the medical staff, who needed the patients for teaching purposes anyway and could admit their own private patients to Presbyterian Hospital a few blocks away.

But in 1973 the State took two actions which threaten to end UH's role as hospital of last resort for the poor. Early in the year the State Legislature (controlled by rural-based representatives with no love for the urban hotshots at the medical school) voted to divorce UH from the State Board of Regents. This had the effect of ending the state subsidy, leaving UH to fend for itself just like any other voluntary hospital. To mitigate the criticism of wiping out the only existing hospital for indigent patients, the Legislature continued a small subsidy for 1974.

Then in mid-December, the State tightened the noose around UH even tighter. The Oklahoma Constitution makes it illegal for a state facility to run in the red, and UH had a $3-million deficit that was still growing. As a result, Governor David Hall amended the state's contract with UH to forbid UH doctors from admitting private (read income-producing) patients to any private hospital. The effect was to force the doctors to admit their own patients to UH and this, on top of an earlier cutback on the number of beds, may force nonpaying patients out of UH.

There are persistent rumors in Oklahoma City that sooner or later UH will be forced to close. The State Legislature periodically talks of moving it to Tulsa. Meanwhile UH daily becomes less distinguishable from other voluntary hospitals.

Most impressively, UH is beginning to cut its losses by doing what every other private hospital is doing—shafting the poor. For example, emergency room visits fell from about 20,000 for the first three quarters of 1972 to 16,500 for the same period in 1973. More striking was the one-third drop in outpatient visits from the first quarter of 1973 to the third quarter in the same year. It was in this quarter that the economic cuts hit UH. In March 1973 a nine-page memorandum detailing a scheme to charge preadmission deposits was leaked to the press by the Consumer Protection Agency. Confronted by an angry press and furious public, hospital officials lost no time denying any plan to exclude folks who could not pay. But more recent statements from the hospital cast doubt upon this denial. Robert Snyder, MD, head of the long-range planning committee for UH's Department of Medicine, says, "We must compete with the private voluntary hospitals in the City and cannot have Mickey Mouse facilities for people who are paying their way." And another hospital spokesman chimes in, "We are operating as a private hospital with a modest State subsidy. In May when the money runs out we don't expect to admit nonpaying patients."

At the receiving end of all these punches are the medically indigent who now have no place to receive medical care. When a State medical official was asked recently, "Where will the poor receive care?" he replied, "I don't know." Odds are he doesn't care either, just so long as the State or the City doesn't have to spend money for it.

In the meantime, as the poor try not to get sick for fear that they will not be admitted to any hospital, Oklahoma City will have a 1,946-bed surplus by 1975. Those with hospital insurance will be paying higher premiums for beds they cannot possibly use. In suburban Northwest Oklahoma City a new hospital

—Edmund Memorial Hospital—has only 26 of its 100 beds occupied. It's a dandy situation—hospital administrators polish their image and enhance their stature by building bigger, if not better hospitals; the local and state government saves money by denying care to those who cannot pay; and the bankers rake in the money. Only the people lose—but isn't that the way it's supposed to be?

If you're doing any traveling, Oklahoma City is the place to get sick. You will be sure to find a hospital bed. But don't forget your Blue Cross card. And watch your gall bladder.

(Bob Nichols is on the staff of the Health Protection Task Force of the Oklahoma Consumer Protection Agency, Eric Johnson was an intern at UH-Presbyterian Hospital and Deborah Roher was a student intern with the Consumer Protection Agency.)

—From the Health/PAC *Bulletin,* March/April, 1974. (abridged)

II.
Health Workers

Historically, health workers other than doctors have been among the most exploited members of the U.S. workforce. Long hours and shamefully low wages called forth a workforce on the economic margins of society—unskilled, often poorly educated, blacks, women, elderly and handicapped people.

The industrialization of health care after World War II, with the hospital as its base, has affected the health workforce profoundly. The number of health workers in general, and in hospitals in particular, has grown enormously. As medical procedures have become more complex, workers' tasks have become more highly differentiated. Formalized, impersonal relations among different ranks of hospital workers have replaced traditional patterns of paternalism. With their jobs becoming more stable and responsible and the old patterns of social relations changing, hospital workers began to organize against the exploitation that had for so long been their lot.

This section will examine the development of the health workforce and the two main vehicles that health workers have used to further their perceived self-interests—unionism and professionalism. Not only are issues relating to the health workforce intrinsically important to examine (for workers as well as patients are exploited by the health-care system), but it is impossible to conceive of a major reordering of priorities for the system without at least the tacit support of health workers.

Barbara Caress's brief analysis of the health workforce begins our consideration of the subject. This first selection in Chapter 5 chronicles the rapid growth of the health workforce, its increasing concentration in institutions and its increasing fragmentation and stratification within these insti-

tutions. Susan Reverby then examines the role of women; she does so in terms of the unskilled, dead- the three-quarters of the health workforce who are end nature of most hospital jobs and their similarity to women's traditional nurturing and housekeeping functions.

The final selection in Chapter 5 is an examination of social relations within the hospital workforce, by John and Barbara Ehrenreich. It introduces the issues of unionism and professionalism, which are discussed in greater depth in succeeding chapters. After examining those factors that distinguish hospital work from factory work, as well as those characteristics they have in common, the Ehrenreichs conclude that the occupational hierarchy in hospitals is "almost designed to promote conflict"—and, it might be added, is quite irrational in terms of patient care.

What maintains this fragmented structure and keeps it from flying apart? For skilled and semiskilled workers, the answer is professionalism. The extent of professionalism in hospitals is almost unique among American industries. There are over a hundred recognized health occupations other than physician that have become or are in the process of becoming health professions, and these comprise 40 percent of all nonmanagerial hospital workers. And, as all hospital workers are subordinate to doctors, so too are their professions subordinate to the medical profession. All other professions must initially be approved by the medical profession, and all are regulated by the American Medical Association's Council on Medical Education. In return for their unequal pact with doctors, other health professionals are granted a small niche in the hospital hierarchy, which is accompanied by higher pay scales, higher status and improved job security that have been doled out by doctors and hospital administrators. These gains have been won by narrowly dividing up and jealously guarding the hospital turf, pitting different levels of workers against each other rather than uniting the hospital workforce. Meanwhile, doctors and hospital managers continue to rule. This issue of professionalism is the subject of Chapter 6.

For unskilled and semiskilled hospital workers, with no claim to professionalism, the advent of hospital workers' unions during the last decade has brought dramatic change. Unionized workers (still a small minority of hospital workers) have greatly improved their pay and job security and have gained sufficient strength to resist arbitrary exploitation and discrimination by hospital management. At the same time, unions have not addressed the oppressiveness of dead-end jobs within a highly fragmented workforce or challenged the present order of hospital priorities. These issues are discussed in Chapter 7.

5
The Health Workforce

THE HEALTH WORKFORCE: Bigger Pie, Smaller Pieces

Barbara Caress

Health care is one of the largest and fastest-growing sectors of the American economy. In 1971 there were about 4.5 million people working in hospitals, nursing homes, doctors' offices, health departments and clinics.[5] This total represented more workers than those employed by the auto and electronic industries combined.

The continuing shift of focus of health-care delivery from solo-practice doctors to institutional settings provides the framework within which to understand the growth and development of the health-care workforce. Following the course of industrialization in the manufacturing sector, the health-care industry increasingly depends upon semiskilled and unskilled workers. Contrary to popular perceptions, the bulk of health

EMPLOYMENT IN THE PRIVATE SECTOR: SELECTED INDUSTRIES 1960-1972 *(in thousands)*

	1960	1965	1970	1972
Total	54,234	60,815	70,593	72,764
Mining	712	634	623	607
Construction	2,885	3,186	3,381	3,521
Electronics	1,467	1,659	1,917	1,833
Auto	724	843	797	861
Health Services*	1,548	2,080	3,057	3,442

* Does not include those employed by government.

Source: *Statistical Abstract of the United States*, 1973.

workers today are not doctors and nurses but aides, orderlies, attendants, maintenance and kitchen workers. This has not always been the case.

SIZE AND COMPOSITION OF THE HEALTH WORKFORCE

The size and composition of the health workforce has shifted considerably over the last 70 years. It has constituted an ever-increasing share of the civilian labor force. At the turn of the century there were about 331,000 people in the various health occupations, comprising about 1 percent of the civilian labor force.[2] One-third of these were doctors, one-third nurses, attendants and midwives and the remaining third were veterinarians, pharmacists, dentists and lens makers and grinders. (The Census Bureau then included "healers and therapists" in its count of doctors.) Except for the attendants, health workers were self-employed, offering the public treatments and cures of one sort or another.[4] There were few health institutions, and these were reserved for the sick and dying poor with chronic or selected infectious disease. Medical care was disbursed in the home, barber shop, office or sideshow.

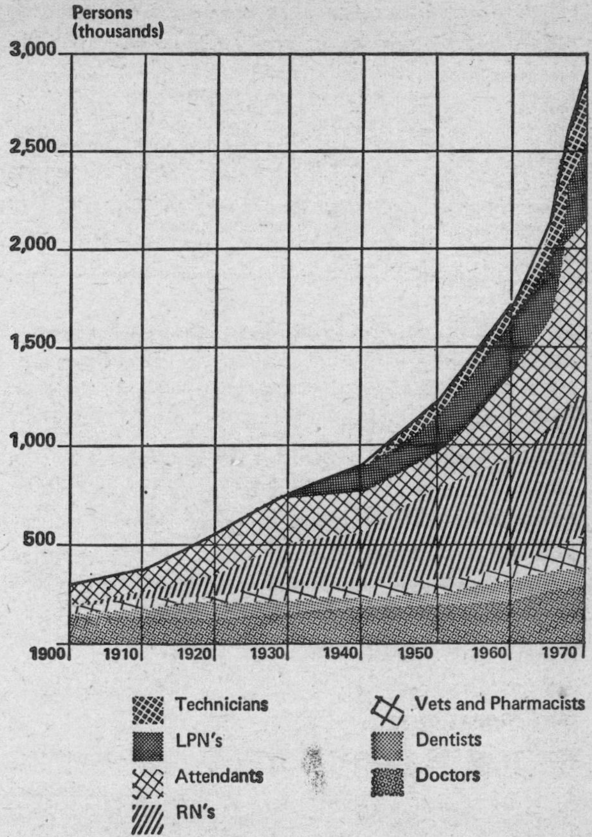

SELECTED HEALTH OCCUPATIONS: 1900-1970
(Cumulative)

By 1930, at the beginning of the Great Depression, employment in health occupations had crept up to about two percent of the labor force.[2] The distribution of health workers had changed radically from the beginning of the century. Doctors dropped from one-third to one-fifth of health workers, while dentists, veterinarians and chiropractors now made up about one-fourth. Nurses comprised the largest group of workers, but they had been split into two categories of about equal size—registered nurses (those licensed by the states) and unlicensed nursing personnel. During the decade of the Depression health employment increased from 815,106 to 879,962 at the same time that the total employed workforce was declining.

Today the health-care workforce is complex and highly stratified, including the highest-paid group of workers in the U.S. and some of the lowest paid. In 1971, health services employed about 5 percent of the civilian labor force.[5] Nursing personnel were the largest single group of health workers, about 2 million. There were about 750,000 registered nurses (RN's), 427,000 licensed practical or vocational nurses (LPN's) and about 800,000 aides, orderlies and attendants. Although the number of physicians tripled between 1900 and 1971, they today comprise only 7.5 percent of the health-care labor force.[2,5]

INDUSTRIALIZING THE HEALTH WORKFORCE

In 1930 less than one-third of the health labor force worked in hospitals or other institutions. Today the proportion is nearly two-thirds.[3,5] The growth of the institutional workforce began accelerating after the Second World War. In 1946 there were 830,000 hospital workers; now there are over 2.5 million.[2,3]

Concomitant with the increase in the numbers of hospital workers has been the proliferation of job categories and professions. Greater New York Blue Cross, for example, recently sent a form to its member hospitals asking them to enter the number of people in different jobs. The form listed 280 titles, excluding physicians. A typical medium-sized general-care hospital with 300 beds employs 1,000 people.[3] If the 280 job titles were equally distributed among this workforce, there would be fewer than four people in each category. Even with the technological complexity of modern medicine, one is hard put to imagine 280 different and distinct tasks to be performed. There is necessarily considerable overlap in the work done by different people with different titles, incomes and status.

Hospitals deliver a qualitatively different product from that of manufacturing plants. Nevertheless, their labor structures demonstrate parallels with that of other industries. Hospital administrators have their counterparts in plant management, maintaining the operation and assigning the workforce. Doctors as salaried employees of health institutions perform similarly to plant engineers in terms of their roles and responsibilities. Like engineers, doctors design the product and generally oversee the work process. Registered nurses, like shop foremen, supervise work at the point of production. Other nursing workers, directly providing patient care, are roughly comparable to skilled assembly-line workers. It is they who are responsible for the day-to-day creation of the product. Finally, the unskilled institutional maintenance people (housekeeping, food services and laundry) are not only drawn from the same labor pool as unskilled manufacturing workers, but do nearly interchangeable tasks. [For some of the important distinctions between jobs in hospitals and traditional factory work, see "Hospital Workers: A Case Study in the 'New Working Class'" later in this chapter.]

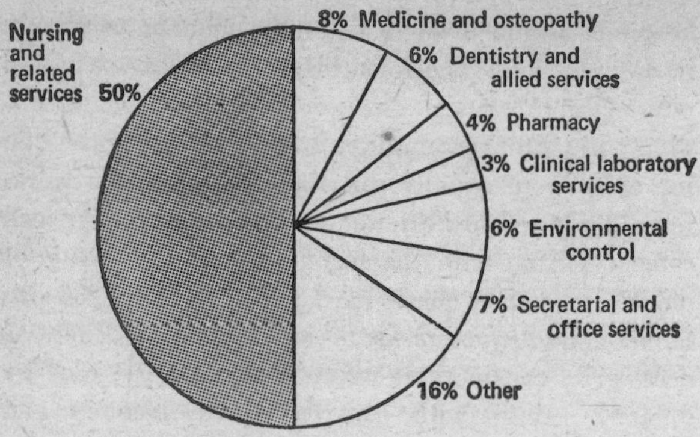

HALF OF ALL HEALTH CARE PERSONNEL PROVIDE NURSE-RELATED SERVICES

Source: *Health Resources Statistics, 1969.* Public Health Service Publication No. 1509 U.S. Department of Health, Education and Welfare

As a service industry, hospitals contain a far greater percentage of highly trained workers than do typical manufacturing enterprises. But a large part of the hospital labor force is relatively unskilled.[5,7] Clerical workers and institutional maintenance people account for nearly 40 percent of employees. Only 4 percent of the hospital workforce are physicians. There are about the same number of physicians as there are maintenance men in American hospitals. The greatest concentration of hospital workers is in nursing services. They run the gamut from skilled (RN's and LPN's) to semiskilled (aides) to unskilled (orderlies and attendants). Of all hospital employees 43.5 percent are either RN's (16.2 percent), LPN's and LVN's (7.4 percent) or aides, orderlies and attendants (19.9 percent). The remainder of hospital workers are in clinical laboratory services (3.5 percent), clinical technology (3.2 percent), pharmacy (0.8 percent), administration (0.6 percent), dentistry (0.6 percent) and even smaller representations in other categories.

THE LAST TEN YEARS

Having created Blue Cross in the 1930's, hospitals assured themselves financial security and laid the foundations for industrial growth. After World War II, the growth of hospital laborpower was constant and steady. Incorporating a similar financing mechanism, Medicare and Medicaid have resulted in a growth rate that has been spectacular. The number of people employed in the health-care industry increased by more than 60 percent in the years 1965–71.[5,6] This is 30 times the rate of growth of the population as a whole and 15 times faster than the growth of the civilian labor force.[1]

Personnel costs have remained a constant percentage of hospital expenditures since 1965, about 60 percent.[3] Although such costs have been increasing, other costs have risen at the same rate. But net hospital income and net assets have increased far more rapidly. The total net assets of nonprofit general hospitals increased by slightly more than 90 percent between 1967 and 1973, compared with 79 percent during the seven years immediately before the implementation of Medicare and Medicaid.[3] Of the $13.5 million increase in hospital net assets $5.5 million was for new equipment.[3]

The introduction of new technology into most industries makes them less labor intensive; more product can be produced with fewer workers. The reverse has generally been the case with hospitals. New technology in hospitals has necessitated the training and hiring of additional workers to operate or monitor the machines, while at the same time a full complement of staff is needed to maintain existing services. As a result the fastest-growing health occupations during the last decade have been technological or support workers. For example, while the total workforce was increasing by 60 percent, the number of electrocardiograph technicians grew by 79 percent.[5]

Thus the last ten years have seen the acceleration of the manpower changes evidenced in earlier decades. Most notable about the recent period has been the enormous expansion in the numbers of people employed in the health-care industry. Secondly, there is increasing concentration in institutional settings. And this institutional labor force is becoming more and more fragmented and stratified into a multitude of professions and titles.

—From the Health/PAC *Bulletin*, January/February, 1975. (abridged)

HEALTH: Women's Work

Susan Reverby

Womanpower is the manpower of the health field: 75 percent of all health workers are women. Control over this workforce is crucial to those who control the health system.

The labor force within the health system is changing rapidly. There has been a vast increase in the number of health workers, from 2.9 million in 1960 to 3.9 million by 1969 to a projected 6.85 million by 1980. The roles they play are also changing: at the turn of the century, 80 percent of all health workers were doctors; today only 7.5 percent are doctors. New occupational divisions have developed to the point where there are now over 375 independent occupations. With their numerical supremacy, women health workers are a powerful potential power for change.

WOMANPOWER

The predominance of women in the health system developed historically because of two factors. Most jobs in health are dead-end, low-wage, semiskilled or unskilled. This kind of work has traditionally gone to women, especially third world women. Also, health-care jobs, with the exception of doctors and administrators, reflect the institutionalization of traditional women's functions: nurturing, caring, cooking, educating, cleaning. In the health system these functions become the jobs of nurse, housekeeper, dietician, clerk, social worker and technician.

Women are 98 percent of registered nurses, 64 percent of cooks, 74 percent of aides and attendants, 96 percent of practical nurses, 94 percent of nutritionists and dieticians, 95 percent of office workers, 80 percent of physical therapists, 75 percent of X-ray technicians, 90 percent of medical technologists and 89 percent of medical social workers. Almost all dental hygienists, medical librarians and clerks are women.

While women fulfill the "feminine functions," men make the decisions. Men are 93 percent of doctors, 90 percent of chiropractors, 98 percent of dentists, and 80 percent of hospital administrators. There is even a feminine role for women doctors. The phrase "a woman's place is in the home" has been changed to "a woman's place is in pediatrics or child psychiatry," according to one woman doctor.

Wage differentials for the same job follow sex lines. In almost every field, especially where women overwhelmingly predominate, the wage difference is great. Thus the 145,942 women practical nurses receive on the average ten dollars less per week than their 3,350 male counterparts. Men's and women's salaries were equal in only one field: medical technology. Women health workers on the top suffer as well. Women doctors tend to take salaried institutional positions rather than go into higher-paying private practice. And they can also expect less advancement.

A 1969 Department of Labor study of hospital wages demonstrates the following weekly wage differentials:

Physical Therapists	
Males	$166.50
Females	155.50
X-ray Technicians	
Males	131.00
Females	116.50
Food Service Supervisors	
Males	137.50
Females	96.00
Housekeeping Chiefs	
Males	154.50
Females	96.00

Practical Nurses	
Males	108.50
Females	98.50
Nurses' Aides	
Males	82.00
Females	75.50

WHY HEALTH WORK?

Columbia University manpower economist Eli Ginzberg describes the predicaments of the health system: "A field which attracts a disproportionate number of women, many of them young, will tend to have the following characteristics: a low wage scale, heavy turnover, excessive training costs, and relatively little accumulation of skill through experience." While the description may be true, Ginzberg puts the burden of blame for these problems on women rather than on the low wages and alienating work conditions of the health system.

The "disproportionate" number of women reflects the fact that women have few other choices. As one medical social worker said, "What do you do as a woman? The options were to be a nurse, teacher or social worker." In interview after interview women health workers in New York City cited economic necessity as the key factor in choosing a health career. One nurse said, "We didn't have the money for me to go to college. My mother was a nurse and had gone to a diploma school, so I decided to become a nurse as well." If society gives women in general few options, it gives even fewer to poor and third world women. "What else could I do?" asked one Harlem Hospital nurses' aide.

TURNOVER

Although most women who worked in the health system do so out of economic necessity, there is nevertheless high job turnover. In 1967, the turnover rate for all workers in nursing (including practical nurses, registered nurses, aides, attendants and orderlies) was 60 percent, compared with 18 percent for women teachers in the public schools. This turnover reflects many factors.

Dual Roles—Women in health face the same tensions that confront women in other fields; they must work to earn money; yet they are expected to have children and care for their families. One ward clerk said, "I have a 15-year-old daughter. She's a good girl, but if she started getting into trouble I guess I'd have to quit and stay home."

Women tend to enter the workforce before their children are born, to leave work while they are growing up and to re-enter after the children are either in school or out of the house. The largest number of non-working nurses are 30 to 34 years old. But both the number of women working and the length of their work experience are increasing. The percentage of mothers who work has risen twice as fast as the rate of all working women between 1940 and 1967.

Yet, the health institutions make very few provisions for a woman's other responsibilities. Child care facilities and paid maternity leave are virtually nonexistent. Some special programs for part-time residencies and internships have been instituted for women doctors who have children; but neither day care nor housing close to the hospital is available for most health workers. In 1969, only 2 percent of the children of all working mothers in the workforce were in the limited number of day care centers; most mothers must find make-shift personal solutions or lose their income to stay home with their children.

Working Conditions—Most women health workers face low-paying jobs and years of frustration and alienation. Low wages are only part of the problem.

In study after study registered nurses stated clearly that if they leave the field, it is because of the vast discrepancy between what they were trained to do and what they are allowed to do. Said one nurse, "We're really like secretaries pushing papers around. All we do is dispense pills to the patients. Giving medications gets to be boring. The aides are the ones who really work with the patients." One nursing educator with twelve years of nursing experience said, "Let's face it, nursing is a rotten job. You have no control over hours, you rotate shifts, work weekends and holidays. You get moved from floor to floor. Sometimes you're the only one with fifty patients and yet the supervisor comes in and yells at you and you think, what do they expect from me?"

Lack of fullfillment is built into all levels of hospital work. Narrow and specific job definitions mean people do the same repetitious tasks day after day: stenographers type medical records, IV technicians start IV's, hematology technicians count blood cells. Doctors, who may do a variety of tasks, have transferred many of the mundane tasks to other workers, mainly women. It is difficult for other health workers to break out of their narrow slots. One cardiology technician said she had not been taught anything about cardiology and that the doctors refused to answer her questions.

Hierarchy and Control—Narrow job definitions is reinforced by hierarchical control in the health system.

Lucille Kinlein, a nurse writing in the January, 1972, issue of *Nursing Outlook*, said, "So often I knew the patient better than the physician and had scientifically based reasons for wanting to initiate a certain action—yet I was prevented from doing so without being given equally valid reasons. The goal seemed to be to keep the institution operating at a smooth pace and to placate the other professional people, rather than to help the patient to meet his needs."

Nor is it just nurses who have no control over their work. The health system is a rigid caste system. Economist Martin Karp noted: "In no other industry is the 'pecking order' more evident." The result is that because workers cannot vent their anger against the people above them, they take it out on those below them or on the patients. Narrow job roles and rigid hierarchy lead to frustrations and divisiveness between health workers.

The caste system in health reflects not only divisions between job categories or sex, but deeper divisions of class and race. This, of course, serves the interest of those who run the health industry. The development of this hierarchy and the concurrent problems it brings for all women health workers is epitomized in the history and current difficulties facing the nursing field.

FLORENCE NIGHTINGALE: GENTLEWOMEN AND DOMESTIC SERVANTS

In the nineteenth century, hospitals were part of poor houses. There was no professional nursing; poor women, many times themselves inmates of the poorhouses, did what little nursing there was. Nursing as a distinct profession began on the battlefield, where disease often killed more soldiers than did bullets. During the Crimean War of the 1850's, Florence Nightingale and a group of dedicated women proved that good nursing care could drastically decrease the mortality rate among soldiers. Nightingale returned to England after the war to introduce her concepts of professional nursing to English hospitals.

Stratification characterized the system from the beginning. The Nightingale system trained women in two categories which reflected English class divisions: "lady probationers" and regular nursing students. The lady probationers were to be gentlewomen of middle- and upper-class backgrounds who would have "those qualifications which will fit them to become superintendents." The regular students were to be ". . . well-educated domestic servants and . . . the daughters of small farmers . . . tradesmen, artisans . . . who have been used to household work." These women would become regular hospital nurses.

Because medicine was still closed to women at this time, many headed for nursing. Nightingale was clear that nursing was to be a separate function, a coprofession to the doctors; but, she was not, she reassured the worried physicians, training "medical women."

U.S. DEVELOPMENTS

Hospitals in America quickly saw the advantages of training nurses. Student nurses could be used to fill the hospitals' nursing needs; and better still, they didn't have to be paid beyond room and board. Between 1880 and 1900 the hospital nursing schools in the U.S. grew from 15 schools with 323 students to 432 schools with 11,000 students. Since cheap student labor provided the bulk of nursing care, hospitals did not hire their students after graduation. Besides, most health care was delivered at home and thus graduating nurses tended to go into private-duty nursing in the home.

As with medicine at this time, there was no uniformity or minimal standard for nurse training. The nursing leadership began to feel the need for uniform admissions standards and curricula in nursing schools. Above all, they sought the legal recognition of nursing through passage of nurse practice laws and the registration of nurses.

Thus, in 1894, leaders of nursing schools organized the Society of Superintendents of Training Schools for Nurses, which in 1912 was to become the National League for Nursing Education (NLN). Recognizing the need for a more broadly based group, a Nurses' Associated Alumnae of United States and Canada was organized in 1896. The NLN was primarily concerned with educational standards; the Nurses' Associated Alumnae with work conditions and the registration of nurses on a state-by-state basis. In 1911, the alumnae group became the American Nurses' Association (ANA). The overarching concern of both organizations was the establishment and upgrading of nursing standards and the recognition of nursing as a defined profession. The result of this professionalization was the creation of an internal hierarchy within nursing.

DIVISIONS BEGIN

Concerned with the increased costs of professional nursing, hospitals supported differentiation within the field. In 1907, the American Hospital Association (AHA) advocated distinction between three grades of nurses: the executive or teaching nurse, the bedside nurse, and the attendant or subsidiary nurse. The AHA suggested that all categories be licensed, but that the first two must be classified as registered nurses, while the third be called by some other title. The AHA study had little influence at the time, but it clearly indicated the hospitals' interest in fostering the divisions within the nursing profession.

World War I increased the need for health workers and raised questions about their training. After the war, the Rockefeller Foundation convened a conference which led to a study of nursing and nursing education. Released in 1923, the study, called the Goldmark Report, suggested that nursing become part of a collegiate program. The report also recommended that auxiliary personnel be trained in shorter periods of time to carry on some of the less important nursing functions. The Goldmark Report attempted to do for nursing what the Flexner Report in 1910 did for medicine. The latter resulted in the upgrading and standardizing of medical training by putting it into a university setting. Following the Goldmark Report, nursing programs at Yale and several other universities were established.

During the Depression, droves of private-duty nurses were unemployed and many hospital-based nursing schools closed. During World War II, hospitals began to hire nurses; the increased cost led to the creation of a new subdivision in nursing—the "practical or vocational" nurse.

By the post-war period, studies by the American Nursing Association recommended that there be a further increase in auxiliary nursing personnel on the one hand, and an upgrading of registered nurses on the other. Thus the hierarchy in nursing became more elaborate and rigid. Bedside nursing was to be done by the practical nurse and later by a new, lower category called the aide. Meanwhile RN's tried to separate themselves from "lower" nursing categories by greater specialization.

PROFESSIONAL VS. TECHNICAL NURSE

By 1964, seeds of the division planted by Florence Nightingale in the nineteenth century had come into full bloom. Indeed, divisions multiplied even within the ranks of registered nurses. The ANA recommended two different kinds of programs to train registered nurses: a four-year baccalaureate college program for "professional" nurses, and two-year community college associate degree with hospital-based diploma programs for "technical" nurses.

The consequences of these new divisions were not long in coming. In the early 1960's 84 percent of all nurses had been trained in hospital-based diploma schools; by 1970 the figure was down to 52 percent. Hospital schools began closing, while new associate degree community college programs expanded. In 1969, 27 percent of all nurses were trained in associate degree programs, 21 percent in the baccalaureate programs.

Nursing authorities see a wide difference in the functions of these two types of nurses. According to Martha Rogers, head of New York University's Division of Nurse Education, "Baccalaureate graduates in nursing are no more interchangeable with associate degree and hospital school graduates than are dentists with dental hygienists or medical doctors with physician assistants." Supervisory and administrative jobs go to baccalaureate nurses, even those fresh out of school. The divisions are racial as well as functional:

In 1968–69, 10 percent of associate degree nursing students were black, while black students were only 5 percent of those in baccalaureate programs. Black graduates of these programs actually dropped from 9.7 percent in 1962 to 4 percent in 1966.

DIVIDED WE FALL

With expanding institutions and developing technology, division of labor in the health field has been irresistible, as it has in other industries. For the majority of health workers, this has meant specialized, alienating, often low-paying jobs. This increasing division has threatened the nursing profession.

Rather than challenging this policy or the hospital hierarchy, the nursing leadership has sought, throughout history, to preserve the power and status of "professional" nursing by creating its own subdivisions and hierarchy. The result has been to divide the interests of all health workers, and to so narrow the functions of professional nursing as to threaten its existence.

Today the nursing profession feels it is being squeezed from all directions. The explosion of "new careers" and manpower training programs is turning thousands of technical and paraprofessional health workers onto the job market. There are now over 250 new job categories, such as medical records technician, dietetic technician, social health technician and family health worker—many of which fill traditional nursing functions. And many are low-paid, dead-end jobs going, by and large, to third world women.

Many nurses are now turning to the gray area between traditional doctor and nurse functions—taking medical histories, screening patients, supervising routine care, etc. Nurses in this role are called nurse practitioners or "extended" nurses. There are now over fifty different training programs for "extended nursing" in pediatrics, obstetrics, anesthesiology, and other specialties.

The only problem with this tack is that it runs headlong into another new medical vocation—the physician assistant. Developed to utilize the experience of ex-military medical corpsmen, physician assistants "provide patient services under the supervision and direction of a licensed physician." [See "The Sorcerer's Apprentice" in Chapter 6.] Rather than advocating that nurses become physician assistants, however, the ANA has attempted to split the hairs that differentiate the two functions. "The term physician assistant should not be applied to any of the nurse practitioners being prepared to function in an extension of the nursing role," stated a December, 1971, ANA position paper.

Meanwhile more sweeping reforms of the nursing field are afoot. Dr. Henry Silver, developer of one of the first nurse practitioner programs, and Patricia McAltee, a nurse, reporting on a study supported by the Carnegie Corporation, advocate dropping the term "nursing," with its feminine connotations, in favor of "health-care practice," to attract men to the field. Schools of health-care practice would offer two curricula. "One would prepare them as providers of care, comfort and nurturing, the other for the expanded scope of health care and services, involving a wide variety of direct care functions and activities" (*American Journal of Nursing*, January, 1972). Although both men and women would attend these schools, it seems clear which curriculum will be set up for whom.

In light of the pressures and threats to the profession, nurses are becoming more militant. Many are now turning to a union approach, although there is ambivalence about whether they should join traditional unions or make the ANA their bargaining agent. [See "RN's Strike: Between the Lines" in Chapter 6.]

UNITED WE STAND

The narrow professionalism of the nursing leadership has boxed nurses into a corner. As they fought for higher wages and more skilled roles, nurses have found themselves threatened from below by unskilled, cheap labor and new technology; and insofar as they have succeeded, they now find themselves threatened from above by men coming into the field to take advantage of the higher wages and status. And the competition and division between job functions, social classes, races and sexes has worked only to the advantage of those who run the health institutions.

It would seem that to achieve job control, status, decent wages, and some measure of job fulfillment, professional nurses must join with health workers at all levels in a struggle which would make these goals possible for all.

(Susan Reverby was a Health/PAC staff member.)

—From the Health/PAC *Bulletin*, April, 1972.

HOSPITAL WORKERS: A Case Study in the "New Working Class"

John and Barbara Ehrenreich

The kind of work most people do has been changing rapidly in the United States and other capitalist countries. Only a few decades ago, most working people performed unskilled or semi-skilled industrial labor, and "the working class" was predominantly the traditional blue-collar proletariat. Today, service workers, white-collar workers, highly educated technical and professional workers—the so-called "new working class"—together make up a majority of the American work force. At the same time, the organization and content of white-collar and service work have also been changing, taking on patterns reminiscent of traditional industrial work.

We have studied the experience of workers in one of the largest and most rapidly expanding of the "new" industries—the hospital industry. The hospital work force spans all the possible definitions of the new working class, from blue-collar service workers, to semi-skilled white-collar workers, to highly educated professional workers. We talked to dozens of workers in each of these categories, and found that they almost all express needs, and experience forms of oppression, which seem to have no exact counterpart in traditional industrial settings, and which cannot be resolved in the context of the existing (capitalist) health system. If they seldom express these needs in the form of collective action to change that system, it is because there are strong countervailing forces which tend to divide the work force and distort the workers' very *experience* of oppression.

I

Before the Second World War, and before the current hospital boom, the hospital work force was made up of doctors and trained nurses, plus a large group of unskilled, semi-differentiated workers. No segment of this work force could be considered in any sense analogous to industrial workers. The doctors and nurses were usually freelancers or students, with no permanent attachment to the hospital. The others were economically marginal people, often handicapped, illiterate, or aged, who were paid barely enough for individual subsistence. With turnover rates for hospital workers in the range of 70 to 80 percent per year, there was no body of American workers who could be said to comprise a stable *hospital* work force.

The explosive growth of the hospital industry in the last two decades has led to the formation of a hospital work force which is increasingly stable, highly differentiated, and in many other ways similar to the industrial work force. Semi-skilled and unskilled hospital workers are no longer transients, or objects of charity, but long-term hospital employees who expect a day's wage for a day's work, and are increasingly turning to unions to make sure they get it. Skilled hospital workers, such as technicians and nurses, are now also almost entirely full-time salaried employees. They too have been joining unions or pressing their professional associations into behavior that is increasingly union-like.

Skilled and unskilled hospital workers alike face working conditions which more and more resemble those in an industrial plant. There is an elaborate division of labor: One New York hospital lists 42 pay categories of service and maintenance workers (nurses' aides, porters, kitchen workers, etc.), 35 types of clerical workers (secretaries, ward clerks, medical-record librarians, etc.) and 38 varieties of technical and professional personnel (registered nurses, lab technicians, X-ray technicians, physical therapists, etc.). And even this understates the fragmentation, for a pay category such as "clinical lab technician" includes technicians specialized in hematology, cytology, urinalysis, etc. As in many industrial settings, workers in hospitals participate in an increasingly small part of the productive process and may tend to lose sight of the final "product."

But despite this apparent "industrialization" of hospital workers, the hospital worker is not just an industrial worker whose "product" happens to be medical care. Hospital work is *different* from industrial work and the hospital worker faces contradictions which have only limited analogies in manufacturing industries or even in other service industries. First, and most obvious, is the fact that the central product of hospital work is not some artifact of questionable value, but a service whose value is *self-evident*. And no amount of automation or specialization can completely obscure this fact. No matter how fragmented or menial their jobs, no matter how bad their working conditions, hospital workers commonly express a degree of commitment to service, to doing one's best, that would be beyond the wildest dreams of an industrial personnel manager. "You still have the patients. You do the best you can," a ward clerk told us. (Indeed, hospital managements have often successfully exploited the workers' "service ethic" to avert strikes and unionization.)

But the hospital workers' service ethic does not guarantee a selfless devotion to the hospital as an institution. To the extent that the modern hospital is not a "mission of mercy," but an expansionist business enterprise, the service ethic is a potentially subversive force. A nurses' aide who is a local union official at New York's Bellevue Hospital summed it up: "Some of our people feel they're not so much in the patient-care area as catering to the comfort of administrators. . . . They [the administration] say they want patient care but they don't make it possible."

The second major peculiarity of hospital work lies in the organization of work. For technological and historical reasons hospital work features a high degree of functional interdependence between workers of extremely different rank within the hospital and extremely different social status outside it. For example, a surgical operation commonly requires the cooperative efforts of a team whose members range in rank from surgeon to aides. The surgeon has had eight or more years of post-college training; he may earn more than $50,000 a year; he may sit on one of the hospital's key management committees, on the almost all-powerful "medical board," or even on the board of directors.* The aide may have no high school educa-

* Hospital management is generally composed of three groups: the doctors, the trustees, and the lay administrators. The trustees play a small role in the day-to-day functioning of the hospital, and have declined in importance altogether in recent years. The lay administrators' importance has grown as hospitals increase in size and complexity, but their role in

tion, earn less than $7,000, and lack even the authority to make a simple suggestion. But in the operation itself, they are both essential participants, as the aide can easily demonstrate by making a small but fatal mistake. There is thus a continual contradiction between the worker's sense of her or his own importance in the productive process and her or his total lack of importance in the institution.

To put it another way, there is a very real contradiction between the doctor's actual functional importance and his inflated status within the hospital. (Here we are not speaking of the doctors-in-training, the interns and residents, whose position is much more ambiguous.) As the division of hospital labor increases and the doctor delegates more and more of his historic functions to members of the nursing and technical staff, he becomes at least as dependent on the skills of other workers as they are on his. "You could imagine a hospital with no doctors. Everything would get done just the same," a nurse in a municipal hospital told us. "But try to imagine a hospital with no nurses. It would be chaos. The patients would all die of neglect." Similarly, the technicians could argue that, without them, the doctor would be virtually unable to diagnose a single case. As his claims to unique functional indispensability are eroded by the division of labor, the doctor becomes, in the eyes of the other hospital workers, more and more clearly, just a *boss*.

The doctor's position has no parallel in industry. On the one hand, he is a top executive in the hospital "corporation." On the other hand, he is simply a highly

---

policy-making is relatively small. In our opinion, the doctors represent the key element in the management of the major "industrialized" hospitals. They lay administrators *are* important in hospital workers' daily experience, but their role does not change our analysis of the contradictions in hospital work.

skilled production worker, working side by side with nurses, aides, and technicians, and subject to their continual surveillance. They are the first, and usually the only, witnesses to his failures—unnecessary postoperative complications, prescriptions for the wrong dosages of drugs, faulty diagnoses, etc. And they are the harshest judges of his ethical standards: Does he discriminate against poor or nonwhite patients? Does he care more about whether he can publish the case than whether he can cure the patient? Insofar as he has become an integral part of hospital management, his individual shortcomings, however minor, serve to discredit the entire authority structure of the institution.

The difference between the doctor-manager and his co-workers is not just one of rank within the hospital, but of absolute social status. In fact, the hospitals' elaborate and militaristic system of rank identifications—uniforms, pins, titles, etc.—is hardly necessary. Everyone knows that in the hospital, white males are likely to be doctors, white women to be nurses or technicians, nonwhites to be aides, janitors, and so on. Doctors *are* 98 percent white, 93 percent male, and predominantly from upper and upper-middle-class families. Nurses and technicians *are* usually lower-middle-class and white; 98 percent of nurses, and about 70 percent of technicians, are women. Aides, cooks, maids, etc., are lower-class men and women—in the big cities of the north, they are usually black, Chicano, or Puerto Rican. (In New York City's municipal hospitals, 80-90 percent are nonwhite.)

This class, race, and sex stratification is due not so much to biased hiring practices, as to the fact that in the hospital virtually everyone remains at his or her entry-level job. Compared to other industries there is an almost complete lack of job mobility, even though there is often a great deal of functional interchangeability between the various types of workers. For example, practical nurses commonly possess the same skills as RNs (Registered Nurses) and are often assigned responsibilities theoretically and legally reserved for RNs (at no extra pay, of course). But the only way a practical nurse can gain the title, the status, and the pay of the RN is by attending school full-time for at least two years. So the practical nurse, like the aide below her and the RN above her, tends to remain where she started, i.e., at exactly the level toward which she was tracked long ago in public school.

The result is an occupational hierarchy which seems to have been almost designed to promote conflict. There is an unbridgeable gap—of both institutional rank and absolute social status—between the technical and managerial elite (doctors and administrators) and the great bulk of the work force. The structural inequity of this hierarchy is made inescapable by a productive process which mixes the two groups in intimate daily contact. Finally, there is a growing substantive antagonism between the two groups over the fundamental issue of the *purpose* of work: human service versus the hospital managers' corporate priorities.

II

To have meaningful work and to be adequately recognized for doing it, both materially and in terms of respect and status within the institution—these are the hospital workers' real and conscious needs. So what prevents the collective expression of these needs? What maintains the hospital hierarchy in the face of the contradictions we have described? There are two main stabilizing forces, operating in part on different sets of hospital workers. For the unskilled and semi-skilled workers, there are forces which lead to a kind of passive alienation from the content of their work. For the skilled workers, there is the ideology of professionalism. The first denies the service ethic and accepts the class division within the hospital. The second denies the class division and diverts the service ethic into a professional "ethic" of institutional loyalty.

Undoubtedly many of the lower-level workers enter hospital work because they can find no other semi-skilled jobs in the cities. But a large majority do start with the expectation that there is some special meaning and dignity to hospital work. Conditions (in even the "best" hospitals), however, are enough to undermine the efforts of even the most dedicated workers—understaffing, inadequate supplies and equipment, obstructive red tape, priorities given to non-patient care functions, etc. In their training or orientation, lower-level workers are warned against taking it all too seriously. "Do not try to achieve perfection in everything, because, admirable as it is, it is an invitation to failure and often is most impracticable," warns one text for practical nurses. (*Personal and Vocational Relationships in Practical Nursing*, by Carmen F. Ross, Philadelphia, 1969, p. 103) Suggestions and innovations from the ranks are not encouraged, and are usually viewed as "troublemaking." An aide told us, "You go to your supervisor [about a patient care problem]. She doesn't do anything. Eventually, *you* stop caring, too." Again and again we heard the refrain. "After a while you just don't give a damn." You become the adjusted, "industrialized" worker, for whom hospital work is just a job.

The recent wave of hospital unionization has done much to reinforce the psychological industrialization of the lower-rank hospital workers. Like unions in other industries, hospital workers' unions do not challenge the nature of the "product" or the organization of work. Their interest in qualitative, service issues has been largely a matter of public relations rhetoric, and their efforts to reform the occupational hierarchy have been minimal. In effect, the unions' message to the workers is, "We can't do anything about the fact that you have a meaningless dead-end job, but we can get you paid more for doing it." In fact, the hospitals pass wage hikes for hospital workers onto consumers, either in the form of higher charges or reduced services. So by concentrating on economic demands, without in any way challenging the hospital hierarchy and its non-service priorities, the unions implicitly place the needs of the workers in conflict with the needs of the consumer—the ultimate alienation.

Professionalism is a factor which is uniquely important in the hospital industry (though it is also present in a number of other "new working class" work settings) and deserves a much more careful examination. Some 40 percent of all non-managerial hospital workers are in job categories which consider themselves "professional." There is no question but that the hospital work force is relatively highly skilled: what is peculiar is that virtually every technically trained category in the hospital has pretensions of professionalism. A technician working for a drug company, for instance, would probably not consider herself a professional; in a hospital, she would. This is not simply a matter of individual self-appraisal, either. X-ray technicians, inhalation therapists, physical therapists, and a host of other job categories boast their own professional associations, complete with ethical codes, publications, conventions, dues, and so on.

Obviously, to make sense out of this rampant professionalism, it is necessary first to clear up what is meant by a "profession." The word calls to mind lengthy, specialized training, high standards of performance, ethics which transcend personal desires, and other worthy attributes. Doctors and lawyers come to mind. The importance of these images is not that they are accurate but that they reflect the special status accorded to professional workers in our society. They usually earn more and are almost always accorded more respect than other workers. But performing what would generally be called "professional" duties in a "professional" manner does not suffice to make a worker a "professional." For example, a practical nurse and a registered nurse may perform exactly the same duties at an identical level of technical and ethical standards. But only the RN is a real professional, i.e., a licensed member of a legally recognized professional group.

Thus the word "professional" has two sets of meanings—one based in popular imagery and the other in legal reality. In the latter sense, a profession is an organized occupational group which has been granted a monopoly over the performance of certain functions and a certain degree of autonomy in carrying them out. For example, the medical profession has a legal monopoly over the prescribing of drugs, surgical practice, the classifying of people as fit or unfit for a variety of functions, etc. It has almost complete autonomy to police its members and to set standards for the admission of new members.

Once we have said that a profession is a legal entity, we have said that it is also a social and political entity. A group does not become a profession by winning a mass vote of confidence, but by winning the recognition of courts and legislatures. In the words of sociologist Eliot Freidson:

> A profession attains and maintains its position by virtue of the protection and patronage of some elite segment of society which has been persuaded that there is some special value in its work. Its position is thus secured by the political and economic influence of the elite which sponsors it—an influence that drives competing occupations out of some areas of work, that discourages others by virtue of the competitive advantages conferred on the chosen occupation, and that requires still others to be subordinated to the profession. (*The Profession of Medicine* [New York: Dodd Mead & Company, 1970], p. 72.)

The American medical profession provides one of the clearest examples. In the mid-nineteenth century there was no American medical profession, only a welter of competing sects. The emergence of one group of doctors as the modern medical profession was due less to their technical superiority (they had little at that time) than to the conscious intervention of the ruling class, and particularly of the Carnegie and Rockefeller Foundations. (See, for example, *Witches, Midwives and Nurses: A History of Women Healers*, by Barbara Ehrenreich and Deirdre English [Glass Mountain Pamphlets, P.O. Box 238, Oyster Bay, New York, 11771].) Today, of course, the medical profession is a political force in its own right, quite capable of defending its own interests without overt ruling-class intervention.

To return to the numerous other health professions: everyone recognizes that they have a much lower status than the medical profession. In fact, there is a definite hierarchy of health professions. At the top is the medical profession, the only completely autonomous health profession, the only one whose authority was derived directly from the ruling class. All the other health professions were sanctioned by, and are to varying degrees supervised by, the medical profession itself. (Sociologists recognize their dependent status by calling them "semi-professions," "paraprofessions," "allied health professions," etc.) The ideologies of these professions reflect their subordinate status and create, in the professional worker, an internalized "sense of one's place."

Consider first the nursing profession. RNs occupy an intermediate position in the hospital hierarchy—subordinate to the doctors, but in a supervisory role with respect to practical nurses, aides, and (depending on the hospital) several other kinds of semi-skilled workers. Ideologically, nursing professionalism combines the authoritarianism necessary for the nurse's supervisory role with the authoritarianism implicit in her relation to the doctors. In a way, this sense of mixed status could be said to come "naturally" to nurses: RNs are women, usually from the lower-middle class. Being women, they have been socialized to be subordinate to the male doctors. Being of high enough economic class to have afforded nursing education, they can easily feel superior to the aides and practical nurses.

This pattern goes back to the origins of the nursing profession in the late nineteenth century. Nursing as we know it was invented by a small number of upper-class reformers, under the intellectual leadership of Florence Nightingale. The Nightingale nurse was defined by her "character," rather than by her skills, and the nursing "character" was modeled after the upper-class Victorian lady: To the doctor, she brought the wifely virtue of absolute obedience; to the patient, she brought the selfless devotion of a mother; to the lower-level hospital employees she brought the firm but kindly discipline of a household manager, accustomed to handling servants. She desired none of the doctor's skills or prerogatives. His professionalism stemmed from the masculine realm of scientific thought, hers from a kind of innate feminine spirituality.

As far as hospital management is concerned, the historic professional self-image of the nurse is as serviceable today as it ever was. Nursing is still a "feminine" profession, and nurses are still trained to be "ladies" (i.e., to imitate the manners and style of upper-class women) and hence to feel a class above the workers they must supervise. Today, however, the four-year liberal arts degree is replacing "character" as the hallmark of class. If the nurses' professional organizations have their way, "professional" nursing, i.e., supervisory roles, will be restricted to the graduates of four-year, college-based, nursing programs. There is still no threat to the doctor, because baccalaureate nursing education is no richer in scientific content than the old hospital training. All it takes is a smattering of high-priced liberal arts courses to make sure that the nurse is a class above her subordinates.

The other sub-medical hospital workers' professions are narrower and more craft-oriented than the nursing and medical professions. Each comprises a narrow set of functions spun off by the medical profession in the last thirty years or so—medical technology, inhalation therapy, physical therapy, medical record keeping, radiation therapy, etc. Organizationally, these relatively new "allied" health professions lack even the dubious independence of the nursing profession. For example, accreditation of schools for training allied health workers is controlled by the AMA Council on Medical Education. Certification of individuals in most occupations is jointly supervised by the allied professional society and its parent medical-specialty society (for example, the American College of Radiologists in the case of X-ray technicians).

The creation of the allied health professions represents a kind of pact between highly unequal parties. The medical profession delegates one of its functions and agrees to recognize the new practitioners as fellow "professionals." (Presumably there is no physician's task so inconsequential as to be entrusted to nonprofessionals.) In practice this means that doctors and hospitals agree to give preference in hiring to certified members of the new occupational grouping, or at least to pay them more than uncertified persons who may have simply acquired the skill in question. Members of the new allied health profession, in turn, agree to "keep in their place": to submit to medical domination of accreditation and certification, to confine their work activities within limits set by physicians, and so forth.

The ideology of the allied health professions is amply illustrated by this credo of the medical technologist:

> As a medical technologist, I am proud, with a pride that is tinctured with a true humility, with a pride in being one of the trio in the medical profession, the physician, the nurse, and the medical technologist, each of whom functions in his distinct way. As a medical technologist, I am independent, with a cooperative spirit working with my fellows in the medical profession. I do not want to encroach upon

anyone else's premises. (From the *American Journal of Medical Technologists*, reprinted in E. Freidson, *op. cit.* p. 68.)

To the hospital, the new allied health professionals are simply workers who do not see themselves as workers. *Workers* are too quickly alienated by fragmented jobs; true *professionals* rejoice in the exercise of their craft. *Workers* identify with other workers in their institution, and can unite on the spot around common grievances. *Professionals* identify only with other members of their profession, and look to a distant professional society for long-term advancement. Finally, *workers* need discipline and close supervision; the true *professional* can be trusted to adhere to the ethics and standards of his profession in any situation. If he should abandon his ethics—by overreaching his narrow responsibilities, criticizing a superior, joining a strike, or whatever—he faces a punishment more severe than firing: he may be decertified by his own professional society, and tossed back into the ranks of mere workers.

III

Conditions of work in the modern industrialized hospital engender a uniquely clear set of class and caste antagonisms. The hospital joins, in the intimacy of its productive processes, members of the upper and upper-middle classes, whose institutional functions are increasingly managerial, with a large body of workers from less privileged strata of society—women, the poor and near-poor, and, in certain localities, nonwhites. It pits these two groups—the managerial elite and the rest of the work force—against each other in conflicts, not all of which can be resolved without a radical recasting of the nature and purpose of hospital work. There is the classic industrial conflict over wages and working conditions, the improvement of which necessarily threatens management spending priorities. There is the worker's need for meaningful, service-oriented jobs, which necessarily threatens the hospital as a business enterprise; there is the worker's need for advancement in skills and for participation as a real "team" member—needs which run headlong into the doctors' defensive monopoly over the scientific underpinnings of the production process.

But, as we have seen, there are forces at work which serve both to obscure these needs and to prevent collective action around them. Lower-level workers are encouraged by management and by their unions to set aside qualitative demands in return for economic gains. Skilled workers are seduced by the ideology of professionalism into forgoing both qualitative and quantitative satisfactions in return for an abstract sense of status. The result is an increasing division of the non-managerial hospital work force into two groups with opposing class identifications: on the one hand, a proletarianized body of unskilled and semi-skilled workers, and, on the other hand, an equally large group of skilled workers who, through the device of professionalism, are allowed to participate—however vicariously—in the very real status of the doctors.

If the hospital were a socially isolated institution, one might expect a stable equilibrium to be achieved between the workers' dissatisfactions and the countervailing forces of alienation and professionalism. But hospitals are not ivory towers—all the less so, in fact, since they have expanding needs for public subsidy, for manpower, for real estate, and for "teaching material." And because the hospital's internal hierarchy so precisely mirrors the stratification of the larger society, it is vulnerable to the slightest egalitarian breezes from the outside. Third world consciousness and, very recently, women's consciousness make the hospital hierarchy appear more palpably unjust every day, and provide a basis for collective workers' action. Even more compelling has been the emergence of consumer groups, especially in poor areas, whose struggles for better care have heightened the contradictions between the hospital's corporate interests and its public "mission" of service and have forced workers to take a stand. As a result, the hospital industry has witnessed a degree of insurgency unparalleled in other sectors. Only in hospitals in recent years have there been even partial plant seizures; only in hospitals have there been explicit demands for workers' control.

For example, in the summer of 1968 workers at Topeka State Hospital demanded pay increases, training programs for unskilled workers, and community control of the hospital. Instead of striking, they seized the administrator's office and briefly ran the services themselves. At New York's Lincoln Hospital, in April 1969, workers in the mental health facility demanded job upgrading and community-worker control. They ousted the administrators and head doctors and operated the services themselves for several weeks (with the cooperation of many of the "professional" workers). Again in the late summer of 1970, there was a major worker and community upheaval at Lincoln around demands for community and worker control of the entire hospital. The insurgent workers' organization, the Health Revolutionary Unity Movement, temporarily established community-worker committees to monitor medical practice and won the ouster of some of the more conservative doctors. There have been dozens of other, less dramatic cases, where hospital workers have transcended the forces which divide them to agitate for worker and consumer control of their institutions.

Straws in the wind or prophetic breakthroughs? There's no way, by dint of sheer analysis, to know. The *contradictions* in hospital work which could lead to further unrest and the *countervailing forces* which seem to mitigate, distort, or deny these contradictions are experienced simultaneously by hospital workers. The hospital workers' very *experience* is contradictory; it leads *both* toward resistance and acceptance of their situation. We cannot put the contradictions on one side, the countervailing forces on the other, try to balance them, and come up with an abstract conclusion such as "hospital workers are potentially revolutionary" or "hospital workers are potentially allies of the bourgeoisie." Only the hospital workers themselves can solve the equation, and only through their *practice*. This practice, in turn, is conditioned by their immediate experiences in the hospital, by the efforts of management to direct the workers' response to that experience, and by external forces which shape their psychological and material responses. Moreover, the answer may turn out to be different for different types of hospital worker.

(John and Barbara Ehrenreich were Health/PAC staff members.)

—From *Monthly Review*, January, 1973. (abridged.)

6

Health Professionalism

Professionalism has been the customary means by which health workers have attempted to protect their interests. With the consent of the powers that be in hospitals, the doctors and administrators, groups of workers have created for themselves a legal monopoly over the performance of certain health-care functions, assuring themselves higher income and improved job security—but at the expense of increasing alienation from other workers. Some of the key issues presented by professionalism are raised by the first selection in this chapter, a short editorial from the Health/PAC *Bulletin* aptly entitled "Fragmentation of Workers: An Anti-Personnel Weapon."

In the next selection Emily Spieler discusses licensure, the process by which new health professions become formally recognized, and its impact on workers. This process is then examined by Susan Reverby in the case of the physician assistants, a rapidly growing new health profession that seeks definition and security by placing itself from the very outset totally under the physician's wing.

Recent strikes by professional groups, such as the RN strike in San Francisco, suggest that some professionals at least are coming to a new perception of their role in the health system and their relation to other health workers. Members of Health/PAC's San Francisco office report on the RN strike there and on the contradictory tendencies within that strike between identification and alliance with other hospital workers on one hand and professionalist assertions of special privilege on the other.

FRAGMENTATION OF WORKERS: An Anti-Personnel Weapon

This chapter examines yet another aspect of the growing industrialization of health care—what it means for the millions who work in these health-care factories. Here we see some familiar historical parallels. The growth of new technology and the need for mass production have created new and more specialized categories of work. In their need for decent wages and job security, hospital workers, who are among the lowest paid in the entire workforce, have begun to organize. Some, particularly those in the lower echelons, have gone the route of unionization [see Chapter 7]. Others, particularly those doing the increasingly specialized tasks, have sought the same ends through professionalization—organizing to claim control of the particular tasks by forming associations which certify members, establish entry requirements, and seek to codify their functions into state law. Since the turn of the century, the "allied health professions" have proliferated tenfold until there are now some 125 recognized health occupations and 250 secondary or specialist designations.

These new health professions follow in the path of their grand predecessor: the doctors and their protective association, the American Medical Association (AMA). There is one major difference, however: each new profession starts with successively less of the turf. Each seizes what it can in terms of power and territory without encroaching on that of the more established and powerful professions, and then joins them in jealously guarding the borders of the new status quo. In fact, most of the emerging health professions are under the indirect control of the AMA and, on the job, the doctors themselves. The differences in power and prestige between the AMA and some of the newcomers are so great that often their only similarity is the claim to professional status.

What does this mean for workers? For those on the inside, professional status does assure some degree of job security, status and higher wages, but at the expense of reinforcing the monotonous, fragmented, alienating nature of the work and rigidifying the job hierarchy within hospitals. For example, the educational requirements thrown up to guard entry to a profession often lock its members into dead-ended, assembly-line-like jobs. For those on the outside, the entry requirements often act to establish the profession as the domain of a particular sex, race or class of workers.

In many respects the development of the allied health professions echoes that of the craft unions of the old AF of L, which organized on the basis of particular skills and, in so doing, set worker against worker, skill against skill and the skilled against the lesser-skilled. And among hospital workers we already see the nurse practitioner vying with the physician assistant and the research technician with the lab technician for crumbs of status, autonomy, and upward mobility, rather than focusing on those who set the context and conditions of hospital employment.

Because the historical parallels are abundant, one would hope that hospital workers might benefit from the rich experience of other industrial workers. Time and again it has been shown that when workers seize on the small bits of privilege which distinguish them from other workers, rather than focusing on the vast majority of conditions which unite them, only management wins. And likewise it has become clear that while decent wages and job security are necessary, they are not sufficient. For hospital workers, perhaps even more than others, it is essential that issues such as job mobility, breaking down the hierarchy, job satisfaction, working conditions and other issues are addressed which might bring an end to the alienation from work.

—Editorial from the Health/PAC *Bulletin*, November, 1972. (abridged)

DIVISION OF LABORERS

Emily Spieler

Licensure, the point at which government steps in to protect the interests of health professional groups, has traditionally been justified as necessary to protect the public from quackery and to ensure quality of care. Workers' groups have seized upon licensure as a means of increasing salaries and ensuring job security. In the last 25 years, as a response to the phenomenal development of medical technology and the increasing demand for services, new categories of workers have proliferated. Tensions have developed among new and old groups of workers as each attempts to guard its set of skills from further encroachment. But the number of "professions" has skyrocketed so that there are now 375 sometimes overlapping job categories each vying for professional status. The result is chaos in the health workforce.

HISTORY: MONOPOLY LEGALIZED

Licensing is merely the final stage in the progression that workers follow in their search for protection. The process is always the same: technology or increased demand creates a new task and a need for on-the-job training. This eventually produces a job category and an identifiable group of workers who form an association in their search for economic security. The association certifies its members, establishes educational criteria, lobbies and propagandizes for state licensing. Finally, educational and experiential criteria are codified into state law and a state board is created, which is usually composed of members of the association.

This pattern was first established by doctors and the American Medical Association (AMA), organized in 1847. While there had been some medical licensing earlier, all laws had been repealed around 1830, as healing sects appeared and it became increasingly difficult to judge their relative worths. Regardless of their quality or lack thereof, the expansion of cults like Thompsonism, electicism, and homeopathy, and the proliferation of schools which provided easy access to the medical profession, meant that women, the poor, and members of minority groups could practice the healing arts. Severe economic competition, coupled with a desire to establish control over their profession, led the emerging AMA to challenge the credibility and power of the schools and cults.

The parallel expansion of scientific knowledge in Western Europe provided the AMA with its ammunition. In 1893 the first European-style, scientifically oriented medical school in the United States was set up at Johns Hopkins. Claims of expertise based on real medical advances, coupled with sometimes valid charges of quackery leveled at sects who lacked the resources to cash in on the new science, gave doctors pre-eminence in the eyes of lawmakers and the public. Consequently, between 1881 and 1900 almost all states enacted licensing laws for physicians. The influence of the doctors was further strengthened by the influx of enormous sums of money from philanthropic foundations set up by nineteenth-century robber barons. After successfully courting their well-to-do clientele for many years, physicians, now almost entirely white, male, and middle class, became the beneficiaries of this new source of income. Starting in 1903, foundations began to pour money into four-year medical schools, which were patterned on the European-Hopkins model. In 1904 the AMA created its Council on Medical Education (CME) to accredit schools and guarantee that control of medical education would never again slip away. The CME immediately sponsored a study of medical schools conducted by Abraham Flexner, a member of the staff of the Carnegie

Foundation. In 1910 the influential Flexner Report was issued, extolling the virtues of the Johns Hopkins model, and graduation from a CME-accredited school became a prerequisite for state licensing. Many of the smaller, less well-endowed schools were forced to close.

Friendly licensing laws, under which the regulated group is made responsible for its own public regulation, proved to be effective tools of economic warfare. Doctors were not the only ones to seek this protection; barbers and horseshoers, also confronted with runaway competition, went the same route during this period. Less powerful occupations were subject to hostile laws which they could not control. But technology made horseshoers obsolete; and barbers, unable to latch onto the public's growing awe of science, were less successful in establishing a monopoly through licensing and later turned to unionism to accomplish the same end.

By achieving friendly legislation, ostensibly enacted to control quality, doctors managed to transform their economic desire for monopoly into economic rights. And in codifying these rights into law, they convinced legislators and consumers that the legislation itself was necessary for public protection. Medicine became a profession, and doctors acquired the legal authority to control the trade without outside interference.

PROFESSIONS PROLIFERATE

This comfortable situation for doctors remained unthreatened until after World War II. Then, the growth of medical technology and the move away from solo practice to complex health institutions expanded the need for categories of allied health workers far beyond the original foursome of physicians, dentists, nurses and pharmacists. Today the workforce includes such groups as radiology technicians, inhalation therapists, medical technologists, laboratory technicians, and occupational therapy assistants. Federal programs have created another, lower category: "new professionals," noncredentialed workers generally drawn from poor minority communities to do social work, e.g., community mental health workers. In contrast to doctors, all of these groups are employees of institutions, not independent practitioners. Yet each new category has attempted to follow the doctor's pattern of establishing itself as a profession. Nurses were the earliest imitators; now as many as 22 different licensed health occupations exist.

Inhalation therapy is a typical example. As heart and chest medicine developed and lung complications arose, hospitals trained orderlies to operate the increasingly sophisticated breathing equipment. The American Association of Inhalation Therapists (AAIT) was formed in 1947, and finally sponsored the first national certification exam for inhalation therapists in September, 1970. In early 1970 there were 56 educational programs in inhalation therapy; by October, 1970 the number had grown to 82. In 1971 hiring practices changed as the supply of certified workers increased; hospitals gave preference to certified workers because they carried a guarantee of minimum training and competence, eliminating expensive-on-the-job training. Characteristically, certified workers' wages increased significantly. Membership in AAIT increased over 100 percent, from 6,000 to 12,500 in the last two-and-a-half years as membership became a prerequisite for certification, and certification became necessary to get a job. Until now two years of experience, successful completion of the test, and membership in the AAIT have been sufficient for certification. At the end of 1973, however, an associate degree from an educational program accredited by the CME in conjunction with the AAIT will be required before taking the exam. State licensing, which will embody the same requirements as those for certification, will probably be required in New York within the year. The regulatory circle is complete.

Even when a worker group achieves licensing, the AMA still maintains control through the accreditation process. Thus the CME, in conjunction with the particular association, accredits 18 categories of allied health training. Moreover, attempts to establish control and security through professionalization backfire by dividing workers into smaller, more easily controllable groups which are forced to bicker among themselves.

THE STATE BOARD: ENFORCING THE BARRIERS

The typical licensing law serves several functions: it establishes entrance criteria for the particular occupation; approves educational programs; ostensibly sets up some system of continuing control over individual practitioners, and defines the scope of practice of each occupation. State boards, which administer the licensing requirements for each occupation, are always composed of practitioners appointed by the state government from lists submitted by the particular professional association. (There are some exceptions. For example, dentists dominate the boards for dental hygienists, and registered nurses run those for practical nurses.) Associations continue to maintain a close working relationship with the boards, which are invariably understaffed and underfunded. Consequently disciplinary and investigatory responsibility are often turned over to the state associations. Office space, employees, and facilities are sometimes shared.

Not surprisingly, the actions of the boards serve the interests of the professional associations. Entrance criteria for the occupations, which mirror the requirements for certification, include membership in the professional association, graduation from an accredited educational program, experience, and successful completion of an exam. Approval of educational programs is turned over to a private accrediting body, usually the CME, and rubber stamped by the state board.

Continuing controls, on the other hand, either do not exist or are ignored. Powers to discipline practitioners through suspension or revocation of licenses are rarely used. Moreover, the boards have created no guarantees against professional obsolescence. Licenses are essentially granted for a lifetime, despite the technicality of relicensing provisions. Yet with no accountability through discipline or relicensing procedures, licensed workers may become institutionalized quacks. Recently, pressure has increased to require continuing education, but professional associations resist substantive changes, claiming that professionals are too busy providing services to undertake further education. Current programs of continuing education are so inadequate as to be meaningless: the Kentucky Board of Dentistry, for example, credits such activities as attendance at local and state dental meetings toward their requirement. Such requirements serve to encourage involvement in the professional association, but do not force practitioners to keep pace with new health science developments.

Finally, scope of practice laws, which are designed to define what tasks a licensed worker can legally perform, are often ignored within institutions without any repercussions. While doctors have unlimited scope of practice, other health occupations have to slice off a narrower piece of the pie—to establish a realm of exclusive expertise—in order to increase their bargaining power with their employers. Registered nurses, for example, cannot legally diagnose and treat; in some states practical nurses cannot administer medications. But behind this legalistic facade, substitutions are constantly made and workers perform tasks for which they are not licensed. "In fact, strict compliance with the law would close many hospitals," asserted E. Martin Egleston in *Hospitals, Journal of the American Hospital Association.* Commenting on a well-known practice, one nurse who works in a large voluntary hospital in NYC said, "The difference between RN's and LPN's is that LPN's do at night what RN's do during the day." While the scope of practice laws appear to have been broken for some workers, LPN's, for example, have no illusions about an increased sense of freedom or power to make administrative decisions. Nor are they financially compensated for the extra duties they perform. When you get right down to it, it's not surprising that institutions don't worry about scope of practice laws, since it is cheaper for them to pay an LPN to do the same work as an RN.

EFFECTS OF LICENSURE ON WORKERS

Clearly licensure laws are not geared to establish quality health services so much as to guarantee a legal monopoly over skills. Thus, licensing increases the economic security of workers in health institutions. Obviously, "the majority of new professionals have to worry about job security and mobility," as Bill Lynch, head of the New Professionals Section of the American Public Health Association, points out. Licensure accomplishes this in two ways.

First, it increases a worker's income. Institutions will accept credentials to avoid the cost of evaluating each applicant for the proper job slot, and to have some assurance of competence without on-the-job training. In exchange, they are forced to pay higher wages, partly because educational levels are most often raised by licensure: "It gives great bargaining power," asserts Lillian Roberts, vice president of the American Federation of State, County and Municipal Employees' District Council 37 (DC 37), which represents hospital workers in New York's municipal hospitals.

Second, credentials, especially licenses, increase the ability of workers to move from job to job and institution to institution, without concern about transferability of skills. On-the-job training, which now varies from 3 to 41 weeks for non-credentialed nurses' aides and orderlies, creates problems for workers who wish to change jobs without losing the benefits of their training. Local 1199 of the Drug and Hospital Workers Union [now called the National Union of Hospital and Health Care Employees] is attempting to establish uniform job descriptions in order to assure its workers mobility within the New York City voluntary hospitals. Meanwhile, the legislative department of DC 37 is developing specific laws, including licensing for new categories like obstetrician's aide. Licensing laws cannot, however, create unlimited geographic mobility, because licenses are issued state by state, not nationally.

Workers must therefore meet requirements in the particular state where they wish to practice.

The advantages for workers are diminished by inflexible requirements for expensive education which have little demonstrable relationship to competence on the job. An inhalation therapist recently complained that the new requirement for accredited education in an academic institution will, in fact, lower the quality of work because such training is less effective than on-the-job training. And by raising entrance barriers, those on the bottom rungs of the economic ladder are effectively excluded from attaining professional status.

Furthermore, licensing nurtures the fragmentation and hierarchical rigidity of the health work force. Educational credit can rarely be obtained for on-the-job training: LPN's must start from scratch, if they want to become RN's. There is little effort toward the creation of core curricula and career ladders; dead-end occupations abound.

Control over skills and specific expertise can guarantee worker security, but does not transform workers into professionals with freedom from outside interference from institutions and other more privileged workers. Rather, it enslaves them to this very expertise, locking them into a structure which discriminates by race, class, and sex. The workers are divided and conquered, while clinging desperately to the small crumbs of security they have managed to wrest from the hierarchy. Meanwhile, white, rich men maintain their monopoly over medicine.

(Emily Spieler, then a law student, was a Health/PAC student intern during the summer of 1972.)

—From the Health/PAC *Bulletin*, November, 1972. (abridged)

THE SORCERER'S APPRENTICE

Susan Reverby

The American health system has given birth to yet another occupation: the physician assistant (PA). So welcome was this new arrival that at a time when there were only ten students in training, the Surgeon General was calling the physician assistant "the hottest thing in health care delivery." A television series has already established the physician assistant as a new American hero.

Despite all the hoopla, controversy has surrounded the PA from its conception. Was the birth of a new occupation necessary? Why not upgrade nurses or produce more doctors? Debate rages over issues as diverse as what sex should she or he be, and how should the PA relate to other groups in the health hierarchy? There are even more fundamental questions: will the PA meet any of the pressing needs for personnel to provide primary health care and will the PA alter, in any way, the structure and control pyramid in the health system?

THE CHRISTENING

The American Medical Association defines the PA broadly as ". . . a skilled person qualified by academic and practical training to provide patient service under the supervision and direction of a licensed physician who is responsible for the performance of that assistant." The concept of an assistant to physicians is obviously not new. Most other members of the health-care team "assist" the physician in some manner. The difference is that the PA was developed to be *totally dependent* upon the doctor for the definition of his scope of practice.

Relieving the physician of his simpler duties, the PA will take medical histories, do physical examinations, instruct patients on specific regimens, write some prescriptions and perform more technical but routine medical tasks like suturing, removing casts, starting IV's, and inserting catheters. The PA will perform even more technical procedures as the assistant to a specialist like a cardiologist or surgeon. Thus, like physicians, PAs can be either specialists or generalists; they can work in private practices or in hospital outpatient departments, in-hospital services, emergency rooms or research labs.

WHY NOT A NURSE, WHY NOT A DOCTOR?

The first PA program was started in 1965 by Dr. Eugene A. Stead, then Chairman of the Department of Medicine at Duke University. The PA was developed to meet two needs: (1) provide specially trained staff to serve the medical center in the face of a nursing shortage, and (2) bring help to the overworked general practitioners of rural North Carolina, where the physician-patient ratio is one-third the national average.

At that time, the Vietnam War was annually producing 6,000 independent, medic-type ex-military corpsmen whose training and experience were being lost to the civilian medical world. Most of these men did not continue in the health field because of educational, licensure, and economic barriers, as well as sexual stereotypes in the health professions. These men were envisioned for the new PA role.

PA advocates at Duke suggested that these men would "stabilize" the predominately female, high-turnover labor situation in the health system. In fact, Dr. Stead asserts that since men are more "aggressive" than women, men would make the best "pioneers" for the new profession as it carved out its new role. Of course a PA would also need "a wife at home to care for him so that he can devote full time to the health field," Stead wrote. Moreover, Dr. E. Harvey Estes of Duke argued that nurses cannot work the long hours required because of their responsibility to "house and home." Furthermore he said at that time nurses were not "interested in expanding their roles." These Duke men did not even consider advanced training and upgrading of nurses or day care centers as a means of "stabilizing" the turnover.

The failure of the originators of the PA to see women or nurses in this role is a result of their sexism, their traditional view of women and nurses as "handmaidens" and "housewives," and their desire to create a new assistant "in their own image" rather than coping with more independent professionals like nurses. The nursing leadership contributed to the male nature of the PA role by refusing to create an alternate to credentialing for the experienced medics, as well as their own drive for supervisory and teaching positions at the expense of developing nurse-clinicians.

While some "aggressive" women have entered the PA field, many from nursing, aide or technician positions, men still outnumber women more than two to one.

But, as is so often the case, sexism cuts several ways: many doctors feel that the PA should, in fact, be a nurse. A woman is less threatening to a doctor's image of control than another male. And, of course, a woman assistant can be paid less than a man. For both these power and economic reasons, the AMA, in 1970, issued a unilateral statement suggesting that at least 100,000 nurses could be upgraded into the PA role.

The angered American Nurses Association (ANA), which was just beginning to develop a more clinically oriented nurse practitioner, responded that the AMA was trying to "rob nursing" to fill in the "doctor shortage." A Joint-Practice Commission is currently attempting to work out a cease-fire.

Meanwhile, the ANA allegation, regardless of the self-protective and hair-splitting motives, raises a good question: Why not more doctors? Once again the answer has to do with economics and control.

To limit competition, the AMA has historically practiced professional "birth control." Because of the increasing societal attacks on this policy, the AMA shifted its line from no more doctors to more assistants (at first more allied health workers and currently the PA), who would increase the doctor's productivity, not to mention his income. The use of assistants doing routine, specialized tasks, serves several functions: it creates a divided workforce on the lower levels, keeps the doctors in control of decision making, maintains the stucture of the health system. All in all it is cheaper and less threatening to both the AMA and the American Hospital Association than the creation of many more doctors. No wonder that after some initial trepidation both groups embraced the PA concept.

THE PROMISE

The PA concept was sold to the medical establishment, the mass media and the public as meeting the following needs:

- It would provide new personnel to increase the quantity and improve access to medical care, without the expense of training new doctors.
- It would bring back the personal, community-minded, family doctor type of medicine.
- It would provide a higher entry point into the health system for people who would normally remain in lower level jobs, or, like corpsmen, don't use their medical skills in civilian settings at all.

The idea caught on: since the inception of the physician assistant program at Duke, with three ex-corpsmen as students, programs have proliferated all over the country. In 1970, there were 67 PA programs. By 1972 the number had climbed to 112, with others in the works as the federal funding fountain was turned on.

Because the term physician assistant can cover almost anybody, diversity has been the name of the game. Programs for PA's are run by hospitals, medical schools and the federal prison system. Some offer baccalaureate degrees; others give only certificates or associate degrees. Some of the programs are tailor-made for ex-corpsmen; others accept people with some health experience, or none at all. Training programs vary. The apprentice-type "Medex" system takes corpsmen for three months of intensive instruction and clinical training at a medical school, followed by a 12-month preceptorship with the primary-care physicians for whom the PA will continue to work. The Duke program consists of one year of clinical and one year of classroom instruction, with both private physicians and hospitals.

GOOD MORNING, OSLER JONES?

Naming the new occupation has become even more difficult than determining its sex. Suggestions range from physician assistant or physician associate and Medex (French for "médcin extension" and used for some of the specifically ex-corpsmen programs) to the even more exotic names out of medical history like Osler, Flexner, Cruzer, Korman or the Greek "syniatrist" ("syn" meaning "along with" and "iatric" for "relating to medicine or physician").

The different names reflect the attempt to sell the rather confused role for the PA as a unique, new and important occupation in the health hierarchy. More critically, the name must make clear that there is a pyramid, and that the doctor on top is in control.

Thus the AMA objected strenuously to the term "physician associate" since an associate might be construed to be another physician. The National Academy of Sciences tried to settle the debate with a definition having three tiers of physician assistants: Type A, B, and C. This definition parallels both the nursing hierarchy (professional, technical and practical nurse) and the recommendations of the American Academy of Pediatrics for associates, assistants and aides. In spite of AMA objections, many of the more academic, generalist programs are moving toward the use of the term "physician associate." But whatever the name, the essential concern is to establish the PA as the dependent assistant.

AN OLD-FASHIONED MARRIAGE

Health professions usually carve out a piece of turf, codify their "independent" skills and right to control their area, and conduct border skirmishes with those who challenge their position. While some of the professions define themselves as independent (nursing being the primary example), in reality they are dependent on the doctor-hospital-administrator hierarchy. Control over decision-making and policy direction, not control over routine technical skills, is the actual difference between dependence and independence.

The PA advocates, in contrast, are not making any pretense of independence. In both the law and practice, the PA is to be made dependent. PA legislation is being written primarily as delegation amendments to the Medical Practice Acts, allowing the doctor the right to entrust work to his assistant. What a PA does is thus legally and practically determined by the physician he works for.

Physician control extends to the state level as well. Medical Boards are being given the responsibility to oversee PA programs and certify and register their graduates. However, Nathan Hershey of the Health Law Center at the University of Pittsburgh points out, "Placing responsibility for implementation in a board other than a medical board may be necessary, unless one believes that foxes protect and foster the interest of chickens."

Reimbursement procedures also reinforce the dependency role. Under current Medicare rulings, the government will reimburse physicians for PA services rendered under the "direct personal supervision" of the physician. But Medicare will *not* reimburse the doctor, if his assistant performs services "in place of" the doctor. Nor will they pay for any services provided by the PA under only "general or remote supervision" of the physician. Similar positions have been taken by some of the private insurance carriers. The Health Insurance Council (which represents 317 independent third-party carriers) is working closely with the AMA to set up compensation guidelines. According to Thomas Crain of the Council, it is clear that "we'll compensate as long as the doctor is in control. He's the boss."

Paradoxically, this dependency may give the PA's more leeway over what they do in terms of a range of skilled technical work. But this privilege is not unlike that granted women in an old-fashioned marriage in exchange for their independence. For after all is said and done, the PA will be hamstrung in terms of control over decisions, patient management and innovative changes. If the PA and the doctor disagree, final authority rests with the physician. There is no alimony. The best a dissatisfied PA can do will be to find a marginally better arrangement with another doctor.

For a few PA's, independence may be guaranteed. Some PA's in rural and inner-city areas are being groomed as the future general practitioners. For example, two PA's, one in Wyoming and another in Alaska, are now working over 100 miles away from their doctor supervisors. In rural areas, where literally no other medical care is available, PA's may be useful and accepted. But in poor and working class urban communities, use of the PA's is seen as the institutionalization of second-class care. Thus many inner-city communities are wary of the new PA.

MS. NIGHTINGALE, RN, MEETS MR. OSLER, PA

Organized nursing and medicine have hit in a head-on collision over the PA role. The collision was caused by the abandonment of the staff nurse by nursing leadership, current changes in roles for some nurses and a push by organized medicine to solidify even further its control over the health labor force.

The nursing profession, especially since the middle sixties, have moved at an increasingly rapid pace in its attempt to create both a hierarchy and an "independent" role for nurses. As the doctor stranglehold and the burgeoning allied health professions were advancing on the clinical front, nursing leadership opted to expand the role of its elite members into supervisory and teaching positions.

Meanwhile, dull and routine housekeeping tasks led to unrest and unhappiness among staff nurses, reflected in the continuing 60 percent a year turnover rates and the perennial nursing shortage. A series of nursing reports began to argue for "the re-establishment of practice as the first and proper end of nursing as a profession."

As a result, over 40 "extended" primary-care-role (nurse practitioner or nurse clinician) programs have developed that prepare the nurse to perform many of the same tasks as are being developed for the PA. The difference between nursing and medicine, at times vague, is becoming even vaguer. As one joint nursing-medical committee put it: "The same act is clearly the practice of medicine when performed by a physician and the practice of nursing when performed by a nurse." While the AMA, clinging to its old definitions, asserts that nurse practitioners are not PA's, the only real difference between the two workers appears to be sex.

As always, behind the sexual politics is the issue of control. The danger that the dependent PA might close the options of the clinically independent nurse is very real. In 1971 New York State's Governor Rockefeller acting on behalf of the state medical and hospital societies rejected the nursing association's bid to expand its scope of practice law. Instead, he signed a law authorizing dependent PA's. In 1972, the nurses were able to get their independent role legislated at the price of agreeing, at least in the legal language, that the nurse *when performing medical regimens* would be dependent on the decisions of the doctor.

Eleanor Lambertson, Dean of Cornell's Nursing School and one of the first directors of a family nurse practitioner program, raised the problem succinctly: "Not who does what but who prescribes and who delegates to whom are at issue." Divisions between PA's and nurses are in store. Staff nurses are already edgy about taking orders from a PA and this feeling is not abated when the president of the ANA declares: "Nurses should not take orders from such assistants because a 'profession' does not take orders from an 'assistant.'" Practitioners are already being given the traditional female roles in pediatrics and obstetrics while male PA's are being used in medicine and surgery.

It may be that the nurse practitioner or PA choice will be settled on an institution-by-institution basis, dependent on the political clout and concerns of the medical boards, the nursing hierarchy and the hospital administrations. The federal officials are trying not to play favorites and have granted $6.5 million for nurse practitioner programs, $6.3 billion for PA's. While nursing has the numbers on its side, the burden of the traditional image and the rigid jurisdictional outlook of the nursing profession may override economic and power concerns. It is still too early to tell. But it is not to early to note that this conflict neatly ties up the energies of the middle-level health workers in border skirmishes, while the doctors continue to reign supreme.

ASSESSING THE PROMISES

Despite the rhetoric, it is becoming apparent, even this early on, that PA's cannot live up to the promises for quality, quantity, access, or lower costs in the delivery of health care.

Quantity—Some of the early public relations pieces on PA's promised that a doctor's ability to see more patients would increase 70 percent with a new assistant. A May, 1972, survey of 29 PA's from the Duke program, however, found that on the whole PA's increased the leisure and reading time for physicians, but did not increase their ability to give additional services. In part the reason is that doctors do not know how to utilize their extra help. As one doctor commented, "After being trained all these years to make decisions myself, how do I begin to trust an assistant and know what to delcgate?" Use of PA's is now beginning to result in a more modest productivity increase for some physicians of between 15 and 30 percent.

Quality and Direction—While PA's were hailed as the future general practitioner, specialization has already begun. PA's are now being trained as assistants in such diverse medical specialties as anesthesiology, pathology, surgery, obstetrics and orthopedics. Even graduates from primary-care programs like Duke are becoming specialists; for example, Duke-trained surgery assistants are now working at Montefiore Hospital in the Bronx.

The AMA supports this trend since it presents no confusion as to who is the doctor and who is the assistant. Among the first guidelines promulgated by the AMA were those for orthopedic assistants. Hospital administrators and surgery chiefs have written to New York area PA programs requesting more surgery assistants, but not more generalists, for whom they have little use anyway. Since the apprentice must follow the sorcerer, and the latter rarely treads in the areas of preventive and general care, PA's will tend to go with the prevailing norms and salary lures of the specialists.

Location—PA's are not going back to the rural scene. Instead the drift appears to be toward non-rural group settings or institutions where the rewards are greater. Recent Medicare rulings accentuate the trend toward institutions. Medicare now allows hospitals, as opposed to private physicians, to bill for all the physician assistants' services as part of the "reasonable cost" of doing business.

An HEW survey of the graduates of 24 PA programs, taken at the end of 1971, demonstrated this trend. Out of 152 graduates, only 40 were working in private practices. Over one-quarter (44) were not working as PA's or were teaching or doing graduate work. And the largest number, 68, were based in hospitals and medical centers.

Naturally, some of the larger hospitals are delighted. PA's are already envisioned as the future housestaff because they are cheaper than doctors, do the scut work that is usually reserved for interns, will stay in one place longer than an intern or resident, and can be more easily controlled by the hospital administration and doctors.

Costs—At the private practice level, PA's will not lower medical costs to the consumer. Doctors can use PA's to increase their practice, then charge their regular fees and pocket the increase.

In contrast to the Medicare administrators (who are sensitive to political outcries about increasing Medicare costs), the more protected Blue Cross-Blue Shield reimbursers are taking a "let's not look behind the billing" attitude, according to HEW officials. If the doctor signs the claim forms, no one is asking who really performed the services. The doctors are being reimbursed as if they, rather than their assistants, performed the tasks. Fees will not be lowered, while doctors' incomes may rise. Fearful of this, many state legislatures have limited the number of assistants one doctor or group can have.

Entry Point—PA programs have made it possible for small numbers of lower level health workers, ex-corpsmen, aides, LPN's, and technicians to build upon their skills and upgrade their training—a rarity in the dead-ended, lock-stepped health hierarchy. PA programs may provide a way for even smaller numbers of qualified people to get the base-level education necessary for medical schools. Even these gains, however, may be cut by the exclusionary process already at work. For like the other health professions, the PA's are beginning to follow the doctor model in the development of their "profession."

Thus an Association of Physician Assistants was formed in 1968 before there were even 20 graduates of the Duke program. By 1970, it had changed its name to the American Academy of Physician Associates to include only Type A, Physician Associate students and graduates. At the same time, at least five other professional associations are competing for PA members, including one group which is backed by a Cincinnati insurance company. An association of the physician associate programs has also been formed. If the definition of PA continues to be as generic and vague as it is now, it can be expected that they will proceed to raise their requirements and erect barriers around their roles. Even now, many PA programs require two or three years of college before acceptance; some have made their PA programs into four-year, bachelor of science in medicine curriculums. This professionalization process may place PA programs out of the reach of most working-class and minority students.

Even upon acceptance to a training program, the students may be locked forever into the PA category. The director of the Duke program wrote in 1970 that ideal PA candidates should not be frustrated medical students, otherwise "they're not going to get enough job satisfaction or ego satisfaction in doing the type of work that a physician will delegate." Some of the programs in fact discourage students who had originally wanted to go to medical school or, because they are middle-class and upper-middle-class men, look like potential medical students.

The PA's are by no means the new "barefoot" doctors who will revolutionize the delivery of health care. As Dr. Stead so bluntly put it, "They were set up to support the present system." PA's are apprentices, created by the sorcerers to do their bidding. And, ultimately, unless the sorcerer's power is challenged by concerted action of all his apprentices, just creating a new, higher-skilled occupation will not create much in the way of change.

—From the Health/PAC *Bulletin*, November, 1972.

RN's STRIKE: Between the Lines

David Gaynor, Elinor Blake, Thomas Bodenheimer and Carol Mermey

On June 7, 1974, 4,400 registered nurses struck 41 hospitals and clinics in the San Francisco Bay area. The RN's, all members of the California Nurses' Association (CNA), remained on the picket lines for 21 days. With the American Nurses' Association holding its annual national convention in San Francisco during the strike, the issues were discussed and brought back to every state in the nation.

On one level the RN strike differed from typical management-labor disputes. The central demands were not for increased wages and other bread-and-butter gains. Rather, RN's posed their fight in terms of control of working conditions and the quality of patient care. In addition, RN's and their professional association, the CNA, displayed a new level of militancy in their willingness to confront the administration on the picket line.

On the other hand, the strike poses many problems and contradictions with far-reaching relevance for future struggles by hospital workers. Given the existing hierarchical division of labor within the hospital, will bargaining along narrow skill lines by a relatively privileged group of professional nurses serve to create even more tension and divisions? And what is the meaning of the demand for workers' control when that demand is made for the sole benefit of a narrowly defined group? On a more pragmatic level, can any single classification of hospital workers win its demands without uniting with others—that is, can any one group muster enough clout to shut the hospital down and force the administration to capitulate?

NO ORDINARY DEMANDS: THE STAFFING CLAUSE

In 1970 the CNA won a clause in its contract with Bay Area hospitals giving RN's the right to help determine how wards are staffed. The clause called for "participation of Staff Nurses in the assessment of patients' daily needs for nursing care and the basis upon which nursing personnel are assigned. . . ." By the time the contract expired on December 31, 1973, neither the hospitals nor the CNA had moved in a significant way to implement this clause. When negotiations for the 1974 contract opened, management's position on the staffing issue became unequivocal—delete the clause and deny RN's any participation in staffing matters.

The staffing clause became the core of the strike: Who decides how many and what type of personnel should work on each unit? This issue is central to both hospital workers and patients. Understaffing makes workers unable to perform all necessary tasks. Patients find that their needs are ignored for hours, and even then are met in a brusque and hurried manner.

Administration, through the director of nursing, distributes RN's, LVN's (licensed vocational nurses, also called licensed practical nurses in some states) and aides around the hospital according to the number of patients on each floor. Some hospitals use the more sophisticated "acuity" method of staffing, which takes into account that some patients are sicker than others and need more staff time. But in all cases, the number of workers is determined by administration, and if the fiscal picture looks bad, staff can be cut back no matter how full or how busy the wards become.

One RN, for example, tells of working a night on a floor with 30 patients, many acutely ill, staffed with one RN, one LVN and one aide. Thirteen patients had intravenous solution bottles running. Each bottle had to be changed at different times, requiring close watching to prevent bottles from running dry. In addition one patient needed irrigation of the bladder with multiple bottles of fluid. After continued pleas from the beleaguered RN, the nursing office offered only one extra LVN—this despite the fact that hospital regulations do not allow LVN's to perform these tasks.

Management was steadfast in its refusal to allow an RN voice in staffing. Hospital negotiator Arthur Mendelson warned physicians: "If we accede to the demands of the registered staff nurses and the California Nurses' Association in this connection it is only one step away for the registered staff nurses to demand a voice in the way you treat your patients with respect to admissions, discharge, treatment and length of stay." The American Hospital Association, in an alarmist statement, took up the cudgels: "An issue with national implications is at stake here. Under the banner of an interest in the quality of care, the striking nurses are attempting to gain control over the number of nurses employed by each hospital. . . ."

In truth, the staffing demand was not nearly as threatening as all that. The CNA was merely asking for participation in deciding staffing levels, not control over staffing. But the rhetoric of control was taken up by some RN's who defined the strike as a worker control struggle, which in fact it was not.

The staffing issue did, however, have implications for other hospital workers. Why shouldn't all personnel on a unit—including LVN's, orderlies and aides—be involved in staffing decisions? The strike could not deal with this question since the CNA is a professional association separate from the union of other hospital workers, and as such can bargain only on behalf of RN's. Thus the demand for some control over staffing by RN's missed the mark of what real worker control might mean—teams composed of all workers on a floor deciding staffing patterns, division of labor between workers, and engaging in patient diagnosis and treatment.

SPECIALIZED TRAINING

A second strike demand was that administration not assign RN's without appropriate training to specialty units. The technological explosion in health care has brought with it increased specialization. Doctors carve out an organ or two as their exclusive area of concern. Technicians are increasingly split up into narrow functions. And with RN's operating complex devices in intensive care units, coronary care units, renal dialysis, emergency rooms and other specialized areas of the hospital, nursing is following suit.

RN's at Bay Area hospitals flatly stated that administrators were staffing specialty units with unqualified "floating" nurses—nurses who spend different days on different floors. At Mt. Zion Hospital in San Francisco, administration first denied the charge of improper staffing, but later reluctantly admitted to such staffing in case of "emergency." An intensive-care-unit nurse responded, "If Mt. Zion does indeed assign untrained nurses to specialty care areas only in emergency situations, then these areas are in a constant state of emergency."

Not only is this practice dangerous to patients, but it is intolerable to hospital workers. One RN told of an orderly sent to a pediatric unit where he had never been trained to work. The orderly accidentally disconnected a life-supporting device. After some tense moments, the child's condition was restored, but the orderly was distraught by what he had nearly done. Nevertheless, the specialty staffing demand would do nothing for this situation since it applies only to RN's.

Bread-and-butter demands were not altogether ignored. These included demands for every other weekend off for all RN's, a 5.5 percent pay increase and a cost-of-living escalator clause. The CNA also asked for a pension plan separate from other workers and portable from one hospital to another. Pensions were an issue because RN's frequently change jobs and do not benefit from the money they place into hospital-wide pension plans. The demand reflects the high degree of job mobility of RN's vis-à-vis other less mobile and less privileged hospital workers.

WHY A STRIKE?

The precipitating cause of the strike was the hospitals' complete intransigence on the staffing issue. Hospital management had refused to negotiate until a few days before the contract expired at the end of 1973, and had failed to budge during the five months of talks in 1974. Administration not only wanted to delete the gains won by the CNA regarding participation in staffing in the 1971–73 contract, but pushed to include a management's rights clause. According to Burton White, CNA Director of Economic and General Welfare, "Management was trying to turn back the clock. That was too much." The CNA had no choice but to give in or strike.

Woven into the strike decision were several underlying threads. Staffing conditions in hospitals have tightened due to the excess of hospital beds and the federal wage-price controls, both of which have hurt the hospitals' economic position. From management's point of view, there is a critical need to limit staffing—after all, each additional worker costs money. For management it would be unthinkable to allow hospital workers—who have no responsibility for keeping the hospital in the black—to control levels of expenditure. From the workers' point of view, the economic pinch means speed-up—more work for each person to do—and wages that fail to keep up with the rising cost of living. Two other Bay Area hospital strikes in the past year—at Kaiser and San Francisco General hospitals—reflect the workers' refusal to bear the brunt of the economic situation.

At the same time, many RN's have been influenced by the women's liberation movement, acquiring a new self-respect and militancy. Traditionally nursing has been women's work—an extension of their caring, cleaning and serving roles as mothers and housewives. Socialized to be passive and to accept the devaluation of their contributions as workers, women have been reticent to speak up for their rights and push forth their demands at the workplace. Although feminist issues were not at the forefront of this strike, women asserted leadership, self-reliance and self-confidence, taking themselves and their jobs seriously. A Kaiser RN stated, "If it weren't for women's lib, we wouldn't have been striking." Another went on to stay, "It definitely gave us the courage to speak up and express our opinions."

Also underlying the strike was the CNA's response to the new militancy of the rank-and-file RN's. In Los Angeles, 600 public hospital RN's recently switched from the CNA to representation by the Service Employees International Union (AFL-CIO). In San Francisco, the AFL-CIO and the Teamsters are the collective bargaining agents for increasing numbers of public hospital RN's. This year seemed like the CNA's last chance to prevent widespread defection of RN's into labor unions.

A final condition underlying the strike was the fact that the RN's didn't know what they were getting into. The CNA had little experience in conducting strikes and the RN's shared a widespread feeling that "We'll go out for a few days, win and be back on the job next Monday."

PRELUDE TO THE PICKET LINE

In December, 1973, the CNA entered into contract negotiations with three groups of northern California hospitals: Affiliated Hospitals (most of San Francisco's private hospitals, banded together solely for the purposes of collective bargaining), Associated Hospitals (a similar grouping mainly in Oakland and Berkeley) and the Kaiser hospitals and clinics.

In January, 1974, the Bay Area Negotiating Council was created to represent the RN's, with each hospital electing two representatives to serve on it. The Council in turn selected 12 RN's to sit in on the negotiating team. These 12 joined the five paid CNA staff members, led by Burton White, a non-RN and experienced labor negotiator. Thus the CNA leadership (staff plus elected officials) was under the surveillance of rank-and-file RN's at the bargaining table.

During the five months of weekly bargaining sessions, the Negotiating Council served as a communications link between the RN's and the CNA. Information about negotiations and strategies passed from the negotiating team to the Council, and the Council brought questions and concerns from RN's at the individual facilities.

In May, mass meetings attended by 1,300 RN's rejected a management proposal by a 95 percent vote and authorized strike action. On June 7, Negotiating Council member Joyce Boone declared, "We are a new breed of nurses, fighting for our rights and those of our patients." The same day RN's set up picket lines around over 40 health facilities.

Meanwhile, contracts for LVN's, aides, housekeeping and dietary workers, represented by Local 250 of the Service Employees International Union (AFL-CIO), had also expired January 1, 1974. Negotiations dragged on for the first five months of the year. As the CNA prepared for strike action, management became increasingly anxious to settle with Local 250. Hospitals can manage without RN's; after all, LVN's do many RN tasks anyway (even though they are paid much less). But a simultaneous walkout by RN's and other hospital workers would be devastating.

So shortly before the anticipated RN strike, management offered a 40 cent per hour (9–12 percent) across-the-board increase to Local 250 members. The union, which had negotiated without rank-and-file participation, recommended acceptance of the offer. Withholding the terms of the agreement from its members until 45 minutes before the vote, the union achieved ratification and thereby helped management avert a combined strike. No attempts had been made by the CNA and Local 250 to coordinate or combine their strategies. Hospital administrators heaved a sigh of relief: Divide and conquer had worked again.

GOING IT ALONE

Unaware of the import of the Local 250 settlement on their own struggle, the RN's went it alone. Bearing signs declaring, "Patients are our business," "We want to serve what you deserve," "Qualified nurses for specialty units," and "Better staffing equals better patient care," the RN's picketed the entrances to their hospitals. Some 50 to 95 percent of RN's participated in the strike, varying from hospital to hospital, a response far better than expected. The RN's encouraged other workers to wear blue armbands in support of the strike but not to leave their jobs.

The CNA hoped to exert financial pressure on the hospitals by eliminating the profitable elective surgery and non-emergency admissions. But not forgetting the patients, the RN's initially maintained staffing of emergency and intensive care areas. Hospitals reported occupancies running 40 to 50 percent of normal levels. Though these occupancy levels clearly hurt the hospitals financially, they were not low enough to bring the institutions to their knees.

Three days after the strike began, 8,000 RN's gathered in San Francisco for the annual American Nurses'

Association (ANA) convention. ANA delegates joined the picket line, raised funds and overwhelmingly passed a resolution in support of the strike. One nursing administrator at a struck hospital responded, "My spies tell me that this [strike] was planned three months ago in Kansas City" (the ANA headquarters), presumably as a staged show for the convention.

On June 12, 200 Kaiser RN's rallied at the Kaiser Center in Oakland, and the following day several hundred RN's held a spirited demonstration in San Francisco. A week later, a march picking up RN's at each hospital converged on San Francisco's Civic Center Plaza for another major rally. Day after day, the strike was the leading story on local TV news broadcasts, with charges and countercharges flying between the CNA and the hospitals.

On June 20, with negotiations at an impasse, the RN's upped the ante—they withdrew from the emergency and intensive-care areas. Irene Pope, President and Acting Executive Director of the CNA, charged that hospitals were assigning supervisory personnel to non-critical care areas because they had strikers available to staff emergency units. Others observed that patients who did not need critical care were kept in the critical care area.

The pull-out from emergency units was the only tactic available to a professional association that bargains for only a limited number of workers in an institution. Strikes by all workers—closing down profitable but not emergency areas of hospitals—would have been more effective in advancing the RN cause than the emergency unit pull-out. But the CNA did not want support strikes by other workers. At least one group, the X-ray technicians at Herrick Hospital, members of the International Longshoremen's and Warehousemen's Union, were on the verge of a sympathy strike when word came from Herrick RN's that the CNA had rejected the support offer, not wishing to be obligated to honor future X-ray technician strikes. One Herrick X-ray technician said, "We wanted to go out—there was sympathy with the RN's standing up to the doctors and administration. But when the RN's told me they didn't want our strike, I pulled my blue armband right off."

The RN's did gain substantial public support from other groups during the strike. Unable to unite with Local 250 in their own workingplaces, the RN's did receive verbal backing from Local 1199 of the National Union of Hospital and Health Care Employees in New York City. The interns and residents organization at San Francisco's Children Hospital issued a statement of support, as did 63 members of Mt. Zion's house staff. Over 100 unit clerks, lab techs, LVN's, social workers and housekeeping personnel at Mt. Zion Hospital signed a petition of support.

But in several hospitals, the atmosphere was hostile toward non-RN staff who supported the strike. Many workers felt that RN's are the supervisors or the "foremen" on the floor, and the strike demands were seen as potentially increasing RN's power over other workers. Thus workers who donned the blue armbands soon began to feel isolated. In fact, one Local 250 representative even threatened to fine armband wearers $50.

As the strike wore on, RN's began to feel acutely the absence of their paycheks. The CNA leadership, fearing that RN's would straggle back to work, tried to hasten the bargaining process by edging the 12 elected RN's off the negotiating team. Told that they were too inexperienced to participate in this stage of the negotiations, the elected team members were forced to wait outside the negotiating room. CNA staff negotiators justified their moves by instilling a Henry Kissinger aura upon the delicate sessions and convinced the team not to speak with their rank-and-file peers.

On June 23, after several attempts to force management to sit down with third-party mediators, the CNA finally succeeded in securing the services of William J. Usery, Jr., chief federal negotiator and personal labor troubleshooter for then-President Nixon [now U.S. Secretary of Labor—ed.]. Usery immediately called for around-the-clock negotiations and a news blackout that extended to the striking RN's. With the breakdown of the democratic process, some RN's began to shift their anger from management to the CNA.

On June 26 a settlement was announced. At 7 P.M. on June 27 the striking RN's, without having been allowed to see the settlement, assembled at San Francisco's giant Cow Palace. Some of them angrily demanded individual hospital caucuses to discuss the agreement before voting on it. But after a short period of confused debate, a vote was forced. The RN's accepted the package by a vote of 1,670 to 494.

VICTORY OR HOLDING ACTION?

The CNA leadership touted the strike settlement as a major victory for RN's. Most importantly, management failed to delete the key staffing clause from the existing contract. Concerning the specialty units, the new agreement provides that "Except in case of emergency, nurses without appropriate training and/or experience shall not be assigned to such areas." The first five words are those of management, and whether this clause is a victory or defeat for the RN's depends on how "emergency" is defined. Management decides what is an emergency unless the CNA can overturn their definition by filing and winning grievances. The hospitals also agree to provide training for specialty care.

The RN's won a whopping 11 percent pay boost, felt by some to be an overt attempt to buy them off. In fact, the figure represents the 5.5 percent raise asked for plus a one-shot 5.5 percent cost-of-living adjustment to cover inflation since January 1. (The RN's failed to win a continuing cost-of-living escalator clause.) The demand for alternate weekends off was compromised, and the portable pension plan was not granted but was submitted for study. Management conceded to the opening of certain issues for renegotiation on January 1, 1975.

Rather than a victory, the settlement is actually closer to a successful holding action. With the economy in decline, hospitals like all industries are trying to squeeze more work out of their employees at lower cost to themselves. The retention of the staffing clause provides the RN's with at least some leverage to fight against understaffing and speed-up. The pay increase slows the rate at which RN's incomes fall behind inflation. The specialty staffing clause, provided that the RN's fight for its implementation, is the only substantial move ahead. Given management's refusal to yield the slightest decision-making authority to the RN's, the staffing portions of the new contract are of little use without constant grievances and battles for enforcement by the RN's at each hospital.

THE NEW CONSCIOUSNESS

After five months of negotiating and 21 days of striking, the RN's won a holding action but made few advances in changing their objective conditions of work. RN's have returned to find the wards still understaffed and themselves still overworked. And the tensions manifested during the strike between RN's and those who take orders from them, such as LVN's, orderlies and aides, have not magically disappeared.

Nevertheless, for the RN's the strike had significance that went past the bargaining table and changes in objective conditions of work. The most marked achievement was the mobilization of the RN's from the wards to the picket lines and the development of a sense of unity, militancy and self-reliance—the antitheses of the passive role women are socialized into in nursing school.

Equally important was the way the strike served to break down the isolation among RN's. There are many structural organizational reasons for hospital workers to be isolated from one another: wards are physically separate, some jobs are more prestigious than others, some pay more and people on different shifts seldom see each other. Moreover, the assigned workloads are often so heavy that merely getting one's work done is difficult. Working together during the strike gave RN's a chance to get to know and trust one another as well as to develop collective strategies and solutions. An obstetric nurse at Alameda Hospital stated, "The strike has given us a new sense of unity."

The strike also served to show the true face of the CNA. Throughout the five months of negotiations and for the first part of the strike the CNA was remarkably democratic, allowing for participation by rank-and-file RN's. RN's were represented on both the negotiating team and the Negotiating Council, bringing the latest developments and management offers back to RN's at the hospitals they represented. In the last week of the strike, however, the CNA reverted to top-down, heavy-handed tactics, which many RN's found infuriating. Reflecting this anger, a committee of RN's at Mt. Zion Hospital sent the following letter to the CNA:

"We at Mt. Zion feel that we were sold out. . . . The most charitable view expressed has been that the team members had hit a low point in their motivation and energy and that they were afraid to let Usery leave without a settlement. . . . The other, less charitable opinion is that the strike was, from the first, a grand-standing maneuver by the paid officials of the CNA; a tactic to tighten their hold on jurisdiction over RN's in the Bay Area. . . .

"We feel that these questions must be spoken to by the leadership of CNA. We ask for the support of all CNA members in working to ensure that this betrayal of democratic principles in our organization does not repeat itself. We are willing to work within CNA to make the leadership more responsive to our needs and to strengthen their commitment to the democratic process. We are willing to work to use the contract to make whatever progress is possible on the issues of staffing, patient care, and professional self-determination. We hope that our analysis of the situation will provide food for thought for all CNA members returning to work under this contract."

Democracy, however, is far from the central issue regarding the CNA. What is at question is the difference between a professional association and a non-hierarchical, anti-professional organization of workers fighting for their own power and interests. Historically the CNA, while making minimal support gestures in other hospital workers' struggles, has not even honored picket lines during their strikes. By choosing to go it alone, the CNA not only loses a powerful bargaining weapon, but keeps RN's separated from the majority of hospital workers.

THE OLD CONTRADICTIONS

While on the one hand the strike raised the level of consciousness of the RN's, on the other hand it manifested and exacerbated the existing tensions and contradictions found in the hospital workforce—namely the race, class and sex antagonisms upon which the hierarchical division of labor rests. At the top of this hierarchy are the male administrators and physicians, enjoying high status, income and power. Next come RN's, predominantly white, female professionals, who in this case were demanding a piece of the pie. Beneath them are LVN's, aides, orderlies and other low-paid, predominantly Third World workers who make up the majority of the workforce and take their orders from the RN's.

While RN's are in supervisory roles and make more money than other hospital employees, they are still wage workers and are exploited as such. The ideology of professionalism promotes elitism on the part of RN's, but in fact they have more in common with other workers than with doctors or administrators. The RN's are pawns in the hospital hierarchy, placed in positions in which they must assume responsibility for running a floor and give orders to other workers. They are forced to act as a buffer for the doctors and administrators, becoming, whether they like it or not, the most visible authority figures, who do the dirty work of the administrators and boss other workers around.

Reactions of other workers during the strike underscore these tensions and hostilities. An LVN at Alta

Bates Hospital said, "I'm glad they're out, this will give us more space to move." A worker at Children's Hospital in San Francisco added, "We're better off without them here." Another worker characterized the strike, "The attitudes of the nurses during the strike seem to have been taken over from doctors—anti-union, pro-professional, pro-specialization. They were competing with doctors to gain more decisions over patient care by raising their level of professionalism to that of doctors."

In the final analysis, RN's alone cannot shut hospitals down and bring significant change to their workplaces. In the long run, demands for professional upgrading by RN's are made at the expense not only of other workers but of the RN's themselves. The RN strike has made clear the tremendous obstacles to success that exist when different hospital workers' groups fight their own battles in isolation and even opposition to those of other health workers.

(David Gaynor, a hospital administration student at Cornell University, was an intern at Health/PAC's San Francisco office during the summer of 1974. Carol Mermey was a Health/PAC staff member.)

—From the Health/PAC *Bulletin*, September/ October, 1974.

7
Hospital Unions

For many unskilled and semiskilled hospital workers, the organization of trade unions has been a logical response to the increasing industrialization of the health-care system. Since the early 1960's, hospital unions have been gaining momentum throughout the country. The growth of these unions was triggered by a series of major strike actions and by first-time coverage for hospital workers under state and federal collective-bargaining laws. The major hospital workers' union include Local 1199 of the Drug and Hospital Workers Union (now called the National Union of Hospital and Health Care Employees), with members mainly at voluntary hospitals on the East Coast; the Service Employees International Union (SEIU), mainly at voluntary hospitals on the West Coast; and the American Federation of State, County and Municipal Employees (AFSCME), mainly at public hospitals throughout the country. While the organizing struggles of these unions have been quite successful in recent years, it is important to remember that they have a long way to go—even now only a small percentage of hospital workers in this country are union members.

The first article in this chapter is an editorial on hospital unions from the Health/PAC *Bulletin.* It considers two critical questions about the hospital workers' unions: How effective are these unions as workers' defense organizations? And how effective are they as vehicles for changing the priorities of the health system? The editorial suggests that unions play a vital role in assuring higher wages, shorter hours and better job security in an industry notorious for its exploitation of workers, especially those who are unskilled. At the same time, it notes tendencies within hospital unions that direct them away from efforts to reform the health system and away from cooperation with community and patient groups.

The second article, by John Ehrenreich, is a brief history of hospital unions and their expansive growth in the 1960's, when public employee unionization drives were catching fire throughout the country.

The final article is a unique account and analysis of the 1970 collective bargaining between Local 1199 in New York City and the management of the city's major voluntary hospitals, reported by Elinor Langer, then an 1199 staff member. She shows how the dynamics of the bargaining process serve to focus negotiations on wage and job security issues and away from such issues as on-the-job education and working conditions, not to speak of reform of the health-care system.

WHAT COURSE FOR HEALTH WORKERS?

Hospitals have long been the urban employer of last resort. The newcomers, the discriminated-against, those who are excluded from other jobs are likely to end up as porters, nurses' aids, orderlies, kitchen help, housekeepers, and the like, in the immense and rapidly growing hospital industry. Wages for these jobs, in most of the country, are scandalous; $60 a week is still common. Hours are long, duties dirty and boring, job security nonexistent. Anyone who can get out of a hospital into another job does so; turnover rates often approach 90 percent per year.

Throughout the country, the drive to unionize is on. Local 1199 of the Drug and Hospital Workers Union, the Teamsters, the Service Employees International Union (SEIU), and the American Federation of State, County and Municipal Employees (AFSCME) are organizing hospital workers in a score of cities. And despite a rapidly turning over, demoralized, fragmented workforce, despite intense hospital opposition, despite an almost total lack of legislation protecting the rights of hospital workers to organize, unionization is making rapid progress throughout the country. The movement to join unions is the major mass movement taking place among health workers today.

To many politically active health workers and students, a unionization drive seems an ideal opportunity to radicalize workers, to gain allies in the struggle to change the health system. Some have hoped that once unionization has been achieved, the union itself would become a major force in changing the health system. For reasons to be discussed below, this seems unlikely, in the short run at least. Nevertheless, health movement activists cannot remain aloof from the unionization drive.

For one thing, unionization and the gains it can bring are rightly the number one priority of most hospital workers. Demands for higher wages, shorter hours, and job security are their most pressing needs. No one can be a friend to the workers who ignores the fastest route to meeting these needs. For another thing, workers do not necessarily lose interest in other issues once their economic demands are met. In fact, it is just as likely to be true that when workers have escaped from the imminent threat of hunger, when they are not afraid that their jobs will disappear from under them tomorrow, that then they are freed to turn their attention to more distant, more far-reaching issues. In any event, the union, by freeing the workers from the fear of arbitrary dismissal from their jobs, can provide the environment in which effective organizing around non-bread-and-butter issues becomes possible.

This means that, in places where there is no union, health movement activists must wholeheartedly support the drive to unionize. And in places where there already is a union, it is wrong to treat the union in itself as an enemy. Support need not be blind support, of course. Unions can be criticized for their failure to raise non-bread-and-butter issues, for internal lack of democracy, for their unwillingness to ally themselves with other forces for change in the health system. But in being critical, it is necessary to be careful not to be divisive, not to threaten the union's role as an organization that is able to protect the economic well-being of its members.

The potential role of unions in restructuring the overall health system, in addition to meeting the immediate needs of the workers, cannot be understood without a more general discussion of the relation between health workers and consumers of health care. Some activists have suggested natural grounds for unity between health workers and consumers, on the grounds that the workers are typically members of the same poor, black and brown communities that are likely to be demanding community control of hospitals. They draw a contrast to the situation which developed in the schools in New York, where the United Federation of Teachers, made up predominantly of white professionals, found itself aligned in 1968 against the black and brown communities' demand for community control of schools. But the factors forcing service workers and their clients apart seem, in the short run at least, more powerful than the unity of skin color and place of residence.

The situation in which health care is delivered in this country almost naturally pits workers against consumers. First, under American capitalism, health, like other social services, takes a low priority. While defense budgets, highway budgets, and the like flourish, health institutions are starved. Even within the hospitals, high wages for administrators and professionals, expensive research and educational programs, prestigious equipment and fancy new buildings take priority over wages for nonprofessional employees and health service for the public. When the workers ask for higher wages, shorter hours, better fringe benefits, all of which cost money, the hospitals claim they have only two alternatives. They can raise charges which, in turn, increases health insurance premiums paid by the public and forces the costs of tax-supported programs like Medicaid and Medicare to soar. Or they can cut back on services and lay off workers. As long as health care is not a high priority of this society or even of its health institutions, the needs of hospital workers and hospital consumers are in direct conflict. More for one means less for the other.

The second cause for conflict between hospital workers and the community stems from the nature of hospital work in our health system. Most hospital jobs are dirty, low paid, tedious. The stagnant hierarchy, supported by elaborate credentialing requirements and arrogant professionalism, turns most hospital jobs into dead-end jobs: a porter or aide is stuck forever as a porter or aide. It is under these conditions that health worker–patient relations deteriorate, that every patient's endless tales of the rudeness and indifference of hospital workers originate.

It is in the context of this tendency of our health system, in our overall political-economic system, to pit worker against client that the role of the union must be examined. Can the unions overcome this worker-consumer antipathy, or will they make it worse? At first glance, their potential to exacerbate the situation dominates our view.

First, unions, by their very nature, are organizations of workers. They exclude consumers. They are thus organs for the workers to press aggressively for their own interests, which in our health system are often in conflict with the needs of the public for low-cost, high-quality hospital care.

Second, unions are a peculiar kind of institution. By law and custom, their role vis-à-vis management is limited. At contract time, they are the organs of the workers' struggle, trying to force management to give the workers more wages, better working conditions, etc. Once the contract is in effect, however, they become to a significant extent an agent of conciliation. They do administer the contract, trying to make sure that management lives up to its end of the bargain. But in return, the union's role is to supply a disciplined work-force. The contract sets up procedures for disciplining workers who threaten an orderly work relationship (whether in a political way or simply through personal tardiness, not knowing their place, etc.). The union contract often forbids wildcat strikes over workplace issues, and the union is legally bound to help quiet things down if the workers do get restive.

The union-management relationship, defined both in federal and state law and in the contracts themselves, creates roles for union and management, leaving a broad area of management prerogative in which the union must not interfere. In effect, the union and the management have made a deal: the management agrees to be reasonably cooperative in giving the workers improved wages and working conditions and in not being too arbitrary in their dealings with workers. It also agrees to tolerate the union's existence, as the workers' representative in these dealings. In return, the union pledges not to tread upon the management's toes in many vital areas of decision-making and to help management maintain a disciplined workforce.

It is not absolutely necessary for a union to accept this framework, of course. The alternative is to refuse formal recognition under the labor laws, to make no long-term contracts, to bargain issue by issue. The choice facing a workers' organization is a bitter one. To forgo the protection of the labor laws means constant struggle against management and even against the government merely to go on existing. Meanwhile, the organization and its members will lack the elementary protections for their activities which the laws and a contract would provide. In practice, the pressure is very strong for a workers' organization to accept the limitations on it implied by the conventional union-management relationship in order to be able to continue to assure gains for its members.

The need to accept this "arrangement" is particularly pressing for the typical hospital union. These unions are made up of unskilled and therefore easily replaceable, poor and therefore easily starved-out workers. Even the standard union relationship, much less an unconventional, more aggressive one, is difficult to achieve and maintain. And so the hospital unions must be content with the relationship they now have with management: they are not likely to be interested in allying themselves with consumers in a radical assault on the health system.

Finally, the necessity of bonding together a large and diverse group of workers to effectively confront a united and powerful institution such as a hospital has encouraged union leaders to try to centralize their power and to squash dissension. Centralized, unquestioned power in the leadership often becomes stagnant, undemocratic bureaucracy. The continuing power of this bureaucracy is dependent on the existing structure of management-worker relationships. Thus the union leadership often comes to oppose any movements, whether among their own members or from outside the union, which threaten to disrupt those relationships.

For all these reasons, there are tendencies for hospital workers' unions not to become involved in efforts to change the health system and even to try to crush such efforts. Ultimately, however, health workers and consumers do have a common interest in restructuring the health system, and this common interest raises the possibility of common action and even of a positive role for unions in this struggle. Consumers cannot hope for decent, dignified health care if they get it from oppressed, alienated, underpaid workers, from people who do not see themselves as participating in the delivery of health care but only as doing an onerous job. Just as consumers are forced to demand more money for the hospitals in order to get decent health services, they have to demand opportunities for health workers to learn about the function of their jobs, to advance to more complex and interesting and prestigious jobs, to break down the hierarchies that oppress them, and, of course, to be decently paid, decently secure, decently honored. Similarly, for the workers, in the long run, better pay and longer vacations alone will not end their oppression. They need opportunities for advancement, education, an end to the humiliating hierarchies of the present health system. And they need to be able to take pride in their "product," in the services they provide. This would only be possible if those services were something to take pride in—if they were high quality, dignified, and humane for all patients. These are goals which can only be achieved when the health system is no longer run for the power, prestige, and wealth of a handful of doctors and administrators, but rather in the interest of and with the participation of the people who need health care and the people who provide it.

The possibility of this community of interest has been recognized by the new health movement insurgencies which have overflowed union bounds. Groups of radical health workers have come to understand that they cannot depend on hospital unions to uphold the workers' end of the health struggle, that they must go outside the union. At the same time, they are beginning to understand that although the union may not take a leading role in their struggle, it is central to it. They have realized that the union can provide space for struggle, that it can protect workers who are involved in struggle. Alternatively, it can narrow that space or even eliminate it entirely, by cooperating with hospital management to smash dissent. And so many radical health workers are realizing that part of their struggle must be within the union itself, to democratize it, to keep it open as an arena for struggle, a point of contact with other workers, to prevent it from itself turning into an open enemy. They have learned that however much they may see the union itself as an obstacle to change in the health system, they cannot isolate themselves from the union members, their fellow-workers, by openly considering the union as their enemy. Increasingly, the struggle to change the health system may have to become a struggle to change the union as well.

—Editorial from the Health/PAC *Bulletin*, July/August, 1970.

HOSPITAL UNIONS: A Long Time Coming

John Ehrenreich

The most massive and dramatic insurgency going on in the health services world today is the headlong rush of the nation's two million hospital workers into unions. Most Americans have forgotten that there was ever anything "new" or "insurgent" about trade unions. Unions by and large have returned, along with the economy, into comfortable middle-aged respectability, if not stodginess. Hospital unions are not intrinsically different from unions in other sectors of the economy. In cities such as New York and San Francisco, where hospitals have been organized for a decade or more, the hospital unions have been unable to escape the aging process that has turned unions in other industries into defenders of the status quo. They have failed to work basic changes in the system of health-care delivery, and their relationship with the new, less conventional insurgencies in the health world is quite unfriendly. But in hospitals in most of the country, which are still back in the 1930's in terms of labor relations, unions are a new and cataclysmic phenomenon.

In the late 1960's a wave of hospital unionization began to sweep the country. Unions working hand in hand with civil rights organizations have turned cities such as Charleston, South Carolina, into battlefields, complete with mass marches through the streets, mass arrests, and the National Guard. The hospital industry's trade journals month after month run slightly hysterical articles on how to halt the union wave. One hospital labor relations consultant hopefully suggested: "The public is reacting against some of the events which occur when this particular union [Local 1199] appears on the scene, for they bear a resemblance to unpopular and illegal activities engaged in by dissidents in other protest movements in our country." But his words were wasted; tens of thousands of hospital workers surged into unions in 1969. Hospital workers in Baltimore, Pittsburgh and other cities throughout the country were swept with the same dizzying excitement that had New York in an uproar 10 years ago.

The impact of unionization on hospital workers is immediate and profound. In New York, for example, wages for unskilled hospital workers have more than tripled in the eleven years since the first major union breakthrough, and paid vacations, health insurance, workman's compensation, and a pension plan, almost unheard of a decade ago, have become standard. A training and upgrading program is in the works to permit hospital workers to escape from dead-end jobs. And hospital workers are now protected against arbitrary firings, disciplining, or reassignment by the hospital administration.

The effect of unionization on the hospital business other than in the area of labor relations, however, has so far been almost negligible. More than 80 percent of the nation's hospital workers are still ununionized, and the hospital unions remain oriented toward organizing the unorganized and winning bread-and-butter gains. But as the unions grow and consolidate, it seems clear that they could potentially be a major force helping shape the health care system of the future.

The first forty years of hospital unionization make a pretty short story. The beginnings took place in San Francisco, where a union of hospital employees was organized as early as 1919, but it was not until the 1930's that any substantial gains were made. Service and maintenance workers in three San Francisco hospitals were organized into a union in 1936 and other Bay Area hospitals quickly joined the fold. Three years later, after the passage of a state labor relations law protecting their right to organize, hospital workers in Minneapolis unionized. From 1939 to 1959, except for a few scattered drives in such places as Toledo, New York, and Seattle, unionization made no waves in the hospital field. An American Hospital Association survey taken in 1961 revealed that less than 3 percent of the nation's hospitals had collective bargaining agreements covering their employees.

There were several factors accounting for the failure of unions to gain a foothold in hospitals. The hospital workforce was difficult material for unionization, at best. Workers were fragmented into dozens of job categories. The combination of licensure laws and the jealous professionalism of such groups as registered and practical nurses, dieticians, medical technicians, X-ray technicians, and the like, made communication amongst the workers difficult, and the development of a sense of common grievances all but impossible. Even where common cause could be found, the attitude among the more skilled workers that "unions are unprofessional" held sway.

Among the less skilled workers, other factors prevented unity. The low wages of the industry, together with its philanthropic image, led to hospitals being more or less the employer of last resort. The work force was rich in the old, the illiterate, the discriminated against, the disabled, the demoralized. Workers came and went; it was a rare hospital worker who stuck out a job for as long as a year. It was thus hard to develop leadership within the hospital, and hard to maintain a stable membership in a union for even long enough to wage a struggle for recognition.

Another factor inhibiting the growth of unions in hospitals was the exclusion of hospital workers from coverage under the laws protecting bargaining rights of other workers. The 1937 Wagner Act had set up machinery under which workers could force their employer to conduct an election to determine whether the workers wished to be represented by a union. If the union prevailed in the election, the employer was legally bound to recognize it and to bargain in good faith with it. Originally, hospitals were included under the coverage of the law. But in 1947, intensive lobbying by the American Hospital Association (AHA) succeeded in tacking an amendment onto the Taft-Hartley law which exempted nonprofit hospitals from these provisions. The AHA's principal argument, according to Senator Millard Tydings of Maryland, who offered the amendment, was that "this amendment would be very helpful in [the hospitals'] efforts to serve those who have not the means to pay for hospital services." The charity of the underpaid hospital worker, who in the absence of union protection was forced to donate his hopes for an adequate living standard to the hospital's bank account, was to continue to be the main philanthropic underpinning of the hospital's charitable acts for the poor. State labor relations acts in a handful of states did cover hospital workers, but this was the exception, not the rule.

The absence of Wagner Act protection for hospital workers not only denied them access to the representation election procedures, but also denied them protection against unfair labor practices. Hospitals were free to fire or intimidate workers for union activities, to misrepresent the facts in the face of a union drive, to offer selective wage increases to "bribe" workers away from the union, and so forth. This freedom proved to be a potent weapon in the hospitals' hands. Although adherence to the labor relations etiquette provided in the law might be in general advisable for public relations reasons even though it was not required, when faced with the imminent threat of successful unionization, no holds were barred. In the words of A. Samuel Cook, the prominent labor relations advisor who (unsuccessfully) advised Johns Hopkins Hospital how to fight unionization in 1969,

"There are times, however, when deviation from some of the provisions of this federal labor code is advisable and in fact essential."

Even state laws protecting the right of hospital workers to organize did not guarantee an end to virulent hospital opposition. In 1967, the Massachusetts Hospital Association advised its members how to respond to unionization efforts under a new state law. "Consider," the Hospital Association handbook said, "whether a proposed action might be an unfair labor practice." After discussing the consequences of such an act, it concluded: "The issue is a matter of balanced risk, and of analyzing the disadvantages of one course of action . . . against the disadvantages of alternative courses of action." In other words, it's okay if you can get away with it. "If," the handbook continues, "a recently hired employee is suspected of being a union plant," don't summarily fire him without considering whether "martyring" him might not be counterproductive. Consider first whether he "is still in his probationary period and thus more easily terminated under existing hospital rules." But in any case, if all attempts to isolate the employee from other employees and to otherwise limit his effectiveness fail, "Terminate the individual if necessary as a final step."

In New York, in 1969, Columbia University's College of Physicians and Surgeons responded to Local 1199's attempt to organize its employees by using spies to compile a dossier on its employees: "Dr. [X] is a rabid civil rights advocate and very pro-union . . . Mrs. [Y's] thought concerning Dr. [X] is that he may oversell the union and antagonize people. . . . Recently this group of workers signed a petition asking for wages comparable to the Presbyterian Hospital.

At this point it is not certain whether Miss [A's] sympathies lie entirely with the University."

In the face of a fragmented, professionalism-ridden workforce, lack of legal protection, and bitter hospital resistance, few unions even tried to unionize hospitals. The few that did generally failed. But in the early sixties, the picture changed, and unions began to move. For one thing, the whole nature of hospitals had changed since the thirties. Hospitals were no longer poverty-stricken institutions, existing primarily for charity care to the poor. Private philanthropy had collapsed, and hospital finance now rested firmly on a base of third-party payments. Their financial existence was no longer as hand to mouth as it once had been. Moreover, with most patients insured, increased costs stemming from higher wages and fringe benefits paid to workers could be passed along to the patients, with relatively little financial strain on the hospital. The hospitals could thus relax a bit if a union came around; they might not like it but it no longer threatened financial curtains. The passage of Medicare and Medicaid in the mid-sixties vastly accelerated the improvement in the financial condition of the hospitals. (One example of what this meant for union-hospital relations: The day after the 1969 New York State freeze on Medicaid reimbursement rates was overturned by the courts, a high official of New York's League of Voluntary Hospitals told an 1199 vice president, not entirely jokingly, "Ask for anything you want!")

Hospital management, as well as hospital finances, underwent a vast change during the forties and fifties. Hospitals had become far more complex, far more technological, far richer. A new breed of more professional administrators developed, trained by newly created schools for hospital administration and encouraged by the plaudits of the corporate managers who now sat on the boards of trustees in place of the old individualist philanthropists. Gone were the old, philanthropic organization-oriented managers. Hospital management had entered the twentieth century. And with more modern management came more modern management attitudes: Unionization was still to be fought, but if worse came to worst, unions could be lived with.

If the hospitals were changing, so were the workers. Spurred on by the rising utilization and the growing complexity of hospital services, employment in hospitals has soared (up 34 percent in the last five years alone). The growth occurred within a tight labor market, and was concentrated in the relatively skilled areas of hospital work. Hospital workers, once the most expendable of workers, were now in demand. The workers were a different breed, too. The civil rights movement and the war on poverty had aroused the expectations of the poor and the minority groups that made up the great bulk of unskilled and semiskilled hospital employment, and the civil rights movement had taught the techniques of mass struggle to a generation that had not lived through the unionization drives of the thirties. Thousands of hospital workers were moved by the words of Dr. Martin Luther King to 1199: "Your campaign to organize all hospital workers, nonprofessionals and professionals alike, is more than a fight for union rights. It is a part of the larger fight in our nation against discrimination and exploitation, against slums—against all forms of degradation that result from poverty and human misery. It is a fight for human rights and dignity."

Finally, the 1960's saw a great wave of public employee unionization—teachers, office workers, policemen and firemen, etc.—and the pressure of these drives influenced the hospitals. For instance, in 1962 President Kennedy issued an executive order which established the right and conditions of collective bargaining for federal government employees. In the wake of this order, many federal hospitals were rapidly unionized. Similar events aided local and state hospitals to unionize—in New York City, Mayor Wagner's 1958 executive order gave the go-ahead, and a few years later District Council 37 of the American Federation of State, County and Municipal Employees (AFSCME) gained bargaining rights in the municipal hospitals. The example of the government hospitals successfully unionizing may have contributed to the momentum of the unionization drive.

As a result of these factors, the early 1960's marked a turning point in hospital unionization. Progress was greatest in the Middle Atlantic, Pacific Coast and North Central states, where several states had labor legislation which protected the right of workers in hospitals to unionize.

Most celebrated of the unionization efforts was in New York: Local 1199 of the Drug and Hospital Workers Union, a small union representing drug store employees, undertook a drive to organize the New York hospitals. At first their efforts were only partially successful. A 46-day strike against seven hospitals in 1959 failed to win union recognition, although an agreement with the hospitals to improve wages and working conditions was reached. But the fledgling union survived three years without a contract, without recognition, and without dues checkoffs, and in 1962, charging that the hospitals had not lived up to the

1959 agreement, 1199 struck again. This time the impasse was only settled when Governor Rockefeller agreed that in return for an end to the strike, he would press the State Legislature to include nonprofit hospitals under the protection of the State Labor Relations Act. Under protection of the law (which they had won in the streets), 1199 organizing proceeded rapidly. By 1966, for the first time, it was the union that had the upper hand in bargaining, and by 1969, some 60 percent of the hospital workers in New York City voluntary hospitals were represented by the union. Meanwhile, District Council 37 (AFSCME) had won bargaining rights for most of the city's municipal hospital workers. (1199 is the bargaining agent for workers on the affiliation payrolls in city hospitals where the private affiliating hospital is organized by 1199.) And Local 144 of the Service Employees International Union (SEIU) had signed up the workers in many of the city's proprietary hospitals and nursing homes.

In the wake of the much-publicized unionization of New York City hospitals, organizing drives hit such diverse cities as Chicago, Cleveland, Gary, Youngstown, and Detroit. By 1967, AFSCME, 1199, SEIU, and the American Federation of Government Employees (which represented most of the organized workers in federal hospitals), along with a host of other unions (including the Teamsters, Laborers, Mine Workers, Hotel and Restaurant Workers, and Operating Engineers), represented over 200,000 workers. Almost 8 percent of the nation's hospitals reported to the AHA that all or some of their workers were covered by collective bargaining agreements. New York, Minneapolis and San Francisco still had the bulk of the organized.

In 1969, the dam broke. Local 1199 set up a National Organizing Committee, which set out to organize outside of New York City. First stop, more or less by accident, was Charleston, South Carolina. After an epic 110-day strike, featuring weeks of mass demonstrations led by the Southern Christian Leadership Conference, hundreds of arrests, a threatened closing down of the port of Charleston by the Longshoreman's union, support from unions all over the country, and the occupation of the city by the National Guard, the union was victorious. Although formal recognition was not granted, the hospitals established a grievance procedure, pay hikes, agreed to rehire the fired unionists, and established what was in fact, if not in name, a dues checkoff for the union.

The organizing drive then moved on to Baltimore, where Johns Hopkins Hospital agreed to a representation election without a fight (although it was not required by state law), hoping to avoid another Charleston. Local 1199E (out-of-New York locals of the 1199 drive were given letters after the 1199) won the right to represent 1400 Johns Hopkins hospital workers by a two-to-one margin. Other hospitals rapidly fell in line with the prestigious Johns Hopkins, and by early January, 1970, membership in Local 1199E was rapidly passing the 6000 mark. In addition to grievance procedures, fringe benefits, and the like, Baltimore hospital workers won a contract providing for wage increases of $36 to $42 a week—a lot of money when you are earning $1.80 an hour.

With calls for help pouring in from all over the country, 1199 organizers fanned out to Connecticut, Philadelphia, North Carolina, Harrisburg, Pittsburgh, Ohio. Within weeks, close to ten thousand hospital workers signed union cards. Opposition to unionization had not collapsed, however. In early January, 1970, Pittsburgh suffered a hospital strike as Mellon-dominated Presbyterian Hospital and Catholic Mercy Hospital refused to permit a representation election. As in the 1962 New York strike, a temporary peace came when the hospitals agreed to support legislation providing for orderly union-management relations. Meanwhile, the confident 1199 reorganized its National Organizing Committee into the National Union of Hospital and Health Care Employees. Other unions, notably AFSCME and the Service Employees, stepped up their drives as well. The spark had ignited a prairie fire, and it appeared that the long delayed large-scale unionization of American hospital workers was under way.

—From the Health/PAC *Bulletin*, July/August, 1970.

THE HOSPITAL WORKERS: "The Best Contract Anywhere"?

Elinor Langer

I

Unions exist to negotiate contracts, to set out the terms under which workers will supply their services until the next negotiations. The contract justifies the very existence of the union, justifies the building of buildings, the payment of salaries; it justifies the officers and is the excuse for, if not the source of, their power; it also justifies the dues the workers pay to support the structure. A good contract is what holds the union together, giving the blacks and whites, the Puerto Rican porters and the Jewish technicians a common interest. Most important, the contract is the spring of all real gain: it is the source of additional money, of dental insurance, of pensions, of vacations. You have only to be around a union at contract expiration time to feel what an emotional, as well as a political and practical, watershed it is.

During contract negotiation time all the chickens in a union's barnyard come home to roost. The union's history and character come together and are revealed as having a functional, not an arbitrary, source. This was certainly true of 1199 [Local 1199, Drug and Hospital Workers Union in New York City—ed.]. Patterns that seemed abstractly "authoritarian," rooted in power hunger, egotism, or sectarian conceptions of structure, seemed, while the contract was at stake, to make perfect sense. Factionalism or opposition to the leadership, however idealistically inspired, seems when it occurs at this stage to border on treachery: will not disruption risk the unity needed to face down the bosses? As a result the settlement might be unfavorable, a matter not just of loss of credibility for the leadership and the union, but of overwhelming practical consequence to the members: the workers won't get what in fact they desperately need. They won't get it this time, and the power of the union will be compromised in the future. Immediate interests are at stake.

These things are so because of the adversary nature of collective bargaining in America. Capitalism rewards workers not according to need but according to the power of their organizations to threaten or disrupt. There are lights, cameras, smoke-filled rooms, clustering reporters, political machinations, all-night waits, exhaustion. The leaders need endurance, oratorical skill, and technical understanding. They must be equally at home in the bureaucratic regions of the managers and in the field commanding their own troops. During 1199's talks with the hospitals the problems of negotiation were very much exaggerated because of the way hospital services are financed: the dependence of hospitals on state and federal funds made them irresponsible negotiating partners. They never would or could say what resources were in fact available, or how far they might go in meeting the union's demands. Moreover, the tension and infrequency of contact during collective bargaining made it impossible for both sides to discuss real issues or grievances, real ways in which working conditions might be reformed.

Collective bargaining is a grueling, insane, time-consuming experience, full of truth and full of lies. It can also be exhilarating. As an instrument of achieving real progress, this proud invention of the American class struggle seemed to me absurd. But it is the world in which unions live, and in which they must prove themselves or fail.

There were essentially three elements in the 1970 talks between Local 1199 and the League of Voluntary Hospitals. The first was what was happening within the union: the formation of demands, the mobilization of support, the development of tactics. The second was the talks themselves: the interplay between workers and management, the dickering over what it was possible to achieve. The third was the hospitals' side: the strategy that the hospital leadership had adopted and its relation to New York State politics, and specifically to Governor Rockefeller. People in the union sometimes felt, as one of them said, that the negotiations were being manipulated "by forces greater than Leon Davis [President of Local 1199]." I don't know to what extent that is true; perhaps no one does. But certainly the demands on the union officials to provide mass leadership—to inspire, then control their troops—were inseparable from the demands on them for tactical judgment and political skill in dealing with the managers. It was the tension between these demands that defined the entire process.

Within the union, preparations were carefully arranged to reach a climax on July 1. Beginning in March, meetings were held in every hospital, with the Guild and Hospital Divisions meeting separately. The workers were asked what they wanted—a rare occurrence—and at least in the places I visited, there was a spontaneous outpouring of present grievances and visionary hopes for the future. For example, from the basement of a chronic disease hospital in the Bronx: Why can't we take our holidays when we want them? Make the bosses stop calling to check on us when we're home sick. Let's get paid for unused sick leave at the end of the year. We should get paid every week, not every two weeks. Why does my husband at another hospital make more money than I do when we do the same work? We need a locker room with a shower. They've taken away the chairs where we take our breaks. Make the hospitals pay for cleaning uniforms. We need: dental care, $100 take home pay after taxes, $50 a week raises; free meals; hour-long lunch breaks; more respect from the supervisors; differential pay for night and weekend work . . . and so on.

The organizer, the staff member chairing the meeting, takes it all down. We'll see, we'll see. The problem of negotiations exists from the beginning: to determine where there is real need and strong feeling, to mobilize support without making false promises. The organizer then supervises the election of a worker to sit on the negotiating committee. It is clear from the start who the representative will be. It will be the active union delegate, the worker who has already proved his or her reliability to the organizer and the leadership. "I think you should elect Mrs. P. She was on the committee two years ago and she did a great job." Mrs. P. is elected. It is apparent that the process was roughly the same in every hospital because the composition of the negotiating committee was like a who's who of the 1199 rank and file. Dissension was unlikely to afflict its ranks.

The final demands, sifted by the leadership and the committee from these outpourings, seem now, months later, to be somewhat limp or trivial. Yet each one had a concrete meaning for thousands of workers. Each one would have made their lives just a little better: a greater accumulation of sick leave, differentials for weekend work, differentials for Licensed Practical Nurses who act as RNs, longer vacations after shorter periods of employment, payment of laundry costs for uniforms, dental care under the benefit plan. The demands reflected a certain amount of internal pork barreling: LPN differentials, for instance, or a demand to end inequities in reimbursement to social workers were clearly aimed at satisfying the more highly skilled workers in the division of the union known as the Guild. For itself, the union demanded that workers' savings at the Credit Union and contributions to the union's Brotherhood Fund be deducted by the hospitals from the payroll. Then there was Martin Luther King's birthday as a holiday: a little soul, something for everyone.

Money, however, was the critical demand. During the negotiations of 1968 the problem had been simpler: the $100 minimum was plain, dramatic, a good magnet for community support. No one could argue that human beings supporting families should make less than $100 a week. Now the money question was more complicated. The union feared that people would argue—and at one point the hospital managers actually did, incredibly in view of their $75,000-a-year salaries—that the workers were no longer so poor. They would point to industries such as retailing where New York workers are still making only $80 or $90 a week.

The committee therefore decided to tie its coattails to the Bureau of Labor Statistics, which in the early summer of 1970 reported that the minimum needed to maintain a family of four in New York City was $139.71 per week, or $7,265. (Try it.) The union accepted this figure, though many of its members are supporting far larger families, and demanded a $140 minimum: a 30 percent increase across the board or a $40 increase, whichever would be higher. It also demanded a cost-of-living escalator clause.

One union demand was more than ameliorative and its fate is significant. This was a demand that appeared on the list simply as "Establishment of Career Ladders Within Each Hospital." I believe this was meant to be an extension of a union-management program which was begun under the 1968 contract. Known as the Training and Upgrading Fund, it trains workers in lower job categories to be technicians or clerical workers. The program is extremely expensive to administer, because under it the hospitals must not only finance the worker's training, but also pay him or her a salary during training and, in addition, pay another employee filling the job the trainee has left. Because of its cost, the program has remained very small and will not become a major factor in changing conditions for a significant number of workers.

The new "Career Ladders" proposal, as I understood it, would have—or more accurately could have—been more effective. It was designed to establish an *automatic* upgrading procedure open to all the workers in the hospitals: a maid would be trained as an aide, an aide as an LPN, a file clerk as a typist, a typist as a technician, a kitchen aide as a dietitian, etc. The proposal might have abolished the worst and most notorious characteristic of hospital jobs: that they are dead ends. It was hardly a revolutionary proposal, unless increasing people's capacities and giving them more mobility are revolutionary. It did not, for example, change the distribution of power between workers and management. But it was a reform which would have made a difference, and that is why the union's inability to work it out is important.

That was how the Career Ladders proposal seemed to me; yet I sometimes felt that I was the only person around who had noticed it at all. It appeared on the list (by what process I do not know), but was never mentioned again. It was never central to the negotiations. No one mourned its passing. The reason for its extinction is not that the leaders of 1199 do not want to improve the lot of hospital workers; they do. But given the structure of collective bargaining, particularly the two-week period in this case in which there was no contact whatever between the antagonists—there was no possible time for the discussion, planning, and argument that would have been needed to consider and implement such a huge administrative program. The negotiations stayed deadlocked on money and were barely able to deal with anything beyond that.

Secondly, the union itself was unprepared to support its idea with the detailed staff work, administrative proposals, funding, arrangements, and so forth that would have helped to make the demand real. Only one person on the union staff could conceivably have been assigned to such a job, and she was at work on another urgent task, an attempt to straighten out job classifications and wage rates and make them uniform throughout the different hospitals. And so "Career Ladders" came and went without leaving a trace. It had no priority.

It is usually said of unions that their structure follows the structure of the industry whose workers they represent. Among New York hospitals the opposite occurred. The voluntary hospitals formed themselves into a unified assembly only after the union became a power. The sole visible function of the League of Voluntary Hospitals is to negotiate with the union. Not all voluntary metropolitan hospitals are members of the League, but most of the major ones are: Beth Israel, Mt. Sinai, Montefiore, Maimonides, and so forth. (Workers in city-financed hospitals belong to another union.) The non-League hospitals generally abide by terms identical to those set by the League, but for various reasons have decided against participation in it.

The men representing the hospitals during the

spring and summer negotiations at the Roosevelt and the Biltmore Hotels were middle-aged, middle-class, white men from White Plains and Great Neck, professional, respectable, serious: clear in their hearts that they are not agents of medical empires (as radicals have charged) but agents of humanity. The union side was a different sight. Everything that was homogeneous about the managers was diverse about the union: color, size, shape, sex, nationality, temperament, language.

In this setting in which the very shapes of the bodies of the people, the difference in the way lines formed in their faces told of the reality of class in America—everything happened. The officers did not, except for one (crucial) moment at the end, have any private dealings with the bosses or the mediator. There were no private conferences, no secret meetings. There was not for one moment the possibility of a sellout or deal, the possibility that the leadership would accept a settlement which would be unacceptable to the workers. What occurred in the strike of the New York postal union, for instance, could not have occurred here. Whatever Davis and the other officers did or said, they did or said in front of the committee. What went on when the officers were alone I don't know, but I never heard the president speak in a staff meeting, for instance, any differently from the way he spoke in front of the members. Because of the loyalty of the members and their faith in Davis there was no need for him to dissemble.

The committee acted chiefly as a chorus, assenting to whatever Davis decided. They were rarely consulted in advance, and never took the initiative in anything but social matters. There came a moment, for example, when it was the union's turn to trade. Davis unilaterally decided to abandon the demand for pay differentials, then turned and asked the committee if that was okay. They agreed that it was.

Nevertheless, it is important to understand what was remarkable and positive about this "participatory collective bargaining." First, I think it put some kind of brake on at least the theoretically possible runaway development of "togetherness" between the top union officials and top management. In reality, of course, there is a good deal of mutual understanding and respect between them. The hospitals do not mind the union—in fact they like it—because it has simplified administration in general and because the resulting wage gains have created job stability where there used to be a tornado-like turnover. The hospitals appreciate the union's role in keeping up its end of the bargain, in contributing to order in the hospitals, in helping to ensure that a disciplined, dependable work force shows up to work every morning.

The union is proud of its contribution as well: this is precisely the symbiosis of non-militant "responsibility" which leads radicals to despair of unions. Nevertheless, the less good feeling at contract time, the less of that characteristic muddle of labor-management harmony, the better it is for the workers. In this sense the constant presence of the workers' committee helped to keep the union negotiators on the right (that is to say, the antagonistic) side of the class war. Davis could never forget that he was bargaining on behalf of workers whom he knew and loved; he could never forget that the items in question were very important to them, or that his strength and power depended ultimately on satisfying them, and not on the esteem of the prestigious people on the other side of the table.

Furthermore, in a roomful of working people—

and partly because of Davis's own bluntness and vulgarity—a lot of the pomp of the proceedings was deflated. Middle-class technicians in American institutions have developed the habit—or skill—of making things seem much more complicated than they are. Hospitals are no exception. League spokesmen entered the negotiations with a list of counter-demands that far outdistanced those of the union, a catalogue of simple threats to workers' privileges disguised as a set of managerial headaches and couched in complex bureaucratic terms. The members of the committee, however, always knew exactly what was going on and they understood the hidden implications of the various positions the hospitals took.

With the committee present the level of bullshit dropped considerably. Everyone knew that "efficiency" meant layoffs, that "contracting out" meant loss of jobs, that the hospitals were trying to use this time to enforce more rigid rules about coffee breaks and marriage leaves. The committee's presence meant that the corporate middle-class jargon of the hospital bureaucrats would not be allowed to triumph.

It quickly became apparent that there would be no substantial negotiations. The hospitals' position was that they were in a severe economic crisis and anticipating huge deficits. They were dependent on the state's reimbursement formula (under Medicaid) to underwrite the added costs of any new settlement with the workers. Unless the state would guarantee to underwrite such a settlement they could not negotiate one because they did not know where the money would come from. Their hands, they said, were tied.

Amid this uncertainty, another deep limitation of the union became apparent. 1199 has never questioned the hospitals' version of their economic situation. Occasionally the union complains that the hospitals keep closed books. But it has never aligned itself with the critics of American medical care, either professional or radical, who contend that hospitals are inefficient, that they are incapable of providing adequate medical care, that they are interested mainly in competitive expansion, and that their practices are creating a deadly medical inflation. Wherever the quality and character of medical care are being challenged by community groups—such as in the case of the Gouverneur Clinic on the Lower East Side or at Lincoln Hospital—the union either overtly or tacitly supports the hospitals. Hovering in the background is the feeling in the union that someday a "policy" on medical care will have to be developed because it is plain from frequent news reports that medical care is in a crisis, and the crisis is of great significance to hospital workers.

So far, however, such a policy has not emerged. The union has no experts in hospital economics or medical care and the instinct of the leadership, even in the heat of battle, is to support the hospitals' own analysis of their condition. As a result, the union was helpless to affect the maneuverings of the hospitals with the state. It had to say, "Look, you boys work things out however you have to. We don't care how you do it. We don't care who runs the hospitals. We are here simply to get what we need and if we don't get it we'll strike."

II

Twice during the few days before the contract expired management came back into the talks with offers: once for a 6 percent increase in each year of a three-year contract, once for an 8 percent, two-year arrangement.

Both times Davis threw them out. Once he threw a microphone at the chief hospital negotiator. Another time he reached new heights—or maybe depths—of earthiness: "You know what you can do with your forty-two demands? Shove one up each of you so there'll be fair and equal distribution. And we have a committee here that's ready to help." Both displays were carefully calculated and of excellent theatrical value. They were designed to bring the talks to an unceremonious close while there was still time for them to be reopened. They permitted both sides to greet the waiting reporters with doleful prophecies meant to intensify the political struggle. "It will be a miracle if a strike can be avoided" was the line of both sides.

On Tuesday evening the delegates assembled at the New Yorker Hotel to begin the long wait to a count-down. The negotiators came over from the Roosevelt to open the meeting. Davis urged discipline, preparation for midnight action. Melody [Phillips, a union representative generally critical of Davis—ed.] got up to speak and chaos erupted. Davis returned to the negotiations. A group of Young Lords [a Puerto Rican organization which had organized a Health Revolutionary Unity Movement at several New York City hospitals—ed.] made an unusual mass appearance distributing copies of their paper stating their case against 1199 and listing their demands. They tried to argue that money gains unaccompanied by long-range plans for upgrading the workers did not offer genuine security in an inflationary period; that hospitals affect their surrounding communities as much in their role of land buyers as in their role as providers of medical services; and that workers needed a stronger role in running the union.

No one would, or could, listen. The Lords got

caught up in the general disruption. Staff members, exhausted, all their energies directed toward protecting the unity they believed the union would need in the hours ahead, became enraged. Screaming matches began. Fistfights were started and barely stopped. By that time all the concentration of the members present was focused on the single issue with which America, and the structure of labor, makes them deal: money. By that time they were totally dependent on the union. It was the only instrument that existed through which they could get not just what they'd been told they needed but what they needed in fact. The vision of the Lords seemed too general and, therefore, irrelevant. The Lords were talking what seemed like rhetoric. The members needed the machinery, the system, the pre-established processes through which gains, however small, could be realized. The Lords were thrown out.

In the New Yorker Hotel people sat playing cards, eating and drinking, sharing their food and drink. Some made tactical plans for shutting down their buildings. A middle-aged white member from Albert Einstein Hospital tried to revive memories of another time, leading the crowd in a lusty version of "We're gonna roll the union on." It fell flat. He was the only one who knew the words. Some of the younger members and staff clustered in a stair well to sing black music. Older people sang: "We Shall Overcome." The spirit was good.

The midnight deadline came and went. Leaders and troops, stationed in different hotels, were in sporadic telephone contact. They kept telling the members to wait. At 5 A.M. union and management were still in separate rooms. A staff member was sent over, a tall, proud black man once described to me as a leading theoretical Marxist in another time. He was gentle, but capable of great anger. He said the talks were "hopelessly deadlocked"; the battle was on. Members from the hospitals where the contract had actually expired should go to the hospitals and set up picket lines. The day shift should be kept from entering. But the members should first check in at the Roosevelt for last minute news before their strike action actually began. The delegates, exhausted from the nearly twelve hours of waiting at the New Yorker, cheered at the news of a strike. They gathered themselves together and set out for the long treks back to their hospitals in Brooklyn, Flushing, Queens.

At 5:25 A.M. a settlement was reached.

III

1199's contract with the hospitals was not a sellout as the opposition within the union charged. Whether it was "the best contract in the country for any group of workers anywhere" only a labor statistician could say. But for the group of workers it involved, and given the history of the industry from which it came, the contract was, as we said in the magazine in enormous type, a "TERRIFIC VICTORY."

Nonetheless, the question remains what it was in the beginning. Is the union making a substantial contribution to change? The leadership's conviction that it is rests chiefly on a trickle-down theory of wage gains. They believe that gains won in the New York hospitals will influence the wage structure of other industries employing unskilled, nonwhite laborers. But this measure, even if correct, is insufficient, it does no good for wages to rise if inflation makes the increments useles, if the skies are so black it is dangerous to breathe, if housing deteriorates and the subways on which the workers ride to work collide, if one son of a worker dies in Vietnam and another of an overdose in Harlem. It does not good to hitch your wagon to a star that is burning itself out.

The answer is not simply, therefore, that the workers should take to the streets. Members of 1199 are not like middle-class radicals who have far greater freedom and other resources stuffed into innumerable hidden crevices of their lives. The workers have lives to lead which they do not have the mobility to change. They have families to sustain. In getting money to support themselves they have made real progress. The problem of evaluation is therefore difficult. Apart from a few propagandists (who fall into every political camp) no one is certain how change will come. No one knows exactly how an institution committed to change should behave. No one can be certain what is real and important or what is "part of the problem." With this uncertainty judgments about effectiveness and relevance should be made with some humility.

One criterion is clear. It makes no difference whether 1199's Executive Council passes resolutions condemning repression, Julius Hoffman, the use of the National Guard in the postal strike, or the murdering of children at Kent State. It makes relatively little difference even that the union gives money for the legal defense of the Panthers. These flourishes so little affect political reality that it is a wonder that people bother to do them at all. The union does them for the reason countless other organizations do; because people feel less trapped if they have devised some vehicle, however inadequate, to express their moral outrage.

But not only do these pronouncements and contributions fail to affect political reality, they are done in a way that cannot serve even to educate the union's members. To the members they appear as resolutions composed in a board room, designed to be echoed. They are occasional statements; short paragraphs in the magazine that convey an attitude without illuminating causes. They float down out of nowhere; they are not connected with any sustained effort of communication or education on the part of the staff.

It does not tell us much, therefore, to leaf through the annals of 1199 and conclude that its stands are progressive, its record honorable. That alone does not make it part of the solution. At the same time, however, conventional radical critiques of the union—including ones which I myself shared and argued about with people when I was there—also seem to me faulty. An example: on the issue of the war, I—and other radicals—condemned the union for failing to make the most of an opportunity presented by the Kent-Cambodia spring to solidify an alliance with New York's striking students into a permanent, labor-student coalition. We saw that such a coalition would be difficult because of the different histories, different styles, different needs, and mutual prejudices of the members of each group—differences in kinds of *apparent* radicalism—and we thought that to overcome the differences by concerted effort and mutual understanding would be a genuine breakthrough, the keystone of an alliance which transcended class and would be in fact . . . what? Make the revolution.

I now think I was mistaken in my criticism that the union leaders were too pressed or too indifferent to develop the alliance when matters became tense (as they did), that I was led by my own susceptibility to rhetoric into ignoring the fact that the student uprising was tame and ephemeral, that it produced no lasting organization with which the leaders on the union side could come to terms. The hard fact is that a year later the union still exists, following its own path toward incremental gains for the workers, and that the students, as students, are hardly in sight.

Much the same point could be made about another tender spot for radicals, the union's difficulties with the Young Lords. It is true that the union resists, persecutes, and tries to destroy the power of its members who are Lords in a relentless, narrow-minded, and overactive way. While I was there, for instance, the union refused to support a group of Lords and others from the Gouverneur Health Clinic of Beth Israel Hospital, who, organized as the Health Revolutionary Unity Movement (HRUM), had staged a demonstration inside the hospital and been fired. 1199 was refusing to petition for their reinstatement. HRUM members found a little-noticed clause in the 1199 constitution which entitled them to present their case against the Executive Council's decision to an appeals board made up of union members. The result was an arduous and prolonged semi-trial worthy of the elders of Salem.

I think I felt most bitter when a union vice-president, who denounced the illegality of the H-RUM demonstration, arguing that "you can't do that" in the hospitals, later came up to me glowing with some remembered spirit of his own radical days. He pointed to a member of the appeals board (who has since joined the staff) and said, with amazing unself-consciousness, "See that guy? We used to break windows together on the picket lines in the Thirties."

Nevertheless, whatever the hypocrisy of the union's language, its disagreeable tactics, and its unconscionable zealotry, its incompatibility with the Lords makes sense. There is no way, given the structure of the union's relations with the hospitals, the omnipresence of the contract which trades off discipline for money to pay a carefully defined number of workers doing specific jobs, that the union could share the Lord's vision of a revolution based in the community. That is simply not a way in which this union, or any other union, can contribute to change in America.

What this suggests is that, in a peculiar way, Samuel Gompers was right. Unions are not political organizations, cannot be, and were in fact shaped by developing corporate America precisely *not* to be. This is why there has continued to be such a gap between the "left" in general and the "labor left"; why Walter Reuther, for all his efforts, was never instrumental in the larger left political movement. Because of their many other functions, because of the limitations of their independence, because of their need for stability (which implies a relation to electoral politics), labor unions can have only a marginal effect on conventionally defined left political issues.

Where they could have an effect, it seems to me, is on the fundamental texture of the industrial system itself. There will probably always be work, and for the foreseeable future at least there are bound to be workers. The job of a radical union should be to reduce the gulf between labor and the managers, between the owning class and the workers. It should not substitute another more genial or benign layer of management between the workers and the power that controls them.

To do this the hospital workers' union would first have to discover (indeed, admit: the cat is already out of the bag) the truth about the organization of medicine in America, the economics of hospitals, the workings of medical administration. Second, it would require a fundamental look at the whole notion of skills and training in this society, since in the hospitals it is the rigid classification of skills and jobs which plays a key role in keeping the workers down. If skills could be demystified and training programs initiated which were realistic (instead of, as at present, immensely costly because they help to reinforce the divisions in the system they are trying to reform), then, finally, there would be a realistic basis on which to begin talking about sharing power, about giving the workers the right, the technical as well as moral capacity, to control their lives and futures. If this were possible collective bargaining, as it functioned in this case, for example, would be a dead process.

The question of what workers would do with their power is the question that links the possibility of larger political change with the importance of industry-based action. But radicalism must begin at home, and the great failure of the 1199 leadership is that it has not told the truth to the workers about the oppression in their working lives or about the union itself. This failure makes the union finally a supporter and not an antagonist of the status quo.

—From *The New York Review of Books*, June 3, 1971. (abridged)

III. Government Intervention in the Health System

National health insurance has been a major issue in the debate over government intervention in the health-care system since the turn of the century. Long proposed by health-care reformers, such a program was first adopted as federal government policy by the New Deal Administration during the 1930's. The initial draft of the Social Security Act of 1935 provided for a federal study of national health insurance, but the provision was withdrawn in response to intense opposition led by the American Medical Association (AMA). A bitter struggle ensued between the AMA and New Deal (later Fair Deal) Democrats until national health insurance was eventually taken off the political agenda after the resounding Democratic defeat in the 1950 congressional elections, in which it had been a major issue. Thus, while the New Deal, with its Keynesian economic policies, was able to regulate many other sectors of the economy in an attempt to head off social unrest, it was defeated in the cottage industry of health care by the doctors/proprietors of fee-for-service medicine.

Meanwhile, events were overtaking this struggle. Hospitals started to grow and become technologically sophisticated after World War II, aided by federal construction grants and loans under the 1946 Hill-Burton Act. In the flush of major advances in medical science and technology, federal research grants began to pour into universities and academic medical centers. This infusion of funds not only aided in the development of medical empires, but also encouraged a general expansion among all hospitals of physical facilities, staff, salaries and equipment. By the early 1960's the resulting increase in hospital costs had far outstripped both the swollen federal research grants and the consumers' ability to pay. The hospitals turned to the federal government for more aid.

By now members of the so-called permanent

government within the federal bureaucracy, especially in the Social Security Administration, had rebounded from their earlier defeat on national health insurance to propose a limited form of national health insurance for the elderly, later called Medicare. They saw in the hospitals' request for federal aid a golden opportunity. The 1964 Democratic landslide brought in a Congress much more open than its predecessors to federal funding of health care, as well as a politically strengthened President looking for potentially popular, New Society programs. The results were Medicare, health insurance for the elderly, and Medicaid, a welfare program of health benefits for the poor, passed in 1965. (The latter bill was the congressional brainchild of then Chairman Wilbur Mills of the powerful House Ways and Means Committee.) These programs were a bonanza for the health-care system, the largest federal health programs ever. Like the Hill-Burton and medical research programs, they were long on financing but short on cost controls and performance standards. (This should come as no surprise since they were shaped by the now-powerful American Hospital Association precisely to relieve the hospitals' financial crisis.)

The programs may have been a windfall for the providers, but they have been something less for the recipients of health care. As discussed in Chapter 8 on Medicare and Medicaid, for all the spending on these programs they have produced little in the way of improved medical care, and they have helped inflate the cost of medical care for everyone. Despite Medicare, elderly people pay more out of their own pockets for medical care today than they did before the program existed. Yet Medicare's main selling point to the public was that it would help relieve the financial plight of the elderly when they are struck down by illness and injury.

By the 1970's federal health costs were nearing $20 billion annually and putting a serious strain on the federal budget, already pinched by a declining economy. But the government needed to do more than just cut the budget; it also needed to regulate the health-care system to contain costs and rationalize the delivery of services. The health-care industry, like other industries, would have to be "responsible" and integrate itself into the capitalist development of the overall economy. The New Deal had introduced this concept of an openly interventionist government that attempts to regulate and stabilize the national economy, and by the 1970's that approach had been accepted by a broad, bipartisan consensus within both the legislative and executive branches of the federal government. The fact that the federal government had financed but not regulated health care prior to the 1970's may well have reflected the organized political clout of the American Medical Association. That impediment was largely removed by the passage of Medicare and the growing importance of the hospital sector that Medicare both reflected and strengthened.

One proposal for federal intervention in health, advocated by the Nixon Administration and supported by most Democrats as well (including Senator Edward Kennedy), was to establish a national network of health maintenance organizations (HMO's). HMO's offered the public a vehicle for the delivery of preventive care: pay the health-care provider a fixed sum of money per patient to treat all medical needs and it will be in the provider's interest to prevent illness, thereby decreasing health-care costs and increasing the provider's profits. HMO's offered the government a way both to cut costs and to establish a rational system for delivering primary (outpatient) and preventive care. To the Nixon Administration and political conservatives HMO's also offered the possibility of a major entry of private investors into the health-care delivery system. HMO's and some of their serious pitfalls are the subject of Chapter 9. One of the main problems of HMO's is that the cost-cutting incentives under which they operate can result in their simply choosing to deliver as few services as possible and to make them as difficult to obtain as possible.

If the economic crisis forced government intervention in the health-care system in the 1970's, the form of intervention was dictated by the political predilections of the Administration, such as the Nixon preference for private enterprise HMO's. An analysis of the Nixon health agenda is presented in Chapter 10. This agenda is still important since it represents a carefully conceived political strategy that has set the framework for Administration discussion of its health-care role ever since. The chapter also discusses various other government regulatory measures, such as Professional Standards Review Organizations (PSRO's) and Comprehensive Health Planning Agencies (CHPA's), and concludes with a discussion of government intervention in the malpractice crisis.

National health insurance, a topic of great political concern in recent years, is discussed in Chapter 11. As in the case of Medicare and Medicaid, the revived interest in national health insurance was triggered in large measure by the financial crisis of hospitals, brought on by the leveling off of Medicare and Medicaid funds and the economic crisis in general. Since national health insurance is a program for financing, not delivering, health care, it cannot directly address such problems as quality and accessibility of care but can only make ineffectual attempts to address these through the back door of financial incentives.

8

Medicare and Medicaid

The enactment of Medicare and Medicaid in 1965 was a response to two major influences—the financial crisis of hospitals in the early 1960's and the internal pressure by New Deal reformers within the federal government to enact some, even if limited, form of national health insurance. The effects of these programs have been a tremendous financial boost for health-care providers, only limited improvement in health care for their nominal beneficiaries and an inflation of health-care costs for all.

The chapter begins with Theodore R. Marmor's short history of federal health insurance legislation, which shows the origins of the Medicare legislation in the long-term effort by New Deal reformers to enact a program of comprehensive national health insurance. The second article, by Godfrey Hodgson, discusses the inflation of health-care costs brought on by Medicare and Medicaid and some of the windfall profits made in their wake.

A brief, poignant news item from *The Washington Post* gives a glimpse of the desperate situation faced by elderly individuals with large medical bills, even after the enactment of Medicare. Barbara Caress's article on so-called Medicaid mills unmasks the operation of one of the many ripoffs (of patients and money) that have been spawned by the Medicaid program, and exposes the unwillingness of local government to investigate and prosecute such abuses.

The final article, by Elinor Blake and Thomas Bodenheimer, shows how California's Medicaid legislation, passed ostensibly to help poor people, has in fact limited their access to medical services, while enriching private hospitals at public expense.

ORIGINS OF THE GOVERNMENT HEALTH INSURANCE ISSUE

Theodore R. Marmor

Demands in America for government involvement in health insurance date back to the first decade of the twentieth century. The impetus in these early efforts came from academics, lawyers, and other professionals, organized in the American Association for Labor Legislation. During the years 1915–1918, this group made a concerted effort to shepherd its model medical care insurance bill through several state legislatures, but with no success. The American Medical Association, whose officials had initially co-operated with the AALL, found local medical societies adamantly opposed to the state health insurance bills, and in 1920 the AMA House of Delegates announced

> its opposition to the institution of any plan embodying the system of compulsory contributory insurance against illness, or any other plan of compulsory insurance which provides for medical service to be rendered contributors or their dependents, provided, controlled, or regulated by any state or federal government.[1]

Even more disappointing to the labor reformers was the unequivocal opposition of Samuel Gompers, the president of the American Federation of Labor, to the model bills. The strength of the opposition prevented America from following England's example of insuring low-income workers against illness. During the 1920's, a variety of groups undertook studies of health care financing in the United States, and attention turned to the feasibility of group medical practice and of prepayment medical plans. But it was not until the Great Depression began, in an atmosphere of general concern for economic insecurity, that a sustained interest in government health insurance reappeared. The evolution of the 1965 Medicare Act reaches back to this New Deal period. To understand the particular form of the Medicare legislation, and to explain the two decades of controversy and delay at which President Johnson expressed surprise, one must begin the story here.

The source of renewed interest in government health insurance was President Roosevelt's advisory Committee on Economic Security, created in 1934 to draft a social security bill providing a minimum income for the aged, the unemployed, the blind, and the widowed and their children. The result was the Social Security bill of 1935, which, in addition to providing for insurance against potential loss of income, broached the subject of a government health insurance program. Edwin Witte, a former professor of economics at the University of Wisconsin who was executive director of the committee, described the extent of the committee's involvement with health insurance and the response:

> When in 1934 the Committee on Economic Security announced that it was studying health insurance, it was at once subjected to misrepresentation and vilification. In the original social security bill there was one line to the effect that the Social Security Board should study the problem and make a report to Congress. That little line was responsible for so many telegrams to the members of Congress that the entire social security program seemed endangered until the Ways and Means Committee unanimously struck it out of the bill.[2]

Roosevelt's fears that the controversial issue of government health insurance would jeopardize the Social Security bill and, later, his chances for re-election, kept him from vigorously sponsoring the proposal. For many of his advisors in the Committee on Economic Security, however, the discussions in Washington in the mid-thirties marked the beginning of an active interest in the subject. The divorce of compulsory health insurance from the original Social Security program of 1935 had alerted the critics within the medical world to the possibility of attempts to enlarge the partial government program to "get a foot-in-the-door for socialized medicine." In response they reversed their former opposition to private health insurance alternatives; in an effort to forestall federal action, the AMA began to promote Blue Cross and commercial hospital insurance, and, in the case of state Blue Shield plans, actively to organize private insurance plans for surgical and medical expenses. In the meantime, passage of the Social Security Act had freed advocates of compulsory health insurance from their concerns about providing income protection for the aged, the blind, and dependent women and children. Their attention was now directed to the broad social question of how equitably medical care was distributed in post-Depression America. From 1939 onward, their activities were reflected in the annual introduction of congressional bills proposing compulsory health insurance for the entire population. An orphan of the New Deal, government medical care insurance was to become one of the most prominent aspirations of Harry Truman's "Fair Deal."

UNIVERSAL HEALTH INSURANCE PROPOSALS IN THE FAIR DEAL

Although the government health insurance issue was originally raised in conjunction with social security income protection, New Deal-Fair Deal champions of medical care proposals did not view it primarily as a measure to further income security but as a remedy for the inequitable distribution of medical services. The proponents of Truman's compulsory insurance program took for granted that financial means should not determine the quality and quantity of medical services a citizen received. "Access to the means of attainment and preservation of health," flatly stated the 1952 report of Truman's Commission on the Health Needs of the Nation, "is a basic human right." The health insurance problem in this view was the degree to which the use of health services varied with income (and not simply illness). In contrast, for those who considered minimum accessibility of health services a standard of adequacy, the provision of charity medicine in doctors' offices and general hospitals represented a solution, and the problem was to fill in where present charity care was unavailable.

The Truman solution to the problem of unequal accessibility to health services was to remove the financial barriers to care through government action. As set forth in his State of the Union message in 1948, his goal was "to enact a comprehensive insurance system which would remove the money barrier between illness and therapy . . . [and thus] protect all our people equally . . . against ill health." Bills embracing such goals had been introduced as early as 1935, but the first to receive widespread public attention was S. 1620, introduced by Senator Robert Wagner (D., N.Y.) in 1939. A decade later, in Truman's term, it was S. 1679 which Senator Wagner, Senator Murray (D., Mont.) and Representative Dingell (D., Mich.) presented for congressional consideration. By 1949, the introduction of a Wagner-Murray-Dingell bill had become an annual event which was invariably followed by congressional refusal to hold hearings on the bill.

Throughout the decade, public opinion polls continued to report favorable reactions to federal involvement in health insurance. However, although from 1939 to 1946 the Democrats controlled both houses of Congress, the partisan majority did not make up an issue majority. There were too few legislative supporters to bring the repeatedly introduced bills through the stages of committee hearings, committee approval, and congressional passage. By 1945, officials within the Federal Security Agency * had secured presidential

* The three key officials—Arthur Altmeyer, Wilbur Cohen, and I. S. Falk—worked for the Social Security Board, a division of the Federal Security Agency. The FSA, created in 1939 to oversee the Board, the Public Health Service, and the Office of Education, was in 1953 replaced by the Cabinet-rank Department of Health, Education and Welfare.

endorsement for the Wagner-Murray-Dingell proposal, but the advantage of Truman's support was offset by the congressional elections the following year, which returned Republican majorities in both the House and the Senate. This Congress, it has been observed, "was generally at loggerheads with Truman in domestic affairs," and in the campaign of 1948, the President used its inaction, on health insurance and other domestic issues, to berate the "do-nothing Republican 80th Congress." The election of 1948, returning the presidency to Truman and control of the Congress to the Democrats, left Truman and his advisors with high hopes for enactment of the domestic proposals that had highlighted his "Fair Deal" campaign against Dewey.[3]

Early in 1949, in keeping with his recent campaign pledges, the President requested congressional action on medical care insurance. The specifications of the proposal repeated those of previous Wagner-Murray-Dingell bills:

> the insurance benefits would cover all medical, dental, hospital and nursing care expenses.
>
> beneficiaries would include all contributors to the plan and their dependents, and for the medical needs of a destitute minority which would not be reached by the contributory plan, provisions were made for federal grants to the states.
>
> the financing mechanism would be a compulsory 3 per cent payroll tax divided equally between employee and employer.
>
> administration would be in the hands of a national health insurance board within the Federal Security Agency.
>
> to minimize the degree of federal control over doctors and patients, it was specified that doctors and hospitals would be free not to join the plan; patients

> would be free to choose their own doctors and doctors would reserve the right to reject patients whom they did not want; doctors who agreed to treat patients under the plan would be paid for their services by the national health board, and the question of whether they would be paid on a stated-fee, per capita, or salary basis would be left to the majority decision of the participating practitioners in each health service area.

The bill's reception in the 81st Congress was bitterly disappointing to the Truman administration. Although the Democrats had gained 75 seats in the House, a coalition of anti-Truman southern Democrats and Republicans blocked most of Truman's major domestic proposals. Despite some success in housing and social security legislation, the federal aid to education bill floundered, and the administration's health insurance plan was not reported out of committee in either house.

The Democrats had their House majority reduced from 263–171 to 235–199 in the elections of 1950, and barely maintained control of the Senate by a margin of two. Attempts to have doctors' participation in the national health insurance plan voluntary had failed to placate the American Medical Association. The organization had been roused by a nationwide propaganda campaign, directed by the California public relations firm, Whitaker and Baxter, and financed by taxing every AMA member $25. The doctors had enlisted hundreds of voluntary organizations and pressure groups to oppose compulsory health insurance, holding out horrific visions of a socialized America ruled by an autocratic federal government. Ignoring the stipulations that doctors would remain free to choose their own patients, and patients to choose their own doctors, the AMA campaign pictured an impersonal medical world under the national health plan in which patients and doctors were forced unwillingly upon each other. In 1950, the AMA took the issue of "socialized medicine" to both the primary and general elections, and their propaganda was credited with the defeat of some of the Senate's firmest supporters of health insurance, including Claude Pepper (D., Fla.), Frank Graham (D., N.C.), Elbert Thomas (D., Utah), and Glen Taylor (D., Idaho).

Although Truman persisted in requesting compulsory health insurance in 1950, 1951, and 1952, his advisors agreed that after 1949 the prospects for such a broad program were bleak. Among those advisors were two Federal Security Agency officials, Wilbur J. Cohen and I. S. Falk, who had the most to do with the drafting of health insurance proposals since 1935. Wilbur J. Cohen, who in 1965 was Under-Secretary of the Department of Health, Education and Welfare, became HEW Secretary in March, 1968. Cohen was a member of the staff of the original committee that drafted the Social Security Act of 1935. He was, in 1950–52, on the staff of the Social Security Board with the Federal Security Agency, as was I. S. Falk. (Falk recently retired as Professor of Public Health at Yale University.) Recognizing the need to "resurrect health insurance" in a dramatically new and narrower form, Cohen and Falk worked out a plan that would limit health insurance to the beneficiaries of the Old Age and Survivors Insurance program. Oscar Ewing, head of the Federal Security Agency, considered this approach "terrific," and it shaped the entire strategy of health insurance advocates in the period after 1951. Thus the stage was set in early 1951 for the programs that have come to be called "Medicare." Millions of dollars spent on propaganda, the activation of a broad cleavage in American politics, the framing of choice in health insurance between socialism and "the voluntary way," the bitter, personally vindictive battle between Truman's supporters and the AMA-led opposition—these comprised the legacy of the fight over general health insurance and provided the setting for the emergence of Medicare as an issue.

THE POLITICS OF INCREMENTALISM: TURNING TOWARD THE AGED

Major shifts in the demands brought to the Congress seldom derive from dispassionate analysis of contemporary social conditions. The decision to pare down President Truman's health insurance aims to a more modest hospitalization insurance program for the aged was no exception to this pattern. In 1951 and 1952 extended discussions took place among Truman's social security advisors about how to deal with congressional reluctance to enact his administration's health program. In October of 1951 presidential assistant David Stowe outlined for Truman three ways of responding to the bleak legislative prospects for general health insurance: "softpedal the general health issue; push some peripheral programs in the area but not general insurance; or appoint a study commission to go over the whole problem." Three days later Truman accepted his staff's recommendation to create a study commission and charged them with finding "the right people." But the effort to "push some peripheral programs" had already begun, with the President's passive acquiescence. In June, 1951, Oscar Ewing, acting on the suggestions of Cohen and Falk, announced a new plan to insure the 7 million aged social security beneficiaries for 60 days of hospital care a year. "It is difficult for me to see," said Ewing to an assembled corps of reporters, "how anyone with a heart can oppose this [type of program]."

Ewing, Cohen, and Falk assumed the administration could most easily build an issue majority in the Congress by narrowing previous demands and tailoring them to meet the objections of congressmen and critical pressure groups. The major objections to the Truman health program which the Medicare strategists felt they had to meet included charges that: (1) general medical insurance was a "give-away" program which made no distinction between the deserving and undeserving poor; (2) that it would substantially help too many well-off Americans who did not need financial assistance; (3) that it would swell utilization of existing medical services beyond their capacity, and (4) that general medical insurance would produce excessive federal control of physicians, and would constitute a precedent for socialism in America. In connection with the latter objection, there was the widespread fear, grounded in the bitter, hostile propaganda of the AMA, that physicians would refuse to provide services under a national health insurance program.

To meet these objections, the proponents of "peripheral programs" turned from the health problems of the general population to those of the aged. As a group, the aged could be presumed to be both needy and deserving because, through no fault of their own, they had lower earning capacity and higher medical expenses than any other adult age group. Since the proponents wished to avoid imposition of a means test to determine eligibility within the ranks of the aged, they limited the beneficiaries to those persons over 65 (and their spouses) who had contributed to the social security program during their working life. As an additional advance concession to spike the guns of those opponents who could be counted on to assault the program as a "give-away," benefits were limited to 60 days of hospital care. Finally, physician services were excluded entirely from the plan in hopes of softening the hostility of the medical profession. What had begun in the 1930's as a movement to redistribute medical services for the entire population turned into a proposal to help defray some of the hospital costs of social security beneficiaries only.

—Excerpt from Theodore R. Marmor, "The Congress: Medicare Politics and Policy," *American Political Institutions and Public Policy: Five Contemporary Studies*, Allan P. Sindler, ed. (Boston: Little, Brown and Company, 1969), pp. 8–15.

Enacted in 1965, Medicare is a federal health insurance program for the aged, regardless of income, administered by the Social Security Administration and financed by a portion of the social security tax. It helps pay hospital costs for people age sixty-five and over (Part A) and, if the beneficiary pays a monthly premium, helps pay physicians' fees as well (Part B).

Medicaid, a health program for the poor modeled after the federal-state welfare programs, was passed, almost without notice, simultaneously with Medicare. Medicaid is administered separately by each of the fifty states, with different benefits and eligibility criteria within general federal guidelines, and paid for out of federal, state and, in some cases, local funds.

THE POLITICS OF HEALTH CARE: What Is It Costing You?

Godfrey Hodgson

Why did the field of debate about national health policy and the role of the federal government shift so sharply to the left after 1968?

In a single word, the answer given by all the experts I talked to was: Medicare. The impact of the enactment of Medicare and Medicaid in 1965 was both financial and psychological.

The fact that hospitals and doctors were reimbursed on a cost basis, under both programs, accelerated the inflation of medical costs. Medicare and Medicaid went into effect in 1966. Within two years, cost inflation had reached the proportions of a crisis. And that steep, sudden inflation exposed other weaknesses in the health system, and triggered a general reassessment of long-accepted assumptions and values.

At the same time, once the federal government was involved in paying for health care, essentially for the first time, it became both possible and necessary to ask how much further it should be involved. As Wilbur Cohen, Secretary of HEW at the time Medicare was enacted in 1965, put it to me: "The passage of Medicare broke the back of the ideological controversy over the government's role, and opened up the possibility of discussing changes in the delivery system." Robert Ball agrees:

> There has been a most remarkable change in atmosphere. I went all through the fight for Medicare, and it would have been unthinkable at that time to get stronger legislation in terms of affecting the delivery of health care. When Medicare came in it was accepted as an economic measure, as something that would protect people against the costs of medical care. It was considered as part of the pension system. The great change which began fairly soon was that people began to feel that there was a real responsibility to do something about cost; to do something about quality; and to do something about organization. Medicare was a terrific catalyst.

It wasn't long before it became plain that the cost overruns on Medicare were going to be spectacular.

Between 1966 and 1968, everything went up: hospital bills, doctors' fees, laboratory charges, insurance premiums, and even—though more modestly—nurses' and orderlies' wages. (At Massachusetts General Hospital in Boston, for example, nurses' wages went up 100 percent between 1959 and 1969; but over the same period interns' salaries went up 1650 percent!) Over the decade of the 1960's, hospital charges rose four times as fast as all other items in the Consumer Price Index; physicians' fees rose twice as fast. And that increase was heavily concentrated in the brief period after the introduction of Medicare. The rate of inflation of hospital costs, for example, increased from an average of 6.9 percent between 1950 and 1960 to an annual average of 14.8 percent between March, 1966, and March, 1970.

Some economists have argued that the primary reason for inflation was increased demand from patients. (For example, Dr. Martin Feldstein, in *The Rising Cost of Hospital Care*, National Center for Health Services Research and Development, 1971.) But the

Nixon Administration's own White Paper in 1971 commented that "while undoubtedly there were improvements in the quality of care for at least some of the population, more than 75% of the increase in expenditures for hospital care, and nearly 70% of the increase for physician services, were the consequence of inflation."

By 1969, some hospitals were charging as much as $150 a day for basic care—in effect for little more than a bed, food, and attention from a nurse when she had a moment. John de Lury, of the New York sanitation workers' union, gave a state legislative hearing a harrowing illustration of what the full cost would come to:

> A ten-year-old boy was admitted to the hospital at 3:20 A.M. The boy died at 10:34 the same night. The family of this child was charged $105.80 for drugs, $184.80 for X-rays, $220.00 for inhalation therapy, $655.50 for laboratory work. The total bill for the child was $1717.80.

With the government reimbursing whatever hospitals and doctors charged, the cost of both Medicare and Medicaid spiraled out of control. Less than *one year* after Medicare came into operation, Congress had to increase by 25 percent the Social Security tax budgeted to pay for it. The actuarial estimates of both utilization and cost presented to Congress by the Administration when the program was under construction proved to be hopelessly understated. Cost overruns, projected over the next twenty-five years, added up to a stupendous $131 billion.

Medicaid was soon in worse trouble than Medicare. Two reporters, generally sympathetic to the program, wrote that "starting in late 1966 Medicaid hit New

York's medical marketplace like a flash-flood." In January, 1967, the federal budget, assuming that Medicaid would be in operation in forty-eight states by the end of the year, predicted that it would cost $2.25 billion. A year later, however, although only thirty-seven states were receiving Medicaid, the actual cost came to $3.54 billion.

In human terms, there is no question that both Medicare and Medicaid have done incalculable good. Medicare, covering about 21 million people, paid portions of bills for roughly half of them last year; allowing for various overlaps among programs, Medicaid paid a part of the bills last year for about 16 million of the many more people who were eligible. No one can put a cash value on the lives that have been prolonged and the suffering saved as a result. But there is no denying that by pouring money into the medical system on a cost reimbursement basis, Medicare and Medicaid set off a wild inflation in costs.

The rise, however, had begun long before Medicare was enacted. The rapid spread of health insurance, both with commercial companies and with Blue Cross/Blue Shield, had been triggering an inflationary effect since the middle 1950's. Private insurance policies worked on a cost reimbursement basis, like Medicare, and far from having any deflationary control over medical practice, often encouraged *expensive* treatment. Many policies, for example, would pay for certain kinds of treatment only in a hospital, a proviso that naturally encouraged needless hospitalization.

Secondly, the acceleration of Medicare-induced inflation coincided with the general inflation of the late 1960's. Half of the inflation of medical costs, Wilbur

Cohen believes, is due to the general inflation, which in turn he blames on the Vietnam War.

In any case, a flood of new money—Medicare and Medicaid are now paying for well over a third of all health care—was poured into the system at a moment when medical costs had been rising more quickly than most other costs. No serious attempt was made either to increase the number of providers or to hold down costs by imposing controls. The result was predictable.

The inflationary effect worked differently in the two cases of doctors' fees and hospital bills. In the case of physicians' fees, what happened was what economists call a "demand-pull" inflation. Since the supply of doctors remained virtually stable, greatly increased demand meant that doctors could increase their fees (sometimes directly, sometimes by splitting procedures and thereby charging more for what would have been one appointment) and still be sure of the same volume of patients.

Some have argued that hospital costs, too, rose mainly in response to demand-pull, as an army of new users descended on overstressed resources. The argument is attractive to hospital administrators, because, if accepted, its logical corollary is that even more money should be spent on hospitals—something administrators approve of for various reasons. But while admissions to hospitals rose by 21 percent over the period from 1961 to 1969, the supply of hospital beds rose even faster, by 25 percent. Medicare and Medicaid did indeed drive hospital costs up, but not by stimulating an excess of demand over supply. In the hospitals, there was cost-push inflation.

In October, 1968, two economists, Paul S. Feldstein and Saul Waldman, correctly summarized what had happened in the *Social Security Bulletin:*

> In Medicare's first year, the financial position of the hospitals improved considerably, possibly as the result of the following factors:
> (a) increases in occupancy rates;
> (b) reimbursement to hospitals for the cost of services to some aged patients, previously provided free or at reduced charges;
> (c) reduction of losses from uncollectibles . . .
> (d) payment to voluntary and government hospitals under Medicare of an allowance amounting to 2% of allowable costs . . .
> (e) receipt of additional revenue from higher charges.

Why did charges go up? Feldstein and Waldman offered two alternative explanations:

> 1. Hospital management may have miscalculated the effect of Medicare and believed higher charges to non-Medicare patients would be needed because it expected less than adequate reimbursement under Medicare.
>
> 2. Hospital management may have decided that the early Medicare period, which was a period of unusual change in hospital finances and accounting, was a convenient time to adjust their charge schedules. (They also added a third point: some large hospitals remained in deficit even after increasing charges.)

That is a gentle way of putting it. Bill Fullerton, in Wilbur Mills's office, spelled it out more bluntly. "After Medicare," he told me, "the hospitals got paid more than before: they got full cost. And that meant that, despite all their protestations to the contrary, for the first time they were really making money. I talk to plenty of hospital administrators, and they say, 'I have a little list of things I want to do for the hospital. When Medicare came along, I could start checking them off.' "

John de Lury put it even less kindly, and still accurately:

> The hospitals with the high patient costs are the newer ones, those on the make, with brilliant reputations, with teaching affiliations. Above all they are the ones with programs of vast expansion and edifice complexes. Their rates are high to support their vast ambitions, and they are making us pay through the nose.

The strategic accommodation accepted by the Johnson Administration in 1965, in order to pass Medicare, was with the hospital people: with the American Hospital Association and with Blue Cross. (In most American cities, hospital trustees, senior medical staff, and Blue Cross boards are so intertwined that it can truthfully be said the deal was made with a single interest: "the hospital people.") Two main concessions were made. Medicare was to be financed by reimbursing costs. And the hospitals were to be allowed to choose their own "fiscal intermediaries" to check, audit, and authorize disbursement. Some chose private insurance companies. More chose Blue Cross. Given the coinciding interests, attitudes, and personal contacts of many hospital administrators and of the Blue Cross people who were supposed to be riding herd on them, it is not too harsh to say that "the hospital people" were given their own ticket to write.

They could, and did, expand their buildings, take on new staff, invest in fancy electronic equipment, make generous settlements with the unions—and could be paid whatever the bill came to by the feds, just as long as the friendly fellows at Blue Cross or at the insurance company said it was OK.

The result was a bonanza not only for doctors and hospitals but for insurers, electronic data processors, surgical dressing manufacturers, drug companies, and all the other interests which feed at the $70-billion trough of the medical-industrial complex. It was no accident that in the years immediately following passage of Medicare, the hottest of the hot stocks on Wall Street were those of profit-making nursing homes for old people. The promoter of the hottest of them all, the tactfully named Four Seasons Nursing Centers, has just pleaded guilty to the biggest stock fraud in American history: $200 million.

What made the Medicare bonanza so attractive was this no-loss proposition: the federal government was footing the bill, and the providers were adding it up. As two Tufts Medical School professors wrote in 1970: "Medicare has proved a better mechanism for insuring the providers than the patients."

Government audits have tightened up recently, and have shown how inadequate both sections of the insurance industry, the profit-making companies and Blue Cross/Blue Shield, proved at controlling costs. Massachusetts Blue Cross, for example, was given a 15 percent increase in premiums by the regulatory authority on December 1, 1970, and then filed for a further 33 percent increase on May 10, 1971. In the previous two years, modest investigation revealed the executive payroll had almost doubled. Blue Cross of Chicago was criticized by HEW auditors for using Medicare money to pay for first-class air travel and entertainment for its executives. And so it went in the commercial companies, too. In certain cases, federal auditors found that insurance companies acting as fiscal intermediaries programmed their computers to omit from cost-control checking procedures hospitals in which the companies had invested.

Two particularly baroque tales illustrate just how free and easy the spending was: the episode of the monogrammed golf balls, and the rags-to-riches saga of the Medicare Billionaire.

In Virginia, Blue Cross was named as the "intermediary" for Medicare, Part A (hospital services), and Blue Shield was the "fiscal agent" on behalf of the state for Medicaid. They were charged by the law with deciding which "providers"—mainly hospitals in this case—should be paid how much, on a "reasonable cost basis." They were then to receive, disburse, and account for the money, and apply safeguards against "unnecessary utilization of services." The government auditors' report suggests that this hardly turned out to be the main problem.

The "Virginia Blues" took on staff until the federal auditors found, two years later, that staffing was "about 23% in excess of requirements." They bought two big IBM machines, so that while the workload increased by 22.3 percent, money spent on data-processing jumped 1409.8 percent. Yet, the auditors found, the system remained "basically ineffective." Other expenditures seemed even harder to justify. Soon after getting the Medicare contract, the Virginia Blues built a new office building, and spent more than a million dollars on new furniture for it . . . from the furniture company whose sales manager was chairman of the state Blue Cross board of trustees' building committee. He did not, however, let that position influence him into giving Blue Cross undue bargains.

With no competitive bidding, Blue Cross paid $1750 each for secretaries' desks.

Medicare was also billed for at least part of the cost of entertainment for Blue Cross executives and their "clients"—it would be interesting to know whether "clients" means insurees or doctors—including "cocktails, beer, wine, alcoholic beverages, tickets for stage plays and football games and golf fees." A portion of the cost of a company picnic was charged to Medicare, including 1050 buffet dinners, two bartenders, bingo prizes, and the rental of six ponies.

The Social Security Administration's auditors commented (dryly) that "since alcoholic beverages are not considered stimulants of production and do not help to disseminate technical information, they cannot be considered allowable costs to the Medicare program."

Finally there were the golf balls. Medicare was charged with one-third of $2138.50 paid for thirteen dozen golf balls imprinted with the Blue Cross/Blue Shield monogram. Teachers and social workers are not the only ones who sometimes benefit more from programs intended to help the poor than the poor themselves do.

Shortly after his first inauguration, President Nixon announced the names of a select group of trustees for the Nixon Foundation. Most of them were either well known to be old friends of the new President, or at least heavy campaign contributors. More than one owed a good deal to the medical-industrial complex; W. Clement Stone, for example, or Elmer Bobst the Vitamin King. But one name was then quite obscure: that of H. Ross Perot.

By the end of 1969, after his elevation to the board

of the Nixon Foundation, H. Ross Perot had become a world celebrity by chartering two jets (one of them modestly christened "Peace on Earth") and flying off to Southeast Asia in a well-publicized attempt to ransom American POW's. By 1970, with stock of the Electronic Data Systems Corporation, which he controlled, selling at over $150 a share on the New York Stock Exchange, Perot's personal wealth was authoritatively estimated at $1.5 billion. No American, *Fortune* magazine guessed admiringly, had ever made so much money so quickly. But then neither Henry Ford nor John D. Rockefeller, nor even Paul Getty, had had federal Medicare funds to help him.

Perot, at one time an IBM software salesman, made his big leap in 1965 when Texas Blue Cross and Blue Shield subcontracted the data-processing work arising under their Medicare contract to the company he had founded in 1962, the Electronic Data Systems Corporation (EDS). Perot was at that time, and remained for almost a year afterwards, a part-time employee of Texas Blue Cross; he was manager of their data-processing department at a salary of $20,000 a year. Until then, EDS had been small beer. Its turnover had never exceeded $500,000 a year. The Blue Cross contract was worth $5 million; the contract ran for three years, even though Blue Cross's contract with the government, on which it depended, was for only one year. There was no competitive bidding, and while the contract between the Social Security Administration and the Texas Blues had a provision for the examination of records, the contract between Blue Cross and EDS did not. To get ready to handle this tempting contract, EDS had enjoyed a vital helping hand: a loan of $8 million from the

Republic National Bank of Dallas, whose chief executive officer was the chairman of Blue Cross.

Once into Medicare and Medicaid work, Perot and EDS never had to look back. The corporation's gross revenue rose from $1.6 million in 1966 to $47.6 million in 1970. The rate of profit on that revenue rose from 15 percent in 1966 to 41 percent in 1969, and then fell back to a mere 29 percent in 1970. By 1971 EDS was doing the electronic data-processing work for Medicare in nine states, including four out of the biggest five. Two-thirds of its gross revenues have come from Medicare and Medicaid. EDS stoutly maintains that it has processed Medicare and Medicaid claims more cheaply than they would otherwise have been processed, and this may be true. In any case, on its own showing, EDS made profits of up to 41 percent on turnover, two-thirds of which came straight out of public funds which were supposed to be disbursed on a "reasonable cost basis." In other words, in a perfectly legal manner, and in less than five years, Ross Perot was able to make himself a very wealthy man in a way that would be regarded in many other countries as incredible: by owning stock in a company that helped other private organizations decide whether the government should or should not pay out public funds for the medical care of the old and the poor.

In an atmosphere where such things were possible, it was probably inevitable that attention should turn from the mechanics of the health care system to its ethics. While the escalation of costs forced even conservatives to concede that the system faced crisis, liberals—who had largely confined themselves to quantitative and economic issues in the past—began to make more searching criticisms.

"The cost question turned the spotlight on the other deficiencies of the system," said Karl Yordy of the National Institute of Medicine. "It was not only the increase in costs produced by the fact that Medicare was on a cost-reimbursing basis," thinks Dr. Jack Geiger of the State University of New York's new medical school at Stony Brook, "it was the rise in costs, plus the failure to deliver health care, that revealed the inadequacies of the system. The push for a reassessment of the system came from the fact that the cost of health care, and the difficulty of finding primary sources of health care, were beginning to hit the white middle class."

Whatever the reason, four new interrelated lines of criticism began to be heard in the late 1960's with increasing force. Each probed more deeply than the last into the substructure of assumptions that underlay the American medical system.

- A new skepticism appeared about the value of technology in medicine; a new willingness to question an equation that had been virtually unchallenged for a generation: the assumption that good medical care means advanced medical technology.
- Institutions, and in particular the dominant institution of modern medicine in America, the hospital, became objects of increased suspicion.
- The physician's professional authority began to be challenged as never before.
- Ultimately, even the traditional ethics of medicine were called into question on issues of social and political responsibility.

—from *The Atlantic*, October, 1973.
(abridged)

REFUSED HOSPITAL BED, MAN HELD IN ROBBERY

William L. Claiborne and Alfred E. Lewis

A 70-year-old man who told police he was refused admission to George Washington University Hospital yesterday for a lack of money, was arrested 45 minutes later during a holdup of a nearby bank.

Clarence Christian Hayes, a retired house painter from Mechanicsburg, Pa., was charged with bank robbery in what police said was an attempt to get money needed for treatment of a blood disease.

Detectives said that when Hayes was told he could not be admitted unless his was an emergency case, he told a receptionist at the hospital, "I've got the money, I'll go get it."

Shortly afterward, police said, a thin, aged man walked up to a teller at the National Savings and Trust Co., 20th and K Streets NW, and handed her a note demanding $2,500 in cash.

The man, identified as Hayes, did not get out of the bank before being captured.

An FBI check on Hayes revealed that he had been arrested in a Harrisburg, Pa., hospital on Feb. 5 and charged with a $5,000 bank robbery three days earlier.

Hayes, who was freed on personal bond in that case, had used part of the $5,000 to pay hospital bills in Harrisburg, police said. About $3,500 was recovered.

Detective Sgt. Harry Noone, of the metropolitan police department's bank squad, said Hayes told him yesterday he had been hospitalized off and on over the last four years for a blood clotting condition. He came here by bus early yesterday from Harrisburg to see a physician he knew at GW.

When told the physician was not on duty, Hayes asked to be admitted to the hospital. Police said Hayes was unable to produce evidence of ability to pay hospital costs and said he was not covered by a private health insurance or enrolled in a public Medicare program.

A receptionist, police said, told Hayes that since his admission would be on a nonemergency basis, he would have to prove ability to pay.

A hospital spokesman confirmed last night that those conditions apply to nonemergency cases. But he said he was unable to explain how Hayes could not be covered by Medicare.

After telling the receptionist he would obtain the money, Hayes walked out of the hospital and was not seen there again. (The physician named by Hayes would not comment on whether he knew Hayes, saying that would violate the doctor-patient relationship.)

Police said that, aside from the Harrisburg charge, Hayes' only other known offense had been an arrest for disorderly conduct in the 1940's.

—from *The Washington Post*, March 22, 1972. (cited in *Materials on Health Law . . . Medicare*, Volume 6, Part A, Health Law Project, University of Pennsylvania Law School, 1972)

MEDICAID MILLS: Ping Pong Rebounds

Barbara Caress

"What is exhilaratingly revolutionary about Medicaid is neither the program's more generous enrollment of the medically indigent, nor even its delightful smorgasbord of comprehensive health services. No, Medicaid's critical innovation lurks elsewhere—in its exclusively assigning to the Health Department the heady tasks of standard setting, surveillance, and enforcement of quality in every aspect and every locus of publicly funded, personal health care."

—Dr. Lowell E. Bellin
Former Executive Medical Director,
Medicaid
New York City Department of Health
At American Public Health
Association convention, Nov. 1968

Mrs. Gloria King went to the Davidson Medicaid Building for treatment of migraine headaches. She saw a doctor. "He told me to stop taking the birth control pill I was using. Then he referred me to a podiatrist." The podiatrist took X-rays of her feet and diagnosed the cause of her headaches as ingrown toenails. He removed the toenails from both her big toes and Mrs. King has been in pain ever since.

Nine years after the inception of the Medicaid program, Mrs. King and other patients in the Bronx have tired of waiting for Dr. Bellin's "exhilarating revolution." They have joined the Morris Heights Ad Hoc Committee for Better Health Care.

Since the beginning of the Medicaid program in 1966, newspaper reports documenting instances of malpractice and outright fraud at neighborhood Medicaid clinics have made headlines. From time to time, local health and welfare officials have announced new programs to curb abuses. But the Morris Heights Committee is the first to attempt to organize patients to challenge such abuses.

MEDICAID FINANCING

The problems of neighborhood Medicaid clinics stem from the way New York City finances medical care for the poor. Last year the City reimbursed providers $1.3 billion. Three-quarters of this impressive sum went to hospitals and nursing homes. Only eleven percent, $145 million, was paid to private doctors, dentists, podiatrists and optometrists.

Most Medicaid payments for ambulatory care are on a fee-for-service basis—the more patients seen, the more money received. In New York City Medicaid pays private doctors $7.40 for the patient's first visit and $6.00 for every visit thereafter. In contrast, outpatient clinics at voluntary hospitals are typically reimbursed at more than five times this rate. For example, Montefiore Hospital in the Bronx is paid $40.24 for each visit and Mount Sinai in Manhattan $46.66. True to form, the municipal hospitals receive a lower rate than most voluntaries ($33.71), although much more than the private doctors. Thus Medicaid's ambulatory program is primarily a funding mechanism for hospital outpatient departments, helping them to cut their losses on outpatient care. At the same time, though, it does provide a way for a few doctors willing to practice bad medicine in poor neighborhoods to reap a financial windfall.

MEDICAID MILLS

These inequities in reimbursement schedules when combined with a fee-for-service system produce Medicaid mills—privately owned, profit-making neighborhood health facilities. The system puts a premium on quantity, not quality. A solo practitioner who must pay all of his costs from Medicaid payments—rent, equipment, salaries, etc.—can hardly be expected to deliver decent care at the rates currently in effect. A Medicaid doctor would have to see over 10,000 patients a year to earn a salary of $40,000 per year, the average for a U.S. doctor. As a result, doctors cut costs by turning to group practices in poor neighborhoods, which in turn become Medicaid mills.

Medicaid mills are usually organized by one or two enterprising individuals who buy or lease a building, often a storefront, and rent space to other practitioners. In some cases the tenants pay a fixed monthly rent, as is customary in New York City. But, typical of the spirit which permeates these operations, many landlord-doctors charge rents on a sliding scale based on the number of patients their tenant-doctors see. The more patients seen or recruited, the lower the rent.

Another way Medicaid doctors increase their income is through a practice graphically called "ping-ponging." One doctor in a clinic refers a patient to another, whether the referral is medically necessary or not; the second doctor then sends the patient back and so on. This practice of I'll scratch your back, you scratch mine drives up the volume of patient visits, resulting in Medicaid money for the doctors and many unnecessary appointments for the patient. For example, in the Bronx, nearly every patient entering the Davidson building, regardless of complaint, was sent to the podiatrists.

Medicaid patients use these facilities because they are all that is available to them. Only 2,000 of the 19,000 practicing physicians in New York City earned any appreciable amount of income from Medicaid (see chart). Nearly all of these doctors practice out of one of the 362 profit-making neighborhood clinics. Of these doctors, 280 (about 10 percent) made over $50,000 last year from Medicaid alone.

PHYSICIANS IN N.Y.C. RECEIVING SUBSTANTIAL AMOUNTS FROM MEDICAID, 1973

Number	Amount
580	$ 5,000–$ 10,000
560	10,000– 20,000
567	20,000– 50,000
220	50,000– 100,000
60	over $100,000

New York Medicine—March 1974, page 96

THE MORRIS HEIGHTS AD HOC COMMITTEE

Within the last half dozen years Morris Heights, a neighborhood in the Bronx, has changed from middle-class Irish and Jewish to predominantly Third World—45 percent Puerto Rican and 45 percent Black. A substantial minority of the residents are welfare recipients and slightly more are covered by publicly funded health programs (Medicaid and Medicare). The 45,000 people of Morris Heights are served poorly by two municipal hospitals, Fordham and Morrisania. Both hospitals are badly deteriorated and difficult to reach. Thus, because the neighborhood falls between the cracks of the City's public hospital system, it is ideally situated for the establishment of private Medicaid clinics. Twelve have now sprung up.

In March, 1973, the Morris Heights Improvement Association, a coalition of block associations and tenants groups, formed an Ad Hoc Committee to investigate the practices of Medicaid offices. The group was composed of eight people, four of whom were Medicaid patients. One full-time paid organizer from the Improvement Association, Roger Hayes, was assigned to work with them. Surprisingly, their first task was to identify the clinics in their area, a difficult chore because storefront offices are not licensed as group practices (they are called "shared facilities" by the Health Department) and practitioners often have separate billing addresses elsewhere. Even the Health Department does not have a complete list of these facilities.

The Ad Hoc Committee, after locating the eight clinics then in operation, finding out the doctors' names and specialties, their hours and equipment, began interviewing patients: "Do you know what you are being treated for? What drugs were you given? Why? Did you see more than one doctor? Do you know why? Does the clinic keep a record of your health status?" Within two months, the Committee had generated enough community interest to hold a public meeting.

PATIENTS TESTIFY

Two of the local clinic doctors/administrators were invited to the meeting to hear the testimony of their patients. They hesitated, but when the Committee threatened to picket their storefronts, they came. The complaints they heard included:

• Unnecessary referral from one doctor to another (ping-ponging). Mrs. Peggy Pierson went to the Davidson Avenue Center for a backache. "They suggested plastic surgery for my nose. Then they wanted to check my feet, my eyes, the whole works."

• Endless visits for specious medical problems. Mrs. Rose Ann Frey was told to come back every three weeks to have her "tilted uterus" examined.

• Patients poorly examined and given inappropriate drugs. Mrs. Angie Reyes took her son to the University Avenue Medical Group. Dr. Malba examined the child quickly, diagnosed a bad cold and prescribed ampicillin. Since he did not get better, Mrs. Reyes took Daniel to Presbyterian Hospital. After a spinal tap, he was found to have spinal meningitis. He was admitted to the hospital and stayed ten days.

• Incomplete or nonexistent medical records. Mrs. Sally Williams was being treated at the Davidson Avenue clinic for asthma. The same drug was given to her a second time although she had gone into anaphylactoid shock after the first administration. "The next thing I knew, I woke up in the Fordham Hospital emergency room."

• Non-Medicaid patients charged high fees for nonservice. Mr. Henry Leisin went to the University Avenue Medical Group to take care of a mole on his face. The clinic manager collected $15 from Mr. Leisin before he saw a doctor. The visit with the doctor lasted less than one minute. He was referred to Bronx-Lebanon Hospital. On his way out Mr. Leisin asked for a receipt. The manager resisted, saying, "You don't want a receipt." Mr. Leisin left in disgust.

The two doctors present at the meeting were asked to sign an agreement which specifically prohibited the above practices, most of which in any case violate Medicaid regulations. They balked and agreed to sign only if the other clinics in the neighborhood did likewise. By mid-July, the Committee had coerced and cajoled seven of the eight clinics into signing. The one recalcitrant clinic was picketed.

Fundamental to the Committee's strategy was the notion that the clinics were basically business ventures and vulnerable to the same tactics used to influence other neighborhood businesses. Because there were so many clinics in close proximity in Morris Heights, the Committee could exploit competition between them for the patients' benefit. Picketing was viewed as a way of putting economic pressure on the noncomplying clinic. People entering the storefront were asked to boycott it and take their Medicaid business elsewhere. This strategy is, of course, of limited value if none of the available facilities are delivering decent care.

The New York City Department of Health, which had initially encouraged the Ad Hoc Committee, sent medical auditors to check out the clinics. This was pursuant to their responsibility "to develop and maintain a system of continuing review of the quality and extent of care provided Medical Assistance [Medicaid] recipients" (*New York State Medical Handbook*). The City Health Department, however, does not have the capacity to audit Medicaid facilities on a regular basis. In fact, it can only perform two audits a week on New York's 362 Medicaid clinics. So teams are sent out only in response to specific complaints, such as those from Morris Heights.

The auditors found the services in Morris Heights to be about average for such facilities—a devastating comment on the quality of such clinics. Copies of the audits were turned over to the Committee. The Health Department report cited such violations as cockroach infestation, "prescribing in small amounts so as to increase the number of patient visits," illegible and incomplete medical records and "unnecessary referrals."

With the Health Department audits in hand, the Ad Hoc Committee went to see the administrators of several of the clinics. They accused the doctors of violating the agreements signed with the Committee since the audits clearly documented the continuation of abuses. They threatened these clinics with picket lines if the violations were not corrected. Only one of the clinic administrators refused to see the delegation. All of the others cleaned up their clinics and eliminated some of the more glaring conditions. The storefront which refused to discuss the situation with the Committee was picketed every Saturday for several months. In addition, the suburban homes of two of the doctors were picketed.

Later on, the Committee investigated collusion between some of the storefronts and local pharmacies. First they surveyed drug prices. They found enormous discrepancies in prices which seemed related to the location of Medicaid mills. For example, forty 250 mg. tablets of ampicillin cost $16.95 in a drug store adjacent to a Medicaid office and $3.50 at a store further away.

The drug price survey and other informational

leaflets were distributed to people entering and leaving Medicaid offices. One entitled "How Good A Patient Are You?" encourages patients to ask for comprehensive and continuous care. For example, it questions, "Do you ask to see the same doctor on every visit? If the doctor tells you to return to the clinic, do you know why? Do you make sure that the doctor knows your complete medical history?" Other leaflets were information and evaluation sheets for patients to use as a basis for judging the quality of care they were receiving.

ONE YEAR LATER

By March, 1974, the Morris Heights Committee concluded that their strategy of patient education and pressuring clinics with Health Department audits and picket lines was not enough. They felt they had made some inroads into the Medicaid situation and that community people looked to them as a watchdog and complaint bureau. One of the organizers commented that "At least the people identified with the Committee are getting better care. They think twice now about ripping off patients." But, they felt services delivered in storefront clinics were still not very good and could not be made better without the intervention of other forces. They called another public meeting to chart their future course. The group demanded that the Health Department, which had sent representatives to the meeting, follow up its audits and impose sanctions on clinics found in violation of standards of good medical practice.

Dr. Lowell E. Bellin, New York City's Health Commissioner, contends that he does not have the statutory authority to enforce standards of care. He tempers this legal assessment with political hesitancy. "We want to put pressure on sufficiently so we can reform them, if we put too much pressure we can drive them out completely." It is difficult to tell if Dr. Bellin is more concerned about his legal limitations or considerations of political realities. His recent action ordering the Bureau of Standards and Evaluations to stop distributing audit reports to community groups leads one to believe that the "problem" is a political one.

Paul Brandt, chairman of Bronx Community Planning Board 5 and an active supporter of the Ad Hoc Committee, feels Bellin is side-stepping the issue. "The Health Department has a statutory responsibility as administrator of the Medicaid program to assure that the services are of good quality. Besides being a public health menace, the Medicaid mills are a tremendous drain on the taxpayer." The Ad Hoc Committee does not believe that the Health Department has brought all of the authority it currently possesses to bear. Bellin's argument might or might not be accurate, but the City has never behaved in a way to test it out. Despite its rhetoric of good intentions, the Health Department has had only minimal impact on Medicaid mills—witness the audit which found the Morris Heights clinics on a par with other Medicaid practices.

The Ad Hoc Committee does agree with Bellin that some new and strengthened regulations are needed, and they have joined him in lobbying in the State Legislature and City Council. They see this as a major focus of their current program. Some of the changes proposed included expanding the legal definition of group practices so Medicaid mills fall under customary licensing requirements, limiting the number of patients a doctor can bill (currently the City will reimburse for up to 50 patients a day), prohibiting rent agreements based on the number of patients seen, requiring facilities to maintain central records and increasing the penalties for noncompliance.

Of course, all of these changes may be fine, but they are dependent upon the ability and willingness of the Health Department to enforce standards and penalize violators. Dr. Bellin before becoming Health Commissioner was Executive Medical Director of New York City's Medicaid program from 1967 to 1972. A few practitioners were prosecuted for fraud and some claims were disallowed. But for the most part his track record in that job does not inspire confidence in the idea that if a few laws are changed, giving the Health Department more power, Medicaid patients would get better care.

For the time being the Ad Hoc Committee has hitched its star to Bellin's legislative program. Their experience with the Health Department before Bellin's installation was one of close cooperation. But under Bellin, the Department seems to have a different agenda and is responding to political pressures often inimical to consumer interests. The reform of Medicaid mills is not high on the agenda of the Health Department. Of course, public agencies have never been adverse to using community struggles to their own ends. And Bellin has openly advocated this position. In speaking of community boards he has said: "In the 1970's one can hardly begrudge the poor the indulgence of serving on boards. . . . The experienced administrator should theoretically be able to work quite comfortably within the mandates of the board's broad policy and claim quite accurately that he is responsive to the will of the community."

—From the Health/PAC *Bulletin*, May/June, 1974.

HOSPITALS FOR SALE (and Other Ways to Kill a Public Health System)

Elinor Blake and Thomas Bodenheimer

On a cold November day last year, 68-year-old Daniel Gibson—poor, disheveled, unable to walk—was turned away from the emergency room of a privately-owned Medical Center Hospital in Butte County, California. Nineteen hours later Gibson died of pneumonia. If he had gotten sick two and a half months earlier, Gibson would have been welcome at Butte County Hospital, where the indigent traditionally were cared for. But the county had closed its hospital on August 23, 1973, and Gibson became the victim of a new and ominous trend in the nation's collapsing public health system.

County hospitals, long maligned for their endless waiting lines, dirty and crowded wards, and rushed and impersonal treatment, are on the way out. And 20 million "medically indigent" Americans, those who fall in the crack between Medicaid and health insurance, have no place to go. These people—the seasonal farmworkers, the black maid who earns $60 a week, the small owner whose business is failing, the warehouse loader out of work six months a year, the single alcoholic ineligible for welfare—are all dependent on public hospitals.

In California alone, 12 out of 50 county hospitals have recently closed or been sold; 10 or more are likely to disappear within a year. Chicago's Cook County Hospital came within a hairsbreadth in 1970 and '71. New York City has initiated plans to close or lease up to 7 of its 19 municipal hospitals. In Florida, Massachusetts, North Carolina and Wisconsin, public hospitals, formerly open to everyone regardless of ability to pay, have gone private.

Last year, Boston's Mayor Kevin White massively cut the budget at Boston City Hospital and eliminated hundreds of jobs. Facing community protests, the Mayor's response was, "Some of you people may have to die."

Like so many other new trends, you can see it best in California. San Diego's county hospital was turned over to the University of California in 1966, Sacramento went the same route in 1973, and Orange County is scheduled to follow. San Francisco is debating a plan to turn its hospital into a quasi-private corporation. In a number of smaller counties—Butte, Colusa, Kings, Madera, Nevada, Santa Cruz, and Solano—hospitals have already closed down. Profit-making companies are now running the former hospitals of Merced and Siskiyou counties. San Mateo County plans to close its hospital this year. And every other county has tightened up bill collecting, and drastically slashed the number of medical services you can get for free. When the dust settles, California's public hospital system will be largely dismantled.

TWO-CLASS HEALTH CARE

Since 1855, county governments in California have been legally responsible for the health care of the poor. The oft-cited law on the books sounds fine: "Every county and every city and county shall relieve and support all incompetent, poor, indigent persons, and those incapacitated by age, disease, or accident, lawfully resident therein, when such persons are not supported and relieved by their relatives or friends by their own means or by state hospitals or either state or private institutions." But in fact, until recently, county hospitals were open *only* to the medically indigent. Those able to pay were referred to private doctors and private hospitals. This was first established in 1933, when a group of Bakersfield doctors successfully sued Kern County General Hospital for admitting paying patients. In essence, California courts ruled that county hospitals were not to compete with the private ones, but only to fill in the gaps. Doctors' incomes were protected—and public hospitals cut off from a source of much-needed money.

The 1965 Medicaid Law (called Medi-Cal in California) was supposed to provide state and Federal money for the health care of the poor, thus relieving the burden of hard-pressed cities and counties. But for California's counties, it wasn't that simple. First, the counties had to pay a big hunk of the Medi-Cal budget through yearly lump-sum payments to the state. Second, Medi-Cal encouraged patients to gravitate toward private care. This left county hospitals with the poor and unemployed who were ineligible for Medi-Cal.

So in the California legislature, the counties won passage of an all-important clause in the Medi-Cal law: the "county option." The state agreed to pay all expenses for county hospitals above the base year 1964–65. For example, if a county spent $20 million for its hospital in 1964–65 and spent $30 million in 1968–69, the state would pay the additional $10 million. According to Gordon Cumming, former Sacramento County hospital administrator and the law's author, "The county option is the best deal the counties ever got." It meant that the hospitals could buy new equipment and hire new staff, and the state would pick up the tab. The Medi-Cal law also overturned that previous court decision and allowed private patients in county hospitals. For a brief time, everything looked rosy.

SICK PEOPLE, EMPTY BEDS

However, the dream of Medi-Cal's creators never materialized. Governor Ronald Reagan soon limited county options funds so severely that hospitals were never able to make the improvements they had hoped for. And then Reagan ushered in the Seventies by appointing head of Medi-Cal a young, 29-year-old ex-flight surgeon and Vietnam hero by the name of Earl Brian, Jr. To celebrate his first day on the job, Brian announced a package of devastating Medi-Cal cutbacks. He followed up with more radical cuts in December, and masterminded a new restrictive Medi-Cal law in October 1971. Glorified as the "Medi-Cal Reform Act," this law spelled doom for county hospitals.

Although it placed more people on Medi-Cal, the Reform Act at the same time abolished the county option, made counties give more to the Medi-Cal budget, and gave their hospitals back less. Los Angeles County, for example, suddenly found itself having to pay over ten million extra dollars—ten percent of its county hospital's budget. Since hospital costs are shooting up rapidly, the renewed burden is a heavy one. More than anything else, this shift back to local support has made county governments anxious to get rid of their hospitals.

When Brian's Medi-Cal Reform Act forced counties to foot a bigger bill for their hospitals, the counties found surprises. Not only had budgets soared, but many hospitals were half-empty. Kern General had a 1971 occupancy rate of 61 percent, Merced General 51 percent, Santa Clara 59 percent, Santa Rosa 42 percent, Fresno 42 percent, Yolo 32 percent, Kings 24 percent.

What on earth was happening? The main thing, it turns out, is that patients are staying in the hospital less time. Some hospitals have sent their chronic patients back home or to nursing homes, Medicare and Medicaid are pressuring hospitals to get patients out, since these programs have to pay the bills. The average length of stay has dropped dramatically in some county hospitals; San Francisco's fell from 13.2 to 7.1 days in nine years.

The same thing is happening to private hospitals. On May 10, 1971, the *San Francisco Chronicle*'s front page proclaimed an "Empty-Bed Crisis for SF Hospitals." The article could have been written in Boston, Los Angeles, Minneapolis, Seattle or Denver. Everywhere the length of stay is dropping, as is the number of people admitted.

But there is another curious factor behind the crisis in private hospitals: there are too many of them. There was a great wave of private hospital building in the 1960s, far more than the country needed. According to the *Wall Street Journal* (November 2, 1971), "The number of beds in general-care hospitals has grown about three times faster than the nation's population," shooting up 33 percent from 1960 to 1971. Even the former executive director of the American Hospital Association, the private hospitals' own lobbying group, said "There are too many hospital beds in this country, although the Association would never want me to say so publicly."

Private hospitals have always exploited their public counterparts. In the past, when they have had plenty of patients, they have taken the ones who could pay, and sent non-paying and "undesirable" patients to public hospitals. [See Chapter 4.]

With the empty beds now in private hospitals, however, the relationship may be reversed. Rather than using public hospitals to dump non-paying patients, private hospitals are looking to them as a source of money. There is tension between a private hospital's wish for more paying patients and its desire to pick and choose which patients are cared for. In California, some private hospitals are getting out of this dilemma by pressuring county governments to close most or all of their hospitals and to contract with the privates instead for the care of the poor. But the poor are still going to lose.

SIX WAYS TO KILL COUNTY HOSPITALS

With climbing costs and empty beds, public hospitals have become a burden that California counties would like to get rid of. There are several ways this can be effectively done, ways which have been tried in various parts of the country. California is doing them all.

• *Closing Down*: Madera County, in the heart of the agricultural Central Valley, is one of California's poorest. Yet in 1972 the Board of Supervisors closed down the county hospital, declaring, astoundingly, that the county no longer had medical indigents. It was a bit like the proposal once advanced that the U.S. should get out of Vietnam by declaring the war had been won.

About the same time, the new private Madera Community Hospital opened across town, but patients without money or insurance were turned away. In fact Madera Community Hospital actually put patients in ambulances and sent them 25 miles south, across county lines, to a public hospital in Fresno. Madera patients even showed up at Merced General Hospital, 30 miles to the north, prompting Jay Akin, Merced's administrator, to suggest that "Someone ought to sue the hell out of them."

In Tulare County, south of Fresno, the hospital is in limbo. Tulare's Board of Supervisors wanted to close the hospital on February 1, 1973. But in late 1972 hundreds of people stormed a Board meeting to demand the hospital remain open. They presented a petition with several thousand signatures. In response the Supervisors waffled by doing what besieged politicians always do: they created a committee to study the situation. However, they did not commit themselves to improving the hospital's inadequate services, and its fate is uncertain.

Next-door Kings General Hospital was closed in Summer 1973. Dr. Paul Murphy, the hospital's retired medical director, suspects that a private hospital played a role: "Sacred Heart wants the county's money but they don't want the county's patients soiling up their marble floors. They're making the laundry into an out-patient clinic, building little cubicles, you know. They'll have the poor patients go in and out through the back door." And Santa Cruz County, 100 miles south of San Francisco, closed its new $2.5 million hospital in July 1973, just five years after it was built.

• *Contracting Out*: Another way to close a county hospital is to do it in pieces. One of the chief guises for this is called "contracting out"—whereby communities make agreements with private hospitals to take county hospital patients.

In Los Angeles County, contracting out is a hot issue. The county already does it to some extent, but the privates want more patients for their empty beds, and, more important, want the county to guarantee that patients who don't have Medicaid or Medicare will be covered. It's the old story: paying patients or no patients. Dr. John Affeldt, the county's Medical Director, is apprehensive, "Privates will pick and choose patients and reject those they don't want. It could destroy the basic core of the county hospitals. We'll lose our staff and deteriorate. You can destroy the county hospitals little by little and you'll never be able to get them back." However County Health Services Director Liston Witherill claims that total contracting out is many years away because "the county has no money to pay the privates."

Though ideal for private hospitals, contracting out is a problem for money-starved county governments. The private sector is far more expensive than public hospitals, and counties just aren't going to pay for everyone. Again, the poor are squeezed out.

• *Medical School Transfers*: If you've ever been a public hospital patient, you've probably seen doctors going from bed to bed through your ward, stopping at the interesting cases, followed by groups of medical students. Medical schools have traditionally affiliated with county hospitals: the school provides doctors, and the county supplies the hospital, the other staff, and the patients. Although the medical school controls how the patients are treated, it doesn't have to worry about paying for it.

But now things are changing. In San Diego and Sacramento, the University of California is taking over the entire operation of those counties' hospitals. And in both cases, the major reason was the county's desire to get out of the hospital business.

The San Diego transfer took place in 1965, but no one has yet made any provisions for the medically indigent, many of them Mexican-Americans, up to at least ten percent of the county's 1.3 million people. Some patients are simply turned away. Others receive care but are unable to pay the bill. But untold numbers are intimidated and never seek care in the first place. An assistant administrator at University Hospital explains that even on emergency admission, "We negotiate with the patient about how he'll pay." If he doesn't pay within six months to a year, the bill is sent to a collection agency. According to the former county hospital administrator, Dr. W. W. Stadel, the University handles patients "like any other private hospital, making some arrangement for payment. Before Medi-Cal, many private hospitals took some charity cases; now no hospitals do. Those patients are in worse shape than five or ten years ago."

Even though people are treated like private patients when it comes to paying the bill, they don't feel like private patients when they are getting medical care. Almost everyone who goes to University Hospital continues to call it "county hospital." Waiting lines are still long; it takes three weeks to get appointments in the clinics; and patients don't have a personal physician but go to several of the 57 specialty clinics. It is still assembly-line medicine. There is still a two-class medical system, and University Hospital is the one for the poor.

The main problem with Sacramento Medical Center (the county hospital) was that no one wanted to run it. From 1966 through 1973, the nearby medical school of the University of California at Davis had a traditional affiliation with the Center, of the you-provide-the-patients-and-money, we-provide-the-doctors nature. By 1970, however, Administrator Gordon Cumming, anticipating the death of the county option, approached the University about taking over the hospital entirely. But the last thing Davis Dean C. J. Tupper wanted was to run the county hospital in Sacramento. Tupper and his research-minded faculty had been hoping for a superspecialty hospital on the Davis campus. Not only was the Sacramento Medical Center a long drive from the Davis campus but the hospital's image would attract poor people, not specialized private cases from all over the region. But Administrator Cumming had other ideas.

On November 30, 1971, the Board of Supervisors gave notice that its affiliation agreement with the University would be canceled in one year. The University had two choices: either take over the hospital or leave. Fearing financial headaches for the county, Cumming's posture had been: "We'd better kick the University out on the street. They can pack their microscopes and set them up on the curb." While Cummings never really intended to throw the University out, the medical school, with no other teaching facility, couldn't take any chances. So the University agreed to take over a hospital that Dean Tupper claims it didn't really want.

The potential conflict was resolved—at the expense

of poor patients. More than 15 percent of the hospital's patients are unable to pay their bills, and in the past the county wrote them off. But a March 1972 document, part of the transfer arrangement, states that "the University would reserve the right to refuse care to any patients, particularly to patients the cost of whose care is not guaranteed by the county." And University of California Vice-Chancellor Elmer Learn admitted, "We're going to have to operate pretty much like a private hospital; if a patient can't pay he won't be admitted." He added regretfully, "Patients may have to sell their homes to pay for care. We can't deprive a student of his education to finance a patient who can't pay." Since the transfer, non-emergency patients are required to place a cash deposit before admission. There will soon be cash registers in the emergency room.

• *Private Takeovers*: Siskiyou County, on the Oregon border, is sometimes called California's Appalachia. With its closed-down mines, scattered wooden shacks and abandoned cars, it could be eastern Kentucky. In 1968, the county board of supervisors leased its hospital to a nonprofit corporation controlled by some of the hospital's doctors. Oddly enough, the hospital had begun making a profit for the county the year before the lease. The doctors then contracted with Beverly Enterprises, a Los Angeles profit-making hospital chain, to manage the hospital. Rumors are rife that the doctors hold stock in Beverly. Beverly receives $75,000 per year in pure profit from the hospital, and is said to extract another $150,000 from the exploited county through its nursing home, Beverly Manor. And the county is required to perform major repairs on the hospital: $40,000 last year and an expected $50,000 next.

The hospital is widely feared and disliked. Many people will go 50 miles north or south to get treatment elsewhere. There are dozens of examples of patients waiting for hours in the emergency room for a doctor to arrive, and of dangerous and unnecessary surgery performed for money. One county resident observes: "There are plenty of medically indigent people here. They know that treatment at the hospital costs them a lot of money. So they don't go until they absolutely have to."

Four hundred miles to the south, Merced County has just signed a similar management contract with National Medical Enterprises, another profit-making hospital chain.

• *Hospital Corporations*: San Francisco, also anxious to separate its hospital from city/county government, is debating another scheme, the quasi-public corporation. Under this plan, a corporation is formed with directors appointed by city or county government, and that corporation runs the hospital with money from Medicare, Medicaid, private insurance and a contribution from the city for its medically indigent. San Francisco has spent thousands of dollars on a feasibility study—ironically, since everyone regards the model for the corporation idea, New York City, as a failure. Even the blue ribbon State Study Commission for New York City concluded in 1973 that the corporation has made "no substantial progress in improving patient care" since it started three years ago. Top administrators at the corporation's hospitals warn that things are worse than ever. And New York City's financial contribution to the corporation has dwindled so much that the corporation is suing the city for more money.

Since San Francisco General is the only county hospital in California which still provides absolutely free care without bills to significant numbers of poor people, the possibility of a corporation takeover—with its inevitably strict billing and collection practices—is especially pernicious.

• *Tighter Billing*: Free health care—an idea on the rise around the world—is dying in California. In 1957, only 20 out of 47 county hospitals sent bills to all patients however rich or poor; the others only billed patients with incomes above a certain level. But by 1960, a new technique was used: In all but ten counties, new patients were required to sign a property lien. The lien stipulated that, if the patient's house or other property were sold either before or after the patient's death, the county would collect the hospital bill out of any money earned from the sale. The hospitals never were able to collect much from this procedure, because collection from people totally unable to pay does not stand up in court. Moreover, many who signed property liens had no property in the first place.

But in recent years, some county hospitals in California have begun to act more like privates in their billing. Los Angeles County, with 35 percent of California's population, is an example. In the 1950's Los Angeles sent bills only to people above a certain income level. The level was usually determined by an eligibility worker, based on diagnosis, cost of care and the patient's resources. Following Medi-Cal, however, Los Angeles County began to bill everyone and is now studying methods to do so more efficiently. That means gearing up the county collection agency.

WHAT'S TO BE DONE?

Despite its flaws, the public health-care system should be preserved and strengthened. Those 20 million people without Medicare, Medicaid, or private health insurance depend on public hospitals and simply cannot afford private care. Erosion of Medicare and Medicaid programs is continuing, and a truly comprehensive national health insurance law is many years away. Moreover, private hospitals, immune from public pressure, have a history of refusing "undesirable" patients —alcoholics, drug addicts, and the chronically ill—even if they have Medicaid cards. The privates have done this whether or not a public hospital exists in the area. There is little reason to believe that they will change.

Had the 1966 Medi-Cal tax money been used to improve the county hospitals, there would now be new buildings, adequate staff, high occupancy rates, and decentralized out-patient care in neighborhood clinics. Instead, money went to the private sector to care for the poor, supposedly making the public system unnecessary. The result? Private doctors, nursing homes and hospitals extracted every cent they could from Medi-Cal, inflating prices 250 percent in six years. Private hospitals used the money to grossly overbuild, creating white elephant buildings with empty beds. Now the counties are bearing the brunt of the private sector's greed. Not only must they care for the many and expensive rejects from private care, but they have less state and federal money to do so. In self-defense, counties are billing people who can't possibly pay, or, alternatively, are getting out of the hospital business altogether.

Private hospitals have always been richer than the public ones. From the beginning, they have had contributions from rich churches or philanthropists, with private doctors to admit paying patients. It is the usual up-or-down spiral characteristics of an economic system based on private capital: institutions and individuals who start out with money can always attract more money, whereas those without money remain impoverished.

As long as a small, underfinanced public system coexists with a large, wealthy, private one, there will be competition for paying patients, doctors, money and powcr. And the private system will win. Thus the struggle to preserve the public system is more than the preservation of a rundown, half-empty, understaffed city or county hospital. It means fighting to divert resources from private to public control. It means attacking private hospitals when they take public money but leave behind the public responsibility to care for everyone. Eventually it means forcing the new, well-staffed local private hospital to become public.

—From *Ramparts* magazine, February, 1974. (abridged)

9

Health Maintenance Organizations (HMO's)

Health maintenance organizations offer their members comprehensive health services, including physician visits and hospitalization, in return for advance payment of a fixed annual fee. Thus HMO's turn the incentive of the fee-for-service system on its head: whereas under the fee-for-service system more services mean more income, under the prepayment system, fewer services mean more income.

The first selection in this chapter is an excerpt from the original proposal for HMO's by Dr. Paul Ellwood and his associates. As the article makes clear, the Ellwood proposal was frankly an effort to stimulate a free-market economy in health care as an alternative to national health insurance legislation. The second selection, by Michael B. Rothfeld in *Fortune* magazine, surveys the state of development of HMO's and gives them business's stamp of approval as a profitable source of investment income that, through fixed annual patient fees, would "hitch the profit motive toward a new goal in medicine: keeping the cost down." The possibility of increasing the role of private enterprise in the health-care delivery system was certainly a plus for HMO's in the eyes of the Nixon Administration. (To many others their profit-making potential is disturbing in light of the conflict between profits in medicine and decent patient care. See Chapter 4 on "Profiteering in the Health System.")

But the main appeal of HMO's to the government, which has created bipartisan support ranging from Republican former HEW Secretary Caspar Weinberger to Democratic Senator Edward Kennedy, is the possibility they hold out of cutting the federal health budget while establishing a rational system for delivering primary and preventive care to the American people.

The cost-cutting aspect of HMO's, however, is in potential conflict with their patient-care possibilities. HMO's are supposed to encourage providers to cut their costs and raise their income by preventing illness. As the Health/PAC editorial on HMO's points out, however, the payment of fixed fees may not encourage preventive measures, as desired, but rather may encourage providing as few services as possible—hardly a prescription for good medical care.

The editorial thus returns the focus of discussion back to patient care, the critical test of this or any other health proposal. The final selection in this chapter, continuing from this vantage point, is a comprehensive study of the Kaiser-Permanente Medical Plan, the oldest and largest HMO in operation and a prototype of the HMO's proposed in federal legislation. As authors Judy Carnoy, Lee Coffee and Linda Koo point out, the Kaiser Plan does keep costs down slightly—in part by restricting access to its services through understaffing and long waits, and in part by enlisting subscribers who are generally younger and healthier than average. Thus the most serious objection to HMO's points to their fundamental nature as a large corporate institution. With finances foremost among its concerns such an institution is not an appropriate setting for the delivery of high-quality, personalized health care.

HEALTH MAINTENANCE STRATEGY

Paul M. Ellwood, Jr., M.D., Nancy N. Anderson, Ph.D., James E. Billings, M.A., Rick J. Carlson, J.D., Earl J. Hoagberg and Walter McClure, Ph.D.

The Nixon Administration must make a major decision on its strategy for dealing with the much proclaimed health crisis in America. It can either

—Rely on continued or increased Federal intervention through regulation, investment, and planning, or

—Promote a health maintenance industry that is largely self-regulatory and makes its own investment decisions regarding resources such as facilities and manpower.

Presently, the Federal government is following the first strategy with these results:

> The Federal government is the dominant voice in deciding how much money will be invested in medical schools (it pays 60% of the bill), the mix of dollars expended for training different types of health manpower, and how many new hospitals will be built.

> The Federal government is fostering a planning structure at regional, state, and local levels through which panels of citizens can decide where facilities will be located and who will do what in medical care.
>
> An inflation-prone health industry is pushing the Federal government toward increasing regulation of hospital costs and physicians' fees (and perhaps beyond that to wage regulation generally).
>
> Faced with rising demand created by Medicare, Medicaid, and the growth of private insurance coverage, the Federal government is trying to decide how many dollars it can and should invest in expanding the capacity to deliver health care. If the demand for medical care is escalated by inauguration of national health insurance, existing resources for delivery would be severely taxed, leading to additional Federal regulation, and perhaps ultimately to a nationalization of health care delivery, at least to the poor, the aged, and rural residents.

We propose a shift from the present Federal regulatory, investment-planning strategy to a strategy that would promote a health maintenance industry.

The health maintenance strategy envisions a series of government and private actions designed to promote a highly diversified, pluralistic, and competitive health industry in which:

> Many different types of Health Maintenance Organizations would provide comprehensive services needed to keep people healthy, offering consumers—both public and private—a choice between such service and traditional forms of care.
>
> Services would be purchased annually from such organizations through Health Maintenance Contracts (capitation), at rates agreed upon before illness is incurred, with the provider sharing the economic risk of ill health.

NATIONALIZED HEALTH INSURANCE

Two far-reaching proposals for reform are currently being discussed: nationalized health insurance and public ownership and management of health care organizations. National health insurance is compatible with the health maintenance strategy but, while it would remove financial barriers to receiving care, it would not solve problems of cost, availability, and quality. Experience with Medicare and Medicaid has shown that a major increase in demand does not stimulate reorganization of the industry (although it does raise costs). Moreover, the experience of other nations suggests that national health insurance may even reduce the likelihood that basic improvements can be introduced.

Even if public ownership of the health system were politically or philosophically tenable, there is good reason to believe that public ownership would further complicate existing problems of cost and quality. Although public ownership might facilitate a more equitable distribution of services, the industry would still require basic reorganization, and in all likelihood a publicly owned system would produce impersonal and immovable bureaucratic control.

THE NEW STRATEGY: A HEALTH MAINTENANCE INDUSTRY

The alternative proposed here—the health maintenance strategy—is based on the promotion of a highly diversified and competitive health maintenance industry. Internal self-regulation would be encouraged by providing economic and professional incentives directed toward maintaining health rather than merely providing services when illness occurs. It is essentially a market-oriented approach in which medical care is delivered by organizations.

The health maintenance policy is expected to substantially lessen the Federal government's role in the planning and management of health programs, and therefore, should not be regarded as "just another Federal health program." Federal health programs are often based on the premise that it is essential to increase the government's responsibility for making decisions that would otherwise be made in the private sector. The health maintenance policy reverses this process of government intervention by encouraging the evolution of organizations that manage themselves in accord with clear and precise Federal policies. If experience should indicate that regulating certain aspects of the industry is desirable, appropriate measures can be initiated. However, undue initial regulation of the health maintenance industry would frustrate its growth without providing definitive proof of its potential advantages.

HEALTH MAINTENANCE CONTRACTS

The operation of health maintenance organizations is contingent upon the health maintenance contract—the key feature which assures that these organizations will deliver health services more efficiently and effectively than conventional providers. By this contract, the health maintenance organization (HMO) agrees to provide comprehensive health maintenance services to its enrollees in exchange for a fixed annual fee. The consequences of this contract to both the consumer and the provider are vital to this strategy. The economic incentives of both the provider and the consumer are aligned by means of their contractual agreement, which assures that the provider will share the financial risk of ill health with the consumer. Since the economic incentives of the contracting parties are identical, both would have an interest in maintaining health. Moreover, the health maintenance organization guarantees that services will be made available to the consumer, unlike conventional insurance plans which merely guarantee reimbursement for services, if the consumer can find them.

CONCLUSIONS

The health maintenance strategy would apply the economic leverage of the Federal government's purchasing power and its persuasive influence to create a competitive health industry in which health services increasingly would be provided by HMO's. The strategy assumes that HMO's are capable of producing services more economically and effectively than conventional providers by integrating and coordinating the many elements of health care, through the incentive of sharing the economic risk of illness with their subscribers.

The emergence of a free-market economy could stimulate a course of change in the health industry that would have some of the classical aspects of the industrial revolution—conversion to larger units of production, technological innovation, division of labor, substitution of capital for labor, vigorous competition, and profitability as the mandatory condition of survival. Under such conditions, HMO's would have a vested interest in regulating output, performance, and costs in the public interest, with minimal intervention by the Federal government.

Most important, the health maintenance strategy

offers a common cause for the collaboration of the professional, public, and private enterprise sectors of the health industry in alleviating the medical care crisis in a rational and timely manner, as a feasible alternative to a nationalized health system.

—Excerpt from *Medical Care*, Vol. 9, No. 3, May/June, 1971.

SENSIBLE SURGERY FOR SWELLING MEDICAL COSTS

Michael B. Rothfeld

Early on a January evening in 1970, a half dozen physicians and officials of the Department of Health, Education, and Welfare held an urgent private meeting at Washington's Dupont Plaza Hotel. Their concern was the rapidly rising costs of medical care, which already had helped to cause an ominous $2-billion cost overrun in the Medicare and Medicaid programs. When the group broke up at 2:00 A.M., the seed had been planted for a whole new national health strategy, and a new term—Health Maintenance Organization (HMO)—had been coined to identify the key element in the plan. In essence, the idea was simple and sensible: why not give doctors more incentive to keep people well, and especially to treat illness before it requires costly hospitalization, instead of paying them mainly to cure the sick?

In the three years since the meeting, HMO's have expanded and proliferated throughout the nation at an unprecedented rate. They are beginning to introduce modern management methods into an $80-billion business that lacks them. And they are bringing some advantages of competitive enterprise to a field that has long restricted competition in the name of medical ethics. Most important of all, HMO's are demonstrating that they can help reduce the cost of medical care.

A $12.5-BILLION INDUSTRY

Three years ago some thirty medical organizations—basically prepaid medical-group practices—could be classified as HMO's. Today there are nearly sixty with an enrollment of about eight million clients; an additional eighty HMO's are in various stages of development. Provided that Congress and the states adopt favorable enabling legislation, government and private sources figure that as many as 50 million people could be enrolled by the mid-1980's. Blue Cross alone hopes to have 280 HMO's in operation by then—enough to give every policyholder the option to join one. With no allowance for inflation, all this expansion would create a $12.5-billion industry inside what is expected to be a $150-billion health market.

The HMO idea is winning support from a surprisingly wide variety of sources. Both the Committee for Economic Development and the AFL-CIO have strongly endorsed the concept. Major employers, including AT&T, and such unions as the United Auto Workers have begun offering employees and members the option to enroll in an HMO. Thirteen states now permit Medicaid recipients to join. One of them is California, where HMO's expect to enroll nearly 500,-

000 Medicaid patients by this autumn. In California, Arizona, and Minnesota, the organizations are vying with one another to sign up union, government, and employer groups.

Not only Blue Cross but several large commercial insurance companies, particularly Connecticut General Life Insurance Co. and the Equitable Life Assurance Society, have made significant commitments to HMO's. C.G. has established a subsidiary to help operate them in Maryland, New York, and Arizona. Equitable recently helped to organize and recruit clients for a new HMO at the prestigious Lovelace-Bataan medical complex in Albuquerque. Sensing a growing demand for large-scale health-care systems, a few industrial companies are exploring ways to put their financial, legal, and managerial talents to use in HMO's. Westinghouse, for example, is studying the possibility of starting one in Florida.

Perhaps the strongest impetus to the expansion of HMO's has come from Washington. In both his 1971 and 1972 health messages, President Nixon not only endorsed the concept but said HMO's "ought to be everywhere available so that families will have a choice" about their health-care system. Reflecting Nixon's interest, the Department of HEW in 1971 established a Health Maintenance Organization Service. By the end of last year [1972] the service had distributed $26 million in planning and development grants or contracts to some eighty-five potential HMO sponsors. Service officials have also made considerable effort to promote the idea among banks, Wall Street investors, and physicians. Despite the current pressures to cut the federal budget, the Administration wants to increase its grants for HMO development to $60 million during the next fiscal year.

THE LURE OF A FREE CADILLAC

HMO's, as President Nixon has pointed out, "are motivated to function more efficiently." Patients save time because physicians, labs, and pharmacies are organized within a system, often under one roof. Clients choose a family physician, but most HMO's also have night office hours and at least one doctor on duty twenty-four hours a day. The fixed-price contract overcomes the consumer's reluctance to seek medical advice for minor ailments. The HMO also permits doctors to spend more time with patients because the administrative staff copes with much of the paper work that may consume as much as a quarter of a physician's time.

An HMO can be pretty attractive for doctors in other ways, too. Many physicians have a large gross income, but it must cover office rent, clerical and technicians' salaries, malpractice and other insurance, and payments to the bank that has financed expensive medical equipment. Additional money must be set aside to provide for retirement. After business expenses, the median pretax income of physicians is estimated to be about $42,000. Salaries in HMO's average $35,000 to $40,000. However, most HMO's offer $5,000 to $10,000 of fringe benefits such as liberal retirement plans, profit sharing, and life and malpractice insurance. To recruit new doctors, HMO International in Los Angeles even offers them the free use of a company-leased Mercedes or Cadillac.

SHIFTING THE EMPHASIS TO THE DOCTOR'S OFFICE

By far the most important advantage of HMO's is that their fixed annual fees hitch the profit motive toward a new goal in medicine: keeping the cost down. HMO's buy drugs and other supplies in bulk. They pare expenses by operating their own diagnostic labs, having specialists on their staffs and, often, facilities for minor surgery. HMO physicians have a personal incentive to cure ailments before the need arises for expensive hospital treatment. In addition to their salaries, many HMO doctors draw a year-end bonus that depends upon how much profit or surplus the organization earns. One HMO even assesses its doctors penalty payments if there is a deficit.

A $2-MILLION ENTRY FEE

While there are many advantages in an HMO once it is running, reaching that point is always a difficult and at times exasperating process. It often takes an investment of at least $2 million, an effort of two to four years, and an enrollment of at least 20,000 for a completely new HMO to break even. The sponsor usually must hire a staff, acquire facilities, and incur big selling costs before significant numbers will enroll.

The ability to raise large sums of money is crucial. In the past, most of the organizations have been funded initially by physicians, charities, consumer groups, bank loans, or private bond placements. But as a rule, an HMO cannot raise enough money by any of these means to permit quick expansion to an efficient size. Even worse, when borrowing saddles an HMO with big fixed payments, unexpected delays in starting up can lead to serious cash-flow problems. The new interest shown by insurance companies will help to overcome such difficulties, but if HMO's are to spread and grow as rapidly as Washington envisages, they will need to find new sources of capital.

One possibility, so far used by only one major HMO, is the stock market. Dr. Donald K. Kelly's HMO International went public in 1969 through a merger with Medicalab Management Corp. of Los Angeles, whose shares were already traded over the counter. Having expanded rapidly since then, the company and its subsidiaries and affiliates now run twenty-one facilities in southern California, with 110,000 clients. Last fiscal year, consolidated revenues jumped to $8,800,000 from $3,200,000 in 1971, and profits nearly quadrupled to $500,807. In two years the bid price of HMO International shares has jumped from $1 to a recent high of $22.

To attract equity capital, an HMO obviously would have to be a profit-making operation. Unfortunately, this idea becomes quite an emotional issue among otherwise rational people. Some think health care is contaminated by the very idea of profits. Others, such as the AFL-CIO, like to belabor profit-making HMO's with examples of the corner cutting that has occurred in some nursing homes and hospitals run for profit. Critics contend that profit-seeking HMO's would be under pressure from shareholders too interested in making a fast buck. As a result, enacted or pending legislation in several states favors nonprofit HMO organizations, and the Pennsylvania law flatly limits the field to nonprofit corporations.

THE AMA PUTS ON THE PRESSURE

In a move that is even more important than their funding provisions, the HMO bills before Congress (except for the Administration's) would remove such [HMO] groups from the jurisdiction of state insurance departments and would override other restrictive state laws. Financial stability would be left to the marketplace, although periodic reports would be made to the Secretary of HEW. The legislation would also set up quality controls; the Kennedy bill goes so far as to establish a National Commission on Quality Health Care Assurance.

The passage of such federal legislation would open the way for a rapid expansion of HMO's. That legislation has received the endorsement of almost every interested group but organized medicine, which is trying to block or at least to delay passage of these bills. A House committee staff member says: "We've had more pressure from the AMA on this issue than on anything since Medicare."

The AMA is certainly correct when it asserts that not all of the data on HMO's are in. HMO's will indeed be difficult to develop in areas with low population density. Some critics argue that their costs should come down, on the ground that they may provide *too much* care. And it's clear that even if HMO's can decrease hospital admissions, the underlying causes of cost inflation in hospitals would remain to be tamed.

Still, the trend in medicine these days is toward more organized systems, in group practices and in full-time hospital-staff practice. All the serious studies so far support the conclusion that when well managed and properly financed, HMO's can sharply reduce the cost of care at a level of quality at least equal to that of the fee-for-service system, while earning a decent return for lenders and investors. And HMO's will pay an important social dividend: they will provide access to better medical care for millions of Americans who have never had that opportunity.

—From *Fortune*, April, 1973. (abridged)

HEALTH/PAC EDITORIAL: HMO's

When *Forbes* and *Fortune* magazines run successive articles contending that health maintenance organizations (HMO's) are "sensible surgery for swelling medical costs," we know that big business is interested. When the supermarket magazine *Family Circle* publishes a story entitled "Is There An HMO In Your Future?" we realize that the official word is spreading to the American people.

Yet most Americans don't understand the HMO concept. An HMO is a health-care organization which is intended to provide comprehensive services to a voluntarily enrolled membership at a prepaid fixed fee. Usually an HMO is affiliated with one or several hospitals. It may be funded privately, publicly or by a combination of both; it may be for-profit or non-profit. Doctors can practice full-time or part-time within the HMO, and can be salaried or paid fee-for-service.

One of the most successful HMO's is the Kaiser-Permanente medical-care program, a prepaid group practice which has been operating in California for over 30 years. Kaiser's membership in California, Portland, Hawaii, Denver and Cleveland exceeds two and a half million.

Other HMO models have emerged that are different from Kaiser. Most notable are the foundations for medical care, created by private doctors. [See "PSRO:

Doctor Accountability or Consumer Disaster?" in Chapter 10.] A foundation, unlike Kaiser, is not a visible institution but simply a mechanism through which paper and money flow. Care is provided in private doctors' offices and hospitals where the doctors have admitting privileges. Patients pay insurance companies, insurance companies pay the foundation, and the foundation pays the doctor or hospital on a fee-for-service basis.

The main success that HMO's can claim is cost reduction. Kaiser can provide a package of services at lower cost than identical services would cost in "mainstream" medicine. The way in which an HMO reduces cost is by lowering the use of services by its members. Kaiser members, for example, spend half as many days in the hospital as a similar population of Blue Cross/Blue Shield subscribers. And the amount of surgery performed by Kaiser compared to fee-for-service practice is distinctly lower.

In the case of hospitalization and surgery, which most Americans are subjected to in dangerous and costly excess, HMO's can perform a positive service. But HMO's will also tend to lower the availability of services that are not presently performed in excess. At Kaiser, ambulatory care is not easily accessible—large numbers of patients complain of several-week waits for appointments, of rushed impersonal treatment, and of being unable to find and keep a personal physician.

Thus HMO cost reduction goes hand in hand with a general inaccessibility of services. The reason for this is the workings of the profit motive. Whether for-profit or technically nonprofit, private corporations have always committed themselves to maximizing their income, reducing their expenditures, and using the surplus for expansion. The profit incentive leads private HMO's to limit services by hiring an inadequate number of physicians and other personnel so that patients will be discouraged from seeking care. In this way, expenses go down and surplus goes up.

HMO's, then, take the profit incentive of fee-for-service medicine and turn it on its head. Whereas fee-for-service doctors and hospitals make more money by seeing more patients, performing more operations and hospitalizing people longer, HMO's increase their net income by doing less. Either way the situation can be deleterious to people's health.

Besides the conflict between cost reduction and availability of services, private HMO's oriented primarily toward their surplus income are actually unable to cut costs significantly over the long run. For equivalent services, Kaiser costs less than Blue Cross/Blue Shield, but Kaiser's rate of cost increase is just as great as, or greater than, the national rate of increase. Thus HMO cost reduction is a one-shot affair; if the entire health system switched next year from fee-for-service financing to HMO financing, the costs of care might dip down, but would then inflate as rapidly as ever. Within a few years any cost reduction would be virtually canceled out.

Again the reason is profit. Each provider and supplier of service—whether the construction company, the manufacturer of the EKG machine, or the doctor—will raise prices as fast as possible in order to make more money.

If HMO's are no long-term answer to cost rises, do they solve the other components of our health crisis? Here the answer is even simpler—they do not. Even within HMO's, care will be fragmented as long as specialists so heavily outweigh the number of general providers of care. HMO's can do nothing to attract doctors and other health personnel to rural and ghetto areas. HMO's will not open their doors to people unable to pay. And evidence suggests that even when lower-income people are insured, they have a far harder time getting care from the HMO than does the middle class.

Finally comes the myth of health maintenance—that it's cheaper for an HMO to prevent disease than to cure it. In the short run, that's just not true. Annual Pap smears, breast exams, blood pressure checks, glaucoma screening and other valuable early diagnostic procedures cost money and require more medical personnel. The savings—in reduced numbers of seriously ill patients—come only many years later (if then), far beyond the projections of corporate accountants and planners. Only with large federal grants has Kaiser offered multiphasic screening exams to many of its subscribers, and with cutbacks in the grants, Kaiser is reducing the screening. In HMO's as within "mainstream" medicine, acute illness will always take precedence over preventive care.

People who believe that HMO's should be publicly controlled and service-oriented rather than privately run and profit-oriented have two courses of action. They can try to set up local health plans publicly controlled by the users and employees. Community groups across the country are planning or even actually establishing their own HMO's. But the capital requirements needed to start, and the enormous time and energy spent on technical proposals, plans and contracts are almost prohibitive. It is the rare community that will put together a plan that it really controls without being indebted to a lending institution or a group of doctors. The alternative is a struggle for areas of power in private HMO's—for community positions on the board, for employee meetings in specific clinics and hospital wards, and for public airing of planning documents and financial transactions. In either case, HMO's will increasingly be foci of community and health worker action in the health system.

—From the Health/PAC *Bulletin,* November, 1973.

CORPORATE MEDICINE: The Kaiser Health Plan

Judy Carnoy, Lee Coffee and Linda Koo

"I want to see a thousand of these health centers all over the country," declared Henry J. Kaiser in 1950. Well, it would warm Henry J's gravestone if he knew that today his name is linked with the most important health care reform in a troubled America. The Kaiser-Permanente medical-care program operates throughout most of California, up to Portland, out to the Hawaiian Islands, into Denver and east to Cleveland.

Kaiser-Permanente (K-P) has its proponents and its critics. K-P, which is group-practice based, has stopped hospital overutilization and cut costs, supporters claim. Critics counter that Kaiser provides "assembly-line medicine" and, because it cuts cost, care is mediocre. Many California subscribers think "Kaiser's not good, but it's the best around."

Kaiser certainly differs dramatically from traditional American medical care. People buy insurance from the Kaiser Foundation Health Plan usually through their union or place of employment. But the insurance is good only for care offered at K-P's own hospitals and clinics.

When Kaiser members get sick, they call the nearest Kaiser facility and make an appointment—with their personal physician if they have one, or frequently with whatever specialist seems appropriate. Because appointments are often hard to get, people needing immediate treatment can go to the drop-in-clinic or emergency room. Those desiring a physical check-up are referred to the multiphasic screening unit for a battery of tests with a follow-up doctor visit. Generally Kaiser covers many more medical services than most private insurance, and leaves fewer deductibles and other out-of-pocket payments for the patient. Another important and innovative feature at Kaiser is that doctors are paid on a salaried rather than fee-for-service basis.

While Kaiser administrators and researchers have written extensively about Kaiser's positive achievements, a critical study is needed to sort out the successes from the failures and to address certain questions: Why is a large corporation like Kaiser Industries, traditionally engaged in construction, mining and aerospace, associated with a health plan? Is K-P really nonprofit? Does it truly keep down the costs of medical care? And how do its subscribers feel about the care they receive?

KAISER-PERMANENTE'S BEGINNINGS

Kaiser-Permanente sprouted in a field of cement: the colossal dam construction of the '30's. Hoover, Grand

Coulee and Bonneville dams were all built by Kaiser Industries under government contracts.

In 1933, more than 5,000 Kaiser workers were cutting a canal to carry fresh water from the Colorado River's Hoover Dam to Los Angeles. The project spread over 400 square miles of desert, and injuries or sickness meant a 200-mile trip to Los Angeles. Because of the distance, Kaiser built medical facilities in the nearby area.

Henry Kaiser made an agreement with Sidney Garfield, an enterprising young doctor in Desert Center, California, to set up a prepaid medical service. Initially, Kaiser paid the Desert Center Hospital and physicians a certain amount to cover industrial injuries. Later, the workers could voluntarily put in a nickel-a-day payroll deduction for general medical services.

When Kaiser moved on to the Grand Coulee Dam project, Garfield followed and continued his prepaid medical plan. For the first time, workers' families were given full medical coverage, wives for seven cents a day and children for twenty-five cents a week.

The Government Helps Out At the onset of World War II the market for dams slackened, and Henry Kaiser turned to shipbuilding. Again using government contracts, Kaiser organized shipyards in California, Oregon and Washington, employed 200,000 people, and turned out fully 35 percent of all U.S. merchant vessels made during World War II. As a result, Henry J was dubbed by many as "Sir Launchalot."

These shipyards were the basis for the first expansion of the Kaiser medical empire. In order to keep his men healthy, Henry Kaiser built clinics at production sites in Oakland, Richmond, Vancouver and at the Kaiser steel mill in Fontana, California. "The financing of these clinics was provided out of government contracts, since their cost was accepted by the authorities as a bona fide operating expense. After the war the clinics and their equipment were declared surplus war property. The Kaiser Hospital Foundation was established by Kaiser and his wife, Bess, to buy them at 1 percent of cost." [1]

With the shipyards closed and the Kaiser workforce plummeting, the health plan was opened to the public and renamed the Kaiser-Permanente Plan. (The name Permanente was Bess Kaiser's idea; Henry's first cement plant was located on the Permanente Creek.) Thus at government expense, the K-P medical-care plan was begun.

Henry Kaiser's Philosophy Henry Kaiser's expansion into the health field wasn't just "one of his crazy ideas," as many critics thought. During the New Deal years, the air was filled with federal and state proposals advocating compulsory health insurance. This movement was strongest in California where over a dozen progressive health bills were introduced during the late '30's and '40's.

A strong advocate of private enterprise, Henry Kaiser in 1942 publicly warned, "If the doctors fear socialized medicine, if industry is anxious about the widening powers of the state, why not venture now, boldly, into the activity that will forestall the super-planners in their schemes to direct medical services into the channels of distributive bounty?" [2]

In 1945, Henry Kaiser began a national campaign for his new prototype of health insurance. He modestly proposed that the Federal Housing Agency guarantee 10 percent of local bank loans to nonprofit groups that wanted to set up facilities for prepaid hospital care. The AMA called Kaiser's program "socialized medicine." Kaiser countered that his prepaid medical projects would operate as "business enterprises motivated by the impelling force of competition."[3]

But Kaiser did not need any legislation. His visions came true much faster than people expected. By 1955, K-P had over 500,000 subscribers.

KAISER IS BIG BUSINESS

Whether Kaiser physicians or subscribers like it or not, Kaiser-Permanente is part of the Kaiser Industries empire and is largely controlled by it. Kaiser Industries consists of about 100 active companies including Kaiser Aluminum and Chemical, Kaiser Steel, Kaiser Cement and Gypsum, Kaiser Engineers and Kaiser Aerospace and Electronics.

Of the 17 persons on the board of directors of the Kaiser Foundation Health Plan and Hospitals, eight represent Kaiser Industries. Most prominent is Henry Kaiser's son, Edgar, who is chairman of the boards of both organizations. Kaiser Industries' representation on K-P was even stronger a few years ago, but as K-P became more successful and secure in its West Coast position, it began responding to public pressures of the '60's and added non-Kaiser people with little power. As public relations man Dan Scannell quipped, "Now we have a Black, a woman and an Oriental on the board."

Many people ask why a successful business would want to get involved with all the problems of health delivery. Dr. Clifford Keene, president of the Hospitals and the Plan, as well as a board member of Kaiser Industries, sums it up in saying, "the unparalleled corporate interest in health and medical affairs . . . arose out of the needs and interests of the Kaiser companies over the past 30 years."[4] We can only speculate what these needs and interests are.

Kaiser and Taxes In 1948, Henry Kaiser set up the Kaiser Family Foundation which is entirely distinct from the Kaiser Foundation Health Plan. In doing so, Henry "seemed more interested in providing a vehicle for tax planning and estate management than in execution of a charitable program," according to a study by the usually staid Twentieth Century Fund.[5] In fact, the Kaiser Family Foundation, the 27th largest foundation in the U.S., plays a key role in the control of Kaiser Industries by members of the Kaiser family.

The Kaiser Family Foundation is now the single largest owner of Kaiser Industries stock, with a controlling share of 32.7 percent. The next largest block of stock, 8.5 percent, is owned by Edgar Kaiser, chairman of the board of Kaiser Industries. Currently, Edgar is also a trustee of the Family Foundation. The Family Foundation's income from Kaiser Industries' stock is tax-free. So Edgar can make a large, taxable personal income from his own shares, and keep control over Kaiser Industries through the tax-free Family Foundation shares.

Specifically, the Family Foundation provides capital to the Kaiser Foundation Medical Care program to assist its expansion in California and into new regions of the U.S.[6] The Foundation donated $3.5 million to start a Kaiser-Permanente program in Cleveland, and $2 million for one in Denver. Seed money for the Oregon and Hawaii ventures also came from the Foundation. To insure that control of the Family Foundation never leaves Kaiser hands, all of the trustees of the Family Foundation are past or present members of the boards of both Kaiser Industries and Kaiser-Permanente. (Interestingly, for a while K-P directly owned $2 million of Kaiser Industries stock, but sold its shares in 1970.) The Family Foundation has received most of its stock from bequests in the wills of Kaiser family members—in 1951 after the death of Bess Kaiser, in 1961 after the death of Henry's youngest son, and in 1967 following the death of Henry himself.

Kaiser Industries also receives a small, but direct benefit from K-P's continuous hospital and clinic construction. Kaiser Engineers, a wholly owned subsidiary of Kaiser Industries, designs most of the hospitals and many of the materials used for construction are Kaiser's. One example comes from Redwood City, California, where a building inspector explained, "Of course Kaiser Industries builds their hospitals, and they specify in their contracts that it uses their own materials." [7]

Kaiser's Growth "Growth is a way of life for the Kaiser-Permanente Program," states the K-P 1969 annual report. Most subscribers don't even know that 4 percent of their premium plus a minimum of 15 cents per member per month is budgeted for expansion.

Why does K-P expand? One important reason was expressed by a K-P planner: "As long as we keep expanding, our patient population won't get too old. If we remain static, our average patient's age will get older and older and then we'll be in trouble economically. This way every time we get a new union or a new factory, we get only the people who are working now and are in good health; not the retirees and the people who've had to quit because of a disabling disease."[8] This is good "business sense," because the older one gets the more medical services are required. Also at Kaiser, the longer one is a member, the easier it is to know and utilize the system. As one Kaiser nurse explained, "The longer you're at Kaiser the more you realize that you can get immediate care by demanding and shouting either on the phone or in the clinics." Clearly, it is more economical for Kaiser to have a continuous stream of new subscribers who don't know how the system works.

HOW THE KAISER HEALTH PLAN WORKS

Who Subscribes? Two and a half million people belong to Kaiser. The Northern and Southern California regions each account for well over a million, with the remaining 300,000 scattered in Oregon, Hawaii, Ohio and Colorado. Yet, as Kaiser's own analysis shows, its membership by no means resembles the general population.[9]

Kaiser families had an average income of $11,309 in 1967 and 1968, while data show southern California families averaging incomes of $10,421. Kaiser tends to enroll healthier people avoiding the burden of those who need medical care the most—the chronically ill, elderly and poor. In the words of Kaiser's own economists, "we are younger and relatively under-represented in certain population groupings, for example, the unemployed, the indigent, the wealthy, the self-employed, and people living in rural and other non-metropolitan areas."[10] It should be noted that Kaiser is no different than private insurance companies in skimming lower-risk people from the population; commercial insurers in southern California, for example, have an even younger and healthier population than Kaiser.

Comprehensive Benefits Kaiser's benefits are relatively comprehensive compared to other health insurance plans. Generally all subscribers receive hospital services, outpatient care with lab tests and X-rays, drugs, eye exams, physical therapy, ambulance service, emergency care and maternity care (after 10 months of membership). However, different members have different plans, depending on the costs of the monthly premiums. A more expensive plan might include psychiatric service and long-term care; a cheaper plan might charge the patient for certain services and limit the number of hospital days.

Currently the health plan does not cover attempts at "suicide or other intentionally self-inflicted injuries or illnesses [this would include overdosage of pills]; drug addiction; alcoholism; conditions covered by Workmen's Compensation; military-service-connected conditions; custodial, domiciliary or convalescent care; cosmetic surgery; corrective appliances and artificial aids; extensive neuromuscular rehabilitation and conditions resulting from a major disaster or epidemic." Also, if a member is injured or taken ill while temporarily more than 30 miles from a Kaiser hospital, Kaiser will pay for treatment in any hospital.

Low-Income Care By dabbling in small projects for low-income people and publicizing these projects far beyond their worth, Kaiser is trying to change its middle-class image. The best-known effort is the Portland OEO (Office of Economic Opportunity) program for 1,200 low-income families. Similar tiny programs were opened in southern California and Hawaii. Kaiser is rightfully proud of the fact that the poor were cared for on an equal basis with regular Kaiser subscribers. Of course, Kaiser received ample funds for its projects; in addition to paying the premiums, OEO provides money for patient transportation, home care, staff training and other social and outreach services. You can bet that these extras will disappear with OEO.

Charity Begins at Home A very small number of the medically indigent—people without insurance, Medicare or Medicaid—get into Kaiser. On the average, according to a Health Plan representative, only 1 percent of any one hospital's inpatients are non-Plan subscribers and have no insurance coverage. They are financed by the individual facility's Medical Social Assistance Account.

In the past the percentage of charitable cases was much higher. The 1961 K-P Annual Report dedicated a page to charitable care nobly stating, "The Community Service Program places special emphasis on charitable care. . . . This charitable care program is designed to assist persons or families the social service workers describe as 'medically indigent.' They become 'medically indigent' in the face of heavy hospital or medical bills. . . . Any clergyman, community welfare agency representative, doctor or nurse may refer these 'medically indigent' cases to Kaiser Foundation Hospitals."

Today Kaiser is far less generous with community services and rarely talks about the individual medically indigent. The community service funds allotted for "charity, research and education" are largely funneled to physicians for individual research projects. This arrangement enables Kaiser to create a "university atmosphere" for many of the "academically inclined" doctors. As one San Francisco doctor said, "Research money is our sanity money. It gives us a half day or so to be away from patient care."

QUALITY OF CARE

The most important aspects of medical care are most difficult to measure. Only a few studies of Kaiser's quality of care have been done. Most useful are (1) a 1972 study by Milton Roemer and others on comparative utilization rates, costs, attitudes of patients, and quality of care under three major types of health insurance plans (Blue Cross/Blue Shield, private insurance company and Kaiser),[11] (2) an examination by Nolan, Schwartz, and Simonian of social-class differences in the utilization of pediatric services at the Oakland Kaiser clinic,[12] and (3) the California Council for Health Plan Alternatives [CCHPA] (a union-sponsored organization) and the Medical Committee for Human Rights [MCHR] 1973 mail questionnaire study of consumer satisfaction among 10,000 members of the Northern California Carpenters Union who subscribed to the Kaiser Plan. (Because only 24 percent replied to the questionnaire,[13] this study must be viewed only as an indication of consumer feelings.)

The findings of these studies will be discussed below in analyzing whether K-P meets its own standards for quality care. Dr. Clifford Keene, as President of the Kaiser Foundation Health Plan and Hospitals, has stated,

> the criteria for judging quality in medical care are the degree to which it is available, acceptable, com-

prehensive, continuous, and documented; and the extent to which adequate therapy is based on an accurate diagnosis rather than symptomatology. I would add the criterion of dignity—the dignity accorded the recipient of services, and the dignity of style of the providers of services.[14]

Availability Almost everyone agrees that the U.S. suffers from a shortage of doctors. But no one is sure just what the proper ratio of physicians to patients should be for optimal care. Kaiser views one physician per 1,000 members as the ideal, but does not achieve its goal. In fact, Kaiser's physician-to-members ratio is lower than the physician/patient population ratio of the states in which Kaiser is located. The ratio of paramedical personnel to patients is also lower at Kaiser, which employs an estimated two persons per patient compared with 2.8 nationally in "short-term hospitals."

Doctors per 100,000 Population—1969 [15]

	State Ratio	K-P Ratio	Percent Difference
Northern California	161	102	—36
Southern California	161	90	—43
Hawaii	133	83	—38
Oregon	128	67	—49

Understaffing causes limited access for Kaiser subscribers. The usual complaint among Kaiser subscribers is waiting on the phone to make an appointment, waiting until an appointment is available, and waiting at drop-in and emergency clinics. Thirty percent of the CCHPA/MCHR respondents wait over one month for an appointment and 27 percent wait from one to two hours to see a doctor at a drop-in clinic.

The telephone appointment procedure is the crucial entry point into the Kaiser system. All calls for appointments are handled at a circular central appointment desk around which sit a number of clerks. In the center of the desk is a huge electrically controlled lazy-Susan filled with all the physicians' individual schedules so that each clerk can handle any appointment for any patient to any physician.

This all appears rather efficient. So why do subscribers chronically complain about long telephone waits of up to an hour? The answer lies in Kaiser's "numbers game."

In northern California, Kaiser's administration has decided that each appointment clerk should be able to handle 25 calls an hour or an average of five and a half to six physicians' calls. The clerks find this impossible to do. Doing their best, each clerk handles about 150 calls a day. The clerks not only care for the patients' needs, but also shuffle calls to other departments. It is almost as if Kaiser deliberately wishes to make access difficult.

If the appointment procedure is sometimes a problem for patients, it is also no joy for the appointment desk clerks. The supervisors of the appointment clerks, who realize that the administration's goals are unrealistic, attempt to do their best. Each supervisor has a panel with automatic counters and red lights which flash on and off. The panel shows how many calls have been taken every hour by each worker, how many have been lost ("lost" calls are patients who hang up in dismay), and how many are waiting at any particular moment.

Another problem facing many subscribers is that they live too far from the nearest Kaiser facility. Among patients sampled at the Oakland pediatric drop-in clinic, Nolan et al. found 22 percent of patients making daytime visits and 53 percent of those making evening visits had a transportation problem.[16]

Lack of access causes many subscribers to seek, and pay extra for, care outside Kaiser's facilities. Fifty-five percent of those who answered the CCHPA/MCHR questionnaire have used non-Kaiser medical services since joining K-P. Seventy-eight percent of these people must pay for these outside services.

Roemer and his colleagues found that 12 percent of the services used by subscribers in a 12-month period took place outside the Kaiser facilities. However, there is no report on the number of subscribers involved. Certainly far more than 12 percent of the subscribers used these outside services.

When broken down by income, Roemer's study showed that families earning under $11,000 seek more out-of-plan care than do families earning over that amount, especially for maternity care. The researchers suggest that lower-income families may go out of Kaiser more often "because of some dissatisfactions or . . . because they have not learned to 'work the system' efficiently. . . ." [17]

It is difficult for any Kaiser subscriber to "work the system," but the general problems of Kaiser come down hardest on people who have previously never been given the opportunity to navigate the health system. Kaiser's outpatient services are organized with a white, middle-class bias. Blue-collar families utilize K-P services considerably less than do white-collar families. Roemer showed that in a three-month period, members of blue-collar families made only 662 doctor visits per 1,000 subscribers, but for white-collar families the rate is 954 per 1,000.[18]

Utilization also differs considerably between whites and nonwhites. Nolan reports that "more than half the visits made by white children were to the appointment clinics, but only one-third of the visits made by Negro . . . children were to the appointment clinics. . . . Slightly more white patients came for health supervision (school examinations) than for acute conditions . . . among Negroes, for every preventive visit there were two for acute conditions." [19]

Acceptability Kaiser members like the prepayment method of financing health care more than commercial plan holders like the fee-for-service system. But prepayment does not necessarily result in equal use of services by families or in equal sharing of costs. Nonutilization is actually an indirect way of subsidizing the care received by the users of services. If there is a greater degree of nonutilization, as the Nolan and Roemer studies show, by lower-income groups enrolled at Kaiser then they are subsidizing the upper-income groups who use the services more extensively.[20]

Attitudes toward medical care received at Kaiser are less positive than attitudes towards Kaiser's financing. K-P's own study, conducted by the Field Research Company, comes up with some startling figures: "In both past and present surveys," according to Greer Williams, "only half of the members interviewed were satisfied with procedures in K-P clinics, such as getting appointments, promptness of service, and so on." [21]

Comprehensiveness Kaiser's benefits and coverage are comprehensive when compared with other insurance plans, although dental care is not covered and psychiatric services are limited. Kaiser covers a greater proportion of medical-care costs than do other plans, but the coverage is by no means totally comprehensive. Studies show that Kaiser pays between 43 and 76 percent of total medical-care costs.[22]

Continuity of Care Kaiser operates a dual ambulatory system of care: a patient can take the appointment route or the drop-in route. The drop-in clinic is not integrated into the rest of the system. Patients go there primarily because they don't know how to use the appointment system or because they don't feel they can wait the days, weeks, or, for some specialties, even months to get an appointment. Frequently, these clinics (and especially night clinics) are staffed by moonlighting doctors.

Drop-in clinics serve as pressure valves on an understaffed, overworked system. Without them Kaiser would have to hire more full-time physicians and ancillary staff; drop-in physicians are frequently part-time employees, not partners in the group practices.

One reason care at Kaiser is discontinuous is because specialty care is emphasized, and is the core of the Kaiser design. Only half of Kaiser's physicians are classifiable as primary-care physicians (general practitioners, internists, pediatricians). The others are specialists or superspecialists to whom patients are referred for illnesses which often could be treated by a primary-care physician.

Although many Kaiser members are victims of discontinuous care, Black patients fall overwhelmingly into this category. Nolan found that 48 percent of all white pediatric patients visited the drop-in clinic, while 67 percent of all Black patients received care there. Furthermore, 18 percent fewer Black patients have a regular pediatrician than do white patients.[23] The CCHPA/MCHR study suggests that an even larger proportion of the total Kaiser population is without a family physician. That study found 51 percent of respondents without a personal physician, of whom 71 percent expressed a desire to have one.

What are Kaiser physicians' reactions to the lack of continuity? An intra-hospital critique at the Santa Clara facility includes physicians' complaints of fractionated care due to overuse of the specialty clinics and poor screening techniques. They added that patients are scheduled to see a different doctor at each visit, even for routine appointment follow-up. Moreover, they claimed, scheduling did not leave them enough time to see their patients adequately. Some physicians discourage "difficult" patients from returning or "punt" them from one doctor to another.

A major issue the physicians continue to wrestle with is the emphasis of Kaiser management on quantity rather than quality of care. As one physician explained, "The system bases many things on numbers without qualifying these numbers. The problem is pressure from the administration which engenders a crazy paranoid way about numbers."

Every month a data sheet with the count of patients seen in each department and facility in the Northern California region is distributed to physicians-in-chief and department heads. Some doctors have been told by their department heads they were not seeing enough patients and shouldn't take educational leaves.

Some doctors feel their schedules are so rushed and inflexible as to preclude delivering adequate, humane care. The schedules are also nerve-wracking to many physicians, and, as one doctor put it, "they have an ultimately eroding effect on a physician's sense of responsibility for the patient."

DEMOCRACY AT KAISER

Membership Participation As far back as 1957, Henry Kaiser summed up K-P policy by stating, "You don't ask your corner grocer to share his ownership with people who buy at the store." Sixteen years later, K-P's attitude on membership participation remains the same. There are no member representatives or representatives of subscriber groups on the national board of directors. In the late 1960's the unions attempted to get on the board; Kaiser flatly refused them.

Thomas Moore, former executive director of the California Council on Health Plan Alternatives, testified in 1971 before the Senate Subcommittee on Health, that, after two years of complaining about Kaiser's inadequate patient grievance procedures, K-P finally proposed some changes. Kaiser agreed to set up a grievance committee "as long as every patient bringing a grievance deposited $150 to cover the cost of arbitration. . . ." "To us," explained Moore, "it is absurd to put such a heavy burden on a man who is making a complaint so that he can't afford to make it."[24]

Physician Participation K-P always emphasizes the democratic nature of the medical groups, and their autonomy from the health plan. Kaiser considers it a "fundamental principle that the physicians must be involved in responsibility for administrative and operational decisions that affect the quality of care they provide."

Structurally the medical groups each have their

own executive committee. Kaiser states it in its literature that "there is constant input from the partners, both formal and informal. . . . Key decisions are made not just by the board of directors but by the board and the full membership."[25] Interviews with physicians in the Northern California region about the decision-making process reveal a very different picture.

One Kaiser doctor characterized the executive committee as "an autocracy which makes decisions in the guise of 'quality of care.'" Similarly a second physician called them "self-serving, power hungry men with coteries of sycophants who are building personal empires." And a third Kaiser doctor described them as "an oligarchy ruled with an iron fist that makes decisions by fiat." Every day in one Kaiser physician's practice, a scheduling situation would arise in which "decisions were coming down from the top that interfered with how care was delivered."[26]

Within the last two years, with the attrition rate increasing significantly, the physicians whose "opinions were neither sought nor listened to" were so dissatisfied that members of the executive committee were forced to tour the hospitals and tokenly restructure their committee.

Today the committee's board, although it has changed from its original composition of self-appointed lifetime members, is still not elected by or accountable to the full membership of the group. Now the committee consists of at least three old-timers whose power positions are unshakeable, plus the physician-in-chief from each hospital, and one representative from each clinic who is elected every two years by the partners of that facility. Only those representatives from groups of 25 doctors or more who have their own hospital are allowed to vote. (The physicians at the

Sunnyvale Clinic and the South San Francisco Clinic, for example, are not voting members.) The company clique is still there; the physicians-in-chief are appointed by the executive committee and elected representatives are always outnumbered.

Worker Participation If things are difficult for doctors, one can imagine the situation of hospital workers. In all hospitals, Kaiser workers are not involved in decision-making. The bulk of the workers at Northern California Kaiser, including LVN's (LPN's), pharmacists, technicians, dishwashers, housekeepers, etc., are members of Local 250 of the Hospital and Institutional Workers' Union. (AFL-CIO).

This fall Local 250 is negotiating a new contract with K-P. There are three areas that the union considers important: The first is wages. The union wants salary increases that will cover Bay Area cost-of-living increases. The second is health benefits. Kaiser gives its own workers Plan D coverage, which is not the most comprehensive. The union wants Plan SS, a better package. The third concern is that of working conditions. Some of the specific working conditions the union would like to see included, according to one union representative, are on-the-job training, career mobility, and lighter work loads. It should come as no surprise that the union considers this last issue to be the most difficult to negotiate with Kaiser.

UTILIZATION AND COSTS

Four comparative studies are relevant to this discussion: (1) Roemer, et al., *Health Insurance Effects, 1972;*[27] (2) *The Federal Employees Health Benefits Program, 1971;*[28] (3) *The Report of the Medical and*

Hospital Advisory Council to the Board of Administration of the California State Employees' Retirement System;[29] and (4) *Family Medical Care Under Three Types of Health Insurance*, Columbia University.[30]

Utilization Kaiser members have lower hospitalization rates compared with other groups when measured by total days of hospital care per 1,000 members per year. Kaiser's rate is lower in comparison with various commercial insurance plans and certain "individual-practice type plans" such as the San Joaquin Foundation for Medical Care, and about half that of Blue Cross/Blue Shield.[31] Two factors, the rate of admissions and length of stay per admission, are responsible for Kaiser's lower hospitalization rates.

Kaiser also has a much lower rate of hospital admissions for in-hospital surgical procedures, about one-half that of Blue Shield. Specifically, the rate is substantially lower for tonsillectomies, "female surgeries," appendectomies, and gall bladder surgery.[32]

Some authors suggest that one reason hospitalization is lower at Kaiser than with other plans is because more procedures are handled on an outpatient basis. However, studies show Kaiser's rate of ambulatory utilization does not differ greatly from the rate in other plans.[33]

Costs On the average, Kaiser members do pay less for the same benefits than members of other health insurance plans.[34] Although premiums for Kaiser are often higher than for other plans, this is more than offset by smaller out-of-pocket expenses.

Yet families with incomes under $11,000 have higher out-of-pocket expenditures and therefore greater total expenses than families with incomes over $11,-

000. Whereas "higher-income" families (over $11,000) have an average $49 out-of-pocket expenditure, "lower-income" families average $112. This suggests that lower-income families seek more care outside of Kaiser because of dissatisfaction or because they haven't learned to use the Kaiser system.[35]

Although Kaiser is generally cheaper than other health insurance plans, it certainly is not the answer to inflation. Kaiser's costs have inflated faster than the national average (the Consumer Price Index for Medical Care or CPI). For the ten-year period 1960–70, the average medical-care costs at Kaiser (premium and supplemental charges) increased approximately twice as fast as the national average (CPI). Yearly comparisons for this period show that Kaiser's costs increased more rapidly than the CPI in every year except 1964 and 1965.[36] Were all medical care delivered through Kaiser-like plans, health-care costs would continue their inflationary spiral.

Cost Reduction and Patient Control In this society, medical services are like other commodities whose sale reaps profits. Producers/providers at once control the supply and create the demand for the product. Unnecessary goods such as too many specialists, drugs and surgery are foisted upon people while actual needs may go unmet. It is within this context that Kaiser's costs and utilization data must be considered.

In prepaid group practices such as Kaiser, the traditional financial incentives are reversed so that profit or savings for physicians and hospitals alike can be achieved through minimizing, rather than maximizing, utilization of services. Given that there is unnecessary hospitalization and excessive surgery in "mainstream" medicine, Kaiser's lower hospital utilization and surgery rates are commendable. How does Kaiser achieve its lower utilization rates?

The National Advisory Commission on Health Manpower, for example, rejects poor medical care, denial of services or relatively good health of members as explanations of Kaiser's cost-savings. The Commission also rejects as explanations both innovations in the practice of medicine and economies of scale. They conclude that pressuring the physicians to be cost-conscious and "avoiding waste" result in savings.

If the Commission is correct and control of physicians is a major source of the economies of Kaiser, several Kaiser doctors indicate that the methods and degree of pressure have an ultimately deleterious effect on the quality of care because of their negative effects on the physician (see Quality of Care section).

Furthermore, contrary to the Commission's conclusions, it appears there are systematic mechanisms in the Kaiser system other than pressure on physicians which discourage utilization. Roemer and his colleagues discussed the deterring effects of barriers created by the system's bureaucracy. And as a Comprehensive Health Planning official said, "Kaiser uses several recognized methods for deterring utilization: copayments, long telephone waits, inadequate waiting room size, shutting down hours of operation, requiring a series of tasks to obtain a prescription, and long waits for lab results." [37]

In terms of costs to members, Kaiser could economize in two ways. One is to reduce the "profits," for example, by slowing expansion and eliminating the physicians' huge bonuses. The other is to reduce the delivery of services. Kaiser is traveling the second route, one which can be followed only so far before quality of care is jeopardized. As a private business, K-P will never take the first route.

Whether corporate HMO's develop in a significant way will depend on whether profits are made. If Kaiser is any indication, the profits will be substantial. However, problems in the delivery of health care will remain. Others, such as overhospitalization and excessive surgery, may risk over-correction. With incentives favoring these extremes it is not unlikely for many people to go unhospitalized who should be in hospitals.

As seekers of health care, we will continue to pay the costs: monetary, physical and psychological. Budding HMO's will fight out their survival in the arena of competition and the small weaker ones will fail because of the huge initial capital investments. Ultimately health care will be delivered full force into the age of corporation capitalism.

(Judy Carney was a Health/PAC staff member. Lee Coffee and Linda Koo were interns at the San Francisco Health/PAC office during the summer of 1973.)

—From the Health/PAC *Bulletin*, November, 1973. (abridged)

10 More Government Cost-Cutting and Regulation

This chapter begins with an analysis of Richard Nixon's health strategy. Besides being a guide to cutbacks in health-care spending during the Nixon Administration, this selection also provides an alternative strategy to Great Society spending programs, one that is likely to guide future, more conservative administrations, both Democratic and Republican. The three objectives of this strategy are to decrease federal involvement in the health-care system, increase the cost-effectiveness of remaining federal programs and weaken those health constituencies considered politically unfriendly. Government involvement in the health-care system is envisioned as having two functions—to develop model programs in health-care delivery that can attract private enterprise (for example, HMO's), or to help individuals gain access to private markets (for example, the Nixon national health insurance plan, which would make it easier for individuals to buy private health insurance policies). But while these models seek to preserve and strengthen the private sector in health care, regulation of the health-care system is also on the conservative agenda—from the creation of Professional Standards Review Organizations (PSRO's) to the strengthening of Comprehensive Health Planning Agencies (CHPA's).

The next two selections discuss PSRO's and CHPA's, respectively. The first is a critique of PSRO's by Robert McGarrah, Jr., and Patricia Kenney of the Health Research Group and Leda R. Judd of the National Urban Coalition. The PSRO law, written by conservative Republican Senator Wallace Bennett of Utah, is an effort to establish and enforce standards for medical treatment under Medicare and Medicaid in order to keep costs down. From the point of view of consumers, as the article points out, the regulatory program is virtually meaningless: it gives power to the doctors to regulate themselves, which is like having the "fox guarding the chicken coop." The next selection, by Barry Ensminger, also of the Health Research Group, shows how local CHPA's, established for the purpose of containing hospital expansion, have become captives of the very industry that they were supposed to regulate.

Although doctors have resisted a long series of attempts to regulate medical practice, there is one arena in which they have pleaded, requested, demanded and struck for more stringent government regulation—namely, medical malpractice. What they have energetically called for, however, is not regulation of themselves, but of patients, lawyers and insurers. The first selection on malpractice is a brief introduction by Thomas Bodenheimer; it describes how the malpractice system works, chronicles how the crisis developed and relates the crisis to the economics of the malpractice insurance system and the poor quality of care delivered to patients. The second selection dealing with malpractice is a penetrating essay by Louise Lander that digs further back into the roots of the malpractice crisis and uncovers its cause in the transformation of health care from a healing relationship to a marketplace transaction.

FEDERAL HEALTH CUTBACKS: Health Policy at the Crossroads

Ronda Kotelchuck and Howard Levy

(May, 1973) The Watergate affair isn't Richard Nixon's only problem. The President is likely losing sleep, as well, over the crisis of American capitalism. The crisis is far more than an occasional article in the *Wall Street Journal* or a series of conferences by high-level economists. It means life or death for many federally supported health programs, because one of the President's ways of handling the crisis is to slash federal spending on health. To understand the specific spending cuts, a more general appreciation of the crisis is called for.

Fortune magazine (November, 1972), a leading corporate bellwether, warns of "galloping inflation, probably an international monetary crisis of vast proportions and, at the extreme, perhaps even another great economic recession." Six months later *Business Week* (May 12, 1973) called for Nixon to cut $20 billion from the federal budget to avert such a crisis. The *Wall Street Journal* agrees. Behind these warnings lie a panoply of problems plaguing the US economy.

First, the US is losing its competitive edge in the world market. Compared to American industry, European and Japanese factories are more modern, efficient and profitable. They can sell their products to the world's markets, including the US itself, cheaper than can American industrial giants. In sundry fields—electronics, home appliances, shipbuilding and automobile manufacturing—American industry is being outpaced and outsold by more vibrant foreign competitors. The result is that American dollars pour out of the US to buy foreign products, creating a negative US balance of trade and concentrating billions of dollars in foreign countries, especially Europe.

With its enormous wealth and power, the US might absorb these trade losses were it not for the cost of maintaining the "American empire." Troops in Europe, B-52's in Thailand, Navy bases in Japan and, very importantly, the immense cost of the Indochina war contribute to the enormous drain of dollars from the US.

The recent emergence of multinational corporations has also exacerbated the problem. However much money they may ultimately bring into the US, in the short run they pump excessive dollars into the international monetary market.

With all these dollars flowing out of the US, foreign governments and banks hold $60 to $80 billion in US currency. With so many dollars, and with few profitable investment options, the dollars are rapidly losing value. International capitalists have been converting dollars to German marks, French francs, Japanese yen and gold, thereby making the dollars worth even less. If confidence in the dollar as a stable medium of exchange goes much lower, international trade could experience multiple revaluations of currencies, erection of tariff barriers, and a worldwide depression like that of the 1930's.

Foreign investors are scarcely reassured when they look at escalating prices in the US. Inflation makes the dollar worth even less, thus aggravating the crisis. And American inflation is exported to other nations with consequent consumer and worker unease and political instability. So Nixon must act dramatically to reduce inflation and convince world business that America's economy is under control. The easiest thing for him to do is to balance the federal budget.

The federal budget has grown by leaps and bounds during recent years and government expenses have exceeded income at a rate that makes even Keynesians blush. Two solutions are always at hand to deal with the problem: raise taxes or cut spending (or some combination of the two).

The US could certainly increase taxes, since its citizens are taxed less than citizens of many other industrialized countries. And, according to the Brookings Institution, federal taxes have actually been cut three times in the last decade (1964, 1969 and 1971), reducing federal income by $35 billion a year in 1972. This provides little solace for taxpayers, however, since local and state taxes have been increasing, and, more importantly and inequitably, there has been a sharp increase of payroll taxes (ten percent during the past ten years). The latter monies go to mandated social security programs, including health programs like Medicare.

Nixon, however, does not want to raise taxes. Owing his loyalty (as well as campaign income) to corporate interests, increases in these taxes are out of the question. They would only be passed on to the consumer in the form of higher prices anyway, further fueling inflation. And owing his electoral success to millions of working-class men and women who already bear the brunt of most taxation, Nixon is loath to jeopardize this support by increasing personal taxes. (Recent statements indicate that Nixon's hand may be forced on the tax issue anyway.) If tax increases are unpalatable, Nixon still has the option of tax reform or spending cuts.

Tax reform is appealing to many Americans. Unfortunately, the large corporations and wealthy individuals who wrote the tax loopholes to begin with show no sign of rolling over and playing dead while their privileges are taken away. Both Democrats and Republicans are beholden to these groups; therefore significant tax reform is likely to remain a seductive, but utopian vision.

HOLDING THE LINE

The logic of Nixon's position leaves him, so it turns out, only one option: hold the spending line. Even this tactic isn't as easy as it looks. Some programs are beyond the reach of the Executive office and for all practical purposes the Congress (e.g., Social Security). According to *Fortune* magazine (November, 1972), these virtually uncontrollable expenditures will increase by about $77 billion by 1977.

As for the controllable portion of the budget, many point to the fat-laden Defense Department (DOD) as a good place to begin slashing away. But it's not that simple. Even without major new weapons expenditures (inevitable given Nixon's priorities), years of liberal opposition to the military draft have resulted in the "volunteer" Army. Unfortunately, its maintenance and support will cost billions. Military personnel costs already account for 56 percent of the DOD budget and, as recruits begin to get $288 a month starting pay, this figure will rise in the future. As it is, the DOD will spend $12.3 billion more in 1974 for its "volunteers" despite the fact that military manpower has been cut 37 percent. (These figures also include more generous retirement pay.)

The problem is that a large military must be maintained if only to protect America's financial interests abroad; on this issue there is no discernible difference between Republicans and Democrats. The sobering truth is that the largest increases in Defense Department spending in this nation's history occurred during the Kennedy-Johnson era ($44.7 billion in 1961 and $78.0 billion in 1968).

Thus, with large chunks of the budget out of reach of the axe, Nixon had to look for other spending programs to cut. When it comes to matching Nixon's political biases to large, potentially expendable government programs, social welfare programs are hard to miss. Overall the fact is that, at least as a percentage of government spending, aerospace and defense-related spending has decreased from 53 to 34 percent of the federal budget during the last decade. It has been nonmilitary spending which has leaped from 47 to 66 percent. Most of the increases, concentrated in HEW, can be accounted for by Great Society programs. And when it comes to cutting down Health, Education and Welfare to size, health, having grown from $2 billion in 1964 to $22 billion in 1974, is an irresistible target.

Aside from sheer size alone, there are additional reasons for cutting federal health spending. As surely as the average health consumer, Richard Nixon knows that the health industry has been the most inflationary of any major industrial sector. By cutting health spending, Nixon hopes to save scarce treasury dollars as well as curtail health care inflation.

More important perhaps, federal spending on health contains an almost built-in escalator. This factor has already been seen with Medicare and Medicaid. Though less obvious, it also applies to service-oriented health programs. It's almost as difficult for the government to build only one model health center as it is for someone to eat only one potato chip. As soon as one community is satisfied, hundreds of others rightly demand their due. And so it is with most federal health service-oriented programs. Unlike one-shot cuts of other parts of the federal budget, cutting health is a preemptive, as well as an immediate saving. A federal dollar not spent today on a demonstration project may save ten federal dollars a few years hence.

Finally, of course, in the real political world some are favored and some are not. There is little question but that the proponents of missile-bearing nuclear submarines and even construction of new federal prisons carry infinitely more political influence with Nixon than poor people clamoring for better health care.

THE HEALTH VIEW FROM THE WHITE HOUSE

Not only has federal health spending shot from $2 billion to $22 billion in the last ten years (a 1000 percent increase), largely as a result of the liberal Great Society health programs enacted during the mid-sixties, but there is painfully little to show for the investment. Even worse, there is mounting evidence that particular programs, like Medicare and Medicaid, are at the heart of runaway health-care inflation.

The Great Society health programs represented the liberal approach to solving America's health problems. Were there large groups who couldn't afford health care? Give them health insurance in the form of Medicaid for the poor and Medicare for the elderly. Were there other urgent needs going unmet by the existing health system? Create special health service programs to meet them, such as maternal and child health programs, family planning programs, community mental health and neighborhood health centers. Did health care seem irrational and unsystematic? Give it a shot of planning through Comprehensive Health Planning and Regional Medical Programs.

While the liberals prescribed a lot of money gilded with a little planning, the real problem lay in the issue of who controlled the health system and for what ends. After decades of fighting the reactionary AMA, it was hard for many to realize that, by the mid-sixties, power in the medical system had shifted to the liberal, academic, institutionally based medical establishment, or that its self-interests might be as pernicious to the delivery of good health care as those of the AMA.

It was natural for the government to rely heavily on this group, both in the design and the administration of the Great Society health programs. The result, however, was programs that benefited the institutional-academic medical establishment as much if not more than they did the groups for whom they were ostensibly intended—programs that gave away large chunks of money with few, if any, cost controls or performance standards.

MEDICARE AND MEDICAID

This is especially true of Medicaid and Medicare, which account for the vast majority of all federal health spending (see Figure). Medicare and Medicaid costs are often called "uncontrollable" because, on the one hand, these programs are not subject to the congressional appropriations process and, on the other, they are obligated to pay for whomever is eligible and claims their coverage. Medicare and Medicaid reimburse health institutions on the basis of "cost" without stringently specifying what makes up that "cost." Thus it has been possible for hospitals to add staff, compete for big-name researchers, buy exotic equipment, expand facilities, pay lavish doctor and administrative salaries, hire public relations firms and do virtually anything else they wanted, all at the taxpayers' ex-

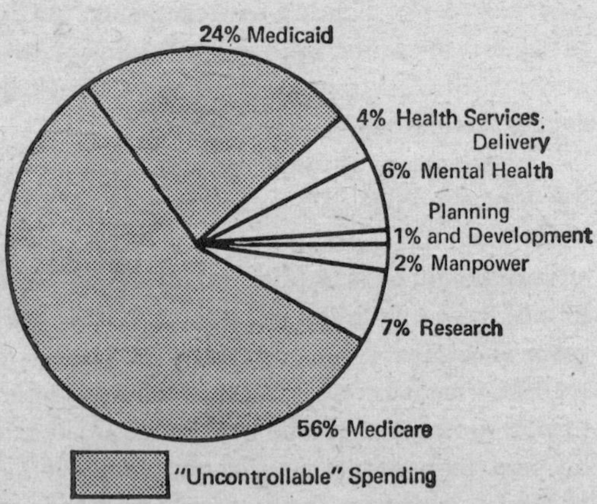

FEDERAL HEALTH SPENDING – F.Y. 1974*
TOTAL EXPENDITURES – $21.7 BILLION

*Excluding health expenditures of DOD, VA, and other non-health agencies which should bring total to $30.3 B.

pense. In the seven short years since their inception, Medicare and Medicaid have come to cost the government $17.3 billion—80 percent of the federal health budget. They now pay over half of all hospital income in the country. Last year alone, Medicare expenditures increased 23 percent and federal contributions to Medicaid rose by 21 percent.

But aside from the increased cost to the government (with little evidence of equivalent improvements in care for the poor and elderly), Medicare and Medicaid, lacking significant controls on spending, have acted to drive up the cost of health care for everyone. In the five years following their passage, medical costs escalated at nearly twice the rate of the previous five years. The cost of the nation's health care reached $83.5 billion last year [1972]—topping for the first time what the country spends for defense. Medical costs have risen so much that today the elderly actually pay more out-of-pocket medical expenses than they did in 1966 when Medicare was passed! The average American last year paid $394 for medical expenses—nearly twice that spent in 1966.

Hardest hit by the legacy of the "Health New Deal" has been the working class. They benefit from none of these programs (except Medicare), yet pay a disproportionate part of the taxes for these (as for all) programs, while suffering under the burden of inflated medical costs.

But what is tax burdens and inflation to some is power, profits and prestige to others. Doctors' fees and hospital fees have risen sharply since 1965. Over 80 percent of Medicare and Medicaid went to institutional providers of health care, consolidating their already growing dominance in the health system and making possible a whole new industry of profit-making providers—Hospital Corporation of America, Extendicare, American Medical International, American Medicorp, etc. Nor did the bonanza stop with institutions. Profits accruing to pharmaceutical companies, hospital supply companies, construction companies, management firms, banks, etc., have made health one of the hottest and surest investments on Wall Street.

HEALTH SERVICE DELIVERY PROGRAMS

Health service delivery programs, such as neighborhood health centers, maternal and child health and family planning programs, have been less inflationary than Medicare and Medicaid, if only because they are small in comparison and are narrowly targeted to meet specific health needs. But they have hardly been more effective. They have been so limited as to constitute a patchwork of tangled, fragmented, bureaucratically encumbered projects and so small as to represent at best a token gesture in the face of the need. While they have made possible some exemplary and much-heralded local projects, these have been at such cost as to make their replication across the country inconceivable.

Many Great Society architects were aware of these shortcomings, but they assumed that the health service delivery programs would serve as demonstrations. When national health insurance—the light at the end of the tunnel—was passed, not only would it pick up their costs, but it would make possible similar models throughout the country. Whether national health insurance could have lived up to such expectations or not is an academic question because, for the time being, the light has faded. And without it these programs were left stranded, demonstrating only that the federal government was getting into a very expensive commitment indeed.

In fact, what the Great Society health programs of the sixties demonstrated best is that money alone, without restructuring the power and priorities of the health system, is no solution. Rather, it may exacerbate the very problems it was intended to solve. Nor has the lesson been lost on Richard Nixon who, having a different political philosophy and facing different economic circumstances, has little interest in solving health problems or restructuring the health care system. His consuming interest is saving money, and health—bloated with often ineffective, exorbitantly expensive, inflation-producing programs—is tailor-made for the Nixon axe.

WHAT IT ALL MEANS

The decision to cut health programs was dictated by the fiscal crisis of the US economy as well as by irreversible commitments by the government to other priorities and interest groups. What to cut within health, however, was dictated by Nixon's own political predilections and what he felt was politically possible. Within health he has moved to do three things: diminish the federal role in health care; efficiently and effectively manage such health commitments as the federal government will retain; and weaken or dismantle what to him are unfriendly constituencies. He accomplishes many of these objectives in the same moves.

Diminishing the Federal Role—Nixon believes that health, like other social services, should be the domain of private enterprise. Where the government must "intervene," there are two appropriate roles: it should develop "models" which can be adopted by private enterprise so that *it* can meet the needs (e.g., health maintenance organizations); and it should enhance individual access to the private market (e.g., national health insurance). In practice, however, it is unclear whether Nixon is serious about these principles, or whether he is using them to simply rationalize reducing the federal commitment to health care.

If the health service delivery programs were intended as "models" for meeting health needs (and there is some doubt), the Administration believes that the time is long since past to decide upon their success or failure and to get them off the books. So by 1976, the federal government will have ceased "intervening" in community mental health and neighborhood health centers, maternal and child health and family planning programs, as well as in hospital construction, the production of health manpower, and a host of other endeavors.

Nixon has a double-pronged strategy for shedding these federal commitments. First, he would like to turn many of the problems of health care delivery over to private enterprise. But the task may be a tough one. HMO's, Nixon's first "model" for making health care delivery into a profit-making investment, failed to immediately convince his hard-nosed business cronies. Nixon is still optimistic about the potential of HMO's (to the tune of $60 million in the FY74 HEW budget), and the concept is gradually being picked up, particularly by private doctors and insurance companies, but on a longer time scale than Nixon would have hoped.

Second, Nixon would like to turn health-care delivery over to states and localities in the form of health revenue sharing, if he can get this measure through Congress. This would mean pooling monies from all the categorical programs (or what's left when he gets through cutting) into one lump sum and turning it over to state and local government to spend as they see fit within the broad confines of health. This strategy is consistent with the more general rubric of Nixon's "New Federalism" in which he would "reverse the flow of money and power from states and localities to the federal government," primarily through the mechanism of revenue sharing. Many suspect revenue sharing is nothing more than a way to reduce expenditures and get the federal government out of its involvement in domestic social issues.

Getting His Money's Worth—Because Nixon feels no obligation to support traditional health constituencies through federal largesse, he would accomplish such commitments as the government has in a single-minded, task-oriented and cost-effective manner. For instance, there is public pressure to increase the production of practicing doctors. So Nixon has reinvested saving from other manpower cuts in medical training and closed off research training funds, the route by which doctors go into research and superspecialties rather than into general practice. This, combined with research cutbacks, will reduce greatly the preclinical scientific orientation of medical education, giving doctors what Nixon considers the bare bone essentials and turning them out as quickly as possible.

Likewise, in the area of research, Nixon wants concrete, publicly salable products. He is through with the old post-Sputnik notion that the more research the better, and with programs whose main function was general support of the medical research establishment.

Dismantling Constituencies—Nixon's use of the cutbacks reveals a clear strategy for dealing with at least three groups in health care. Nixon would use particularly research, research training and health manpower cutbacks to dramatically reduce the size and power of the liberal, academic sector in health which he considers to be expensive, nonproductive and politically unfriendly.

He would deal similarly with the poor, whose organization as a constituency he believes depends on programs such as those in health. But to this objective Nixon brings a more complex strategy than simple cutbacks. For example, by forcing health service delivery projects to become financially self-sufficient, Nixon will not only force them to exclude many poor and medically indigent patients while seeking more affluent clientele, he will force them to drop the less orthodox (and less reimbursable) services such as outreach, community education, etc., which have frequently played an important community organizing role.

Again, Nixon would undercut constituencies organized around health service delivery programs by switching from project grants (which must be specifically applied for and approved) to formula grants. Because formula grants will go automatically to all states (on the basis of a population-income formula), this switch will drastically reduce amounts going to many highly organized, usually urban communities and institutions that applied for and received the bulk of funds in the past. Yet this move is shrewd: no one can argue that the latter group should get an unfair share of the funds.

Health revenue sharing would, of course, extend this policy across the boards. But it is even more insidious to the interests of the poor. Because many state and local governments have been unsympathetic to the problems of poor and minority groups in the past, it is hard to believe that now, with health revenue sharing funds, this policy will change. Furthermore, by pooling monies, health revenue sharing would also pool constituencies and, Nixon assumes, would set constituency fighting against constituency for their particular share of the pool.

Finally, Nixon's actions sound a small warning to health-care providers, particularly institutional providers. The Health New Deal brought them into their heyday of power, prestige and expansionism, and with them the supporting complex of hospital suppliers, drug companies, banks, real estate and construction enterprises, management companies and the like. The Great Society helped to deliver health care full-blown into the age of corporate capitalism. But if the health industry is to take its place among other corporate giants, it must learn the ground rules for "responsible" behavior, and the first ground rule is not breaking the bank. To reinforce this message to the young industry, the Nixon Administration has begun to set forth some regulations—the extension of Phase III price controls for health (one of only three industries for which it was extended), the creation of PSRO's, the strengthening of CHP, the pushing of HMO's. None of these are terribly strong or effective at the moment, but together they may begin to define the outer limits of how "responsible" capitalists in the health system must act.

Nixon may not get away with all his measures for cutting health-care programs, particularly in light of the harm Watergate has done his credibility and power. But it is clear that he will leave an indelible mark on the health system for years to come. Those who attribute this to his personal qualities ignore the larger economic and political realities as well as the contradictions that were built into the Great Society health programs. For given these, it is unlikely that any president would have acted in a substantially different manner.

—From the Health/PAC *Bulletin*, May, 1973. (abridged)

PSRO: Doctor Accountability or Consumer Disaster?

Robert E. McGarrah, Jr., Patricia Kenney and Leda R. Judd

Organized medicine's attitude toward higher costs and poor quality care has always been: "We alone can solve the problem. No one else is qualified."

This "fox guarding the chicken coop" position recently has been enacted into federal law. And unless consumers act quickly to demand full implementation of the legislation's limited public accountability requirements, the American Medical Association will virtually own and control its own new federal agency.

The law (Section 249F of the 1972 Social Security Amendments, PL 92–603) establishes Professional Standards Review Organizations (PSRO's) to review doctors' payment requests under Medicare and Medicaid. In theory this is a commendable idea, but PSRO's are defined as local "nonprofit professional" associations of doctors. Membership, however, must be open to all doctors who are actively practicing in the PSRO's area. With a membership range specified at 300 to 1,000 physicians, this means, in reality, local medical societies.

The job of a PSRO is to establish, after consultation with its member doctors, standards of care, or norms, for the treatment of the different illnesses handled by local doctors. Once these norms are agreed upon, the PSRO can then begin its screening of claims for payment. In other words, the PSRO will then compare the type of medical care shown in the Medicare and Medicaid claims submitted by local doctors with the norms established by the PSRO. If the claims show unnecessary services they *may* be denied payment by the PSRO panel for that medical speciality. Denials probably will be rare, however, since rotating panels of PSRO members will conduct the review. Thus a doctor who has difficulty getting a claim approved by his peers will later be in a position to review their work when his turn comes to sit on the PSRO panel. This will result in typical medical society backscratching.

Consumers are completely excluded from any involvement in local PSRO's just as they are excluded from participating in local medical societies. It will still be virtually impossible for the public to know whether a doctor practices poor medicine. In fact, consumers can only get information on a local doctor when he is actually suspended from receiving Medicare and Medicaid altogether! (If the numbers of doctors barred from practice by medical societies in the past are any indication PSRO suspensions will be rare indeed!) Although there are provisions in the law which permit an appeal of the PSRO's denial of payment to an appeal panel established by the PSRO, anyone who has ever filed a complaint with a local medical society knows how futile this procedure will be. Otherwise, there is simply no way to find out who is practicing good medicine, despite the large volume of information which will be held by the local PSRO.

The local PSRO will be the first level in this new federal structure. There are also state and federal PSRO councils. *Only the statewide PSRO Council permits limited consumer representation. If consumers are to gain any information which will help them reverse the trends in the cost and quality of medical care, it will be from the statewide PSRO Council.*

These state councils will coordinate the activities of all PSRO's in a state where there are three or more local PSRO's. They will have access to extremely valuable information on the cost and quality of medicine in the different regions of a state. For example, a consumer representative on a statewide PSRO Council will be able to pinpoint which hospitals do more unnecessary surgery than others, and which doctors prescribe useless drugs. It also will be possible to determine which PSRO's actually are doing their job, since the statewide councils will evaluate all PSRO's for the Secretary of HEW and recommend those which will receive contract renewals. The value of this information is critical to effective citizen action for changes in medicine.

Each state Governor will nominate at least two "public" representatives to the statewide Council. The law states that these representatives shall be persons "knowledgeable in health care." The Secretary of HEW will confirm these representatives along with two other consumers of his own choosing, making a total of four consumer members of the eleven or more

Council members. (Each local PSRO will have one representative and the state hospital and medical associations will each have two representatives).

The Professional Standards Review Office [of the U.S. Department of Health, Education and Welfare (HEW)] also is in the process of promulgating the regulations which will govern the organization and operation of local PSRO's and is working with the newly appointed National Professional Standards Review Council. This Council is composed of eleven "physicians" (as required by Sec. 1163 of the law). Its duties are to:

1. advise the Secretary in the administration of the Act;
2. provide for the development and distribution, among Statewide Professional Standards Review Councils and Professional Standards Review Organizations of information and data which will assist such review councils and organizations in their work;
3. review the operation of Statewide Professional Standards Review Councils and Professional Standards Review Organizations to determine their effectiveness and comparative performance;
4. make studies and investigations for the Secretary and the Congress to improve and evaluate PSRO's.

The Council also is required to submit at least annually a report to Congress on its findings and to include in this report "comparative data indicating the results of review activities, . . . in each State and in each of the various areas thereof." According to the sponsors of this legislation, this is the provision which will insure "public accountability" in the peer review process.

THE AMERICAN MEDICAL ASSOCIATION AND PSRO

The AMA has stated that it considers PSRO potentially the most significant medical legislation of the 1970's. When the original PSRO concept was proposed, the AMA was vociferously opposed to it. Its view was that it gave the federal government a "strong, intrusive" hand in peer review of Medicare and Medicaid care. And, of course, the law as finally enacted is viewed by them as a compromise. The alternatives to the law as it now stands would have been to have some nonmedical group, perhaps the federal government itself, make the decisions about the quality of care; this would have been clearly more onerous to the AMA than the present law. Already the AMA has had repeated reassurances from HEW that it will play a key role in the organizational process. Because the AMA believes the "stakes are high," it has spent considerable time and effort in gearing up for the implementation of the law. An AMA *ad hoc* Advisory Council on PSRO as well as *eight* subcommittees on a variety of topics have been organized.

These committees have met regularly with HEW officials. (Some HEW people have stated that the AMA has in fact more staff working on PSRO than HEW itself!)

The battle lines already have been drawn between the AMA on one side and Senator Wallace Bennett (R-Utah), author of the PSRO legislation, and HEW on the other. Recent skirmishes include:

> A successful AMA fight to block the Social Security Administration from issuing guidelines outlining the steps a potential PSRO should take in applying for federal approval. The AMA wants PSRO to be di-

rectly controlled by the Secretary of HEW since it apparently has more influence at that level than within the Social Security Administration.

A successful AMA battle to stop the Social Security Administration from controlling, at least until PSRO's are in full operation, the preadmission certification requirements of the law. Had the Social Security Administration been successful, it would have been able to set standards determining whether a doctor could admit a nonemergency patient to the hospital. In this case, the Social Security letter was *recalled*; HEW will issue its own regulations after consultation with the AMA.

A fierce battle by the AMA to gain state medical society control of all local PSRO development. Senator Wallace Bennett was so outraged by the AMA's organized "March on Washington" by members of thirty-six state medical societies that he called the effort "nothing more than a naked power play" that clearly showed the AMA's "obtusiveness and ostrich-like nature." The outcome of this AMA effort is still unknown.

Part of the reason behind this jockeying for power is the view that PSRO will become an important part of any National Health Insurance Program which may be passed by Congress and therefore control of it is important.

All of these seemingly minor skirmishes become important when viewed in the larger context of a National Health Insurance system and who will control it.

BACKGROUND OF THE PSRO LAW

The PSRO concept—where doctors organize themselves to accept responsibility for reviewing cost and quality of practice in their area—was developed through the efforts of Senator Wallace Bennett and the Senate Finance Committee using the Medical Care Foundation model. In recent years medical-care foundations have sprung up all over the country. In the mid-1960's, there were only five of them—today there are well over 100 foundations either operating or starting up. Medical-care foundations are difficult to define because their structure and functioning depends in large measure on the doctors who form them in any given area. There are, however, some basic similarities among all of these foundations. Generally, a group of doctors organize as a foundation to contract with insurance carriers or government programs (Medicaid, for example) to review the cost and quality of services rendered by area practitioners and providers. Failure of participating doctors to comply with the standards set by the foundation can result in ineligibility of the doctor or hospital to collect for the services from the insurance carrier or the government program. Foundations have the right to set ceilings on physicians' fees for particular services. Very often, foundations are an arm of the state or local medical society.

The first foundation, the San Joaquin Foundation for Medical Care, was created in 1958 in California on the initiative of the San Joaquin County Medical Society. Area doctors were reacting to the threat to fee-for-service medical care posed by the Kaiser Foundation Health Plan. Under the Kaiser Plan, a consumer-patient pays a fixed monthly amount and can use the Kaiser Foundation's facilities and medical services. Doctors who work in the Kaiser Foundation clinics and hospitals are salaried and work specified hours. To compete with Kaiser, the San Joaquin County doctors voluntarily organized the Medical

Care Foundation. Through the Foundation, the doctors agreed upon maximum fees for services; they also agreed to monitor one another to avoid unnecessary hospital utilization. Since reducing hospital stays even by one day can save insurance carriers in the neighborhood of $100, the San Joaquin Foundation was able to persuade insurance companies to provide expanded group benefits in return for the monitoring and reviewing of claims by the Foundation. The San Joaquin Foundation claims to save insurance companies 8 to 10 percent of the cost through its performance of peer review. Consumer-patients belonging to groups enrolled with the Foundation can choose any foundation doctor for their medical care.

In 1968, the San Joaquin Foundation signed a contract with the State of California to provide care for all Medicaid (Medi-Cal) patients in its area. The state pays the Foundation a set amount for each Medi-Cal patient and doctors seeing patients submit their bills to the Foundation. Physicians are reimbursed for their services at close to the usual fee. This system provides a foundation approach to the prepaid concept, while still maintaining a fee-for-service mechanism for the individual physician.

Other groups of doctors in other states also have adopted the foundation model. More are likely to do so in the future since they can then qualify as PSRO's and preserve their cherished fee for service practice, free of outside control. In New Mexico, for example, the state Medicaid program was in severe financial straits. In order to bring about the "necessary reform," the medical society organized a foundation.

The New Mexico Foundation for Medical Care has contracted with the state to review all bills from Medicaid recipients for services provided in hospitals or other health-care facilities. The Foundation enlisted the Dikewood Corporation to develop computer programs for reviewing claims based on standards set by physicians using medical practice in the area as a guide. Once in use, the computer will reject those cases in which standards are not met and refer them to physicians working with the Foundation for further review. A doctor disagreeing with the determination of the Foundation that a claim will not be paid can appeal the decision.

The Medical Foundations now in operation and those which are being organized are logical candidates for PSRO's. In fact, many Foundations have expressed interest in adapting themselves to fill the PSRO role. And, of course, the law is specifically written to give these medical society organizations first priority for PSRO grants. The only requirements are that membership, free of charge, be open to all practicing doctors.

Foundations in Arkansas, Tennessee and Mississippi, for example, have applied to HEW to become the PSRO for their state. Their efforts have received support from their state medical societies. Although the AMA opposed PSRO legislation, it is now acting vigorously to insure that it will play a large role in the development of PSRO's. An AMA survey shows that three-quarters of the state medical societies wish to form groups to be designated as the PSRO in their area. PSRO has not received support from all sides, however. For example, the Oklahoma State Medical Association passed a resolution attacking PSRO's and the Association of American Physicians and Surgeons (AAPS) has hired legal counsel to fight the implementation of PSRO's.

Senator Bennett, the "father" of the PSRO, has

stated that if doctors do not take the opportunity to voluntarily organize themselves and impose peer pressure to bring standards up while holding costs down, the federal government will be forced to intervene and develop its own cost and quality standards. Organized medicine is aware of this and is working to insure that it does not happen—*and consumers must work equally hard to insure protection of their interests which are, after all, more significant.*

—From a memorandum by Robert E. McGarrah, Jr., and Patricia Kenney of the Public Citizen's Health Research Group, 2000 P Street, N.W., Washington, D.C. 20036, and Leda R. Judd of the Consumer Health Project, National Urban Coalition, 2100 M Street, N.W., Washington, D.C. 20037. (abridged)

THE $8-BILLION HOSPITAL BED OVERRUN: A Consumer's Guide to Stopping Wasteful Construction

Barry Ensminger

Sporadic attempts have been made for the past decade to stop the runaway proliferation of hospitals through health planning and the regulation of new construction. In 1966, Congress launched the Comprehensive Health Planning Program and federal money began to flow into state and local CHP agencies "to support the marshalling of all health resources—national, state, and local—to assure comprehensive health services of high quality for every person. . . ."[1] This ambitious goal was to be accomplished through voluntary cooperation—everybody concerned would get into the act of planning for better health care. The hope was that hospital representatives, nursing-home operators, doctors, state and local government officials, health and welfare council members, and consumers would all sit down together and work cooperatively for the public good.[2] Proposals for new hospital construction formed a major item on the agenda of the new health planning agencies.[3]

The effort was doomed from the start by a clause inserted in the legislation after last-minute pressure from the American Medical Association. The new CHP's were prohibited from interfering "with existing patterns of private professional practice of medicine. . . ."[4] Since it was these very patterns that lay at the heart of hospital overuse and, in turn, constituted a prime cause of overconstruction, health planning was emasculated from the outset.

HEALTH INDUSTRY DOMINATES HEALTH PLANNING AGENCIES

On Septmber 26, 1974, the Health Research Group sent a survey questionnaire to 218 areawide Comprehensive Health Planning Agencies in order to discover more about their role as reviewers of hospital bed construction proposals. The HRG received 76 responses of which 64 were counted as having sufficient information. These 64 agencies had reviewed a total of 264 hospital projects within the past three fiscal years. The survey results document both the great weight normally attached to local CHP review and the pro-hospital construction bias of these agencies:

> 192 projects or 73% of those considered were approved during the survey period compared with 72 or 27% that were not recommended for approval.
>
> Local agencies approved the building of 9,812 new beds while disfavoring only 6,036.
>
> Only 8 of the 192 recommended projects were later overturned at the state level.
>
> Only 12 of the 72 proposals not recommended at the areawide level were subsequently approved by the state comprehensive health planning agency.

While the participation of consumers is a major feature of the areawide health planning structure on paper, the reality of power in these agencies is quite different. Hospital Associations, administrators, trustees, medical societies, and doctors—the very interests with so much at stake in causing new construction—dominate local decision-making. This domination goes a long way towards explaining the pro-building bias found in areawide CHP's.

Governing boards of local agencies which by law must have consumer majorities all too often fail to reflect the interests of the public:

> The General Accounting Office has found professionals such as retired physicians, administrators of homes for the aged, and directors of social services programs, listed as consumers.[5]

> One quarter of the areawide agencies responding to a recent survey indicated that health professionals had a strong hand in selecting board members.[6]

CONFLICTS OF INTEREST ABOUND

One of the "consumer" members on Oklahoma City's Areawide Health Planning Organization also sits on the Board of Directors of Presbyterian Hospital, now in the process of enlarging its bed capacity from 195 to 412.[7]

In North Carolina, two Duke University professors and the school's architect refused to disqualify themselves from judging the merits of a proposed $90 million hospital expansion project for the University's Medical School.[8]

On March 27, 1974, the President of the Prince George's County Maryland Health and Welfare Council was forced to inform the Attorney General of serious conflicts of interest on the part of the Chairwoman of the Maryland Comprehensive Health Planning Advisory Council: "The supporting information included herein compels a conclusion that Mrs. Spellman's personal relationship, political affiliation with and apparent indebtedness to Dr. Offen, the sponsor of the Parkway Medical Center, dictated her political and governmental support of the Parkway Medical Center." [9]

The control over information is a powerful means of shaping decisions and health planning agencies are dependent on hospitals and medical societies for their information and ideas.

> One-third of all local CHP's have formal arrangements for consultation with medical societies and

> more than one-half actively solicit feedback from these doctors' groups.[10]
>
> Relationships with hospital associations are even closer—60 percent of all areawide planning agencies solicit feedback and well over half have formal agreements with the hospital industry's trade associations.[11]
>
> Statewide agencies also get most of their information from the health industry; only 13% thought that consumers should be the main source of ideas and goals for their program.[12]

Professionals have a strong voice in decisions on new construction since many consumers are hesitant about "intruding on the provider's area of expertise."

A case study of consumer participation in the Puget Sound Health Planning Council gives some important insights into the attitudes of public board members on reviewing new facilities proposals. Nearly all of the dozen consumers interviewed indicated that most of the Council's nonhealth professionals were reluctant to encroach on the expertise of providers.

> . . . even after they have been on the boards and committees for a year or two, many consumers still were somewhat hesitant about "intruding on the provider's area of expertise," as one consumer put it. Part of the reason seemed to be genuine appreciation of the complexities involved in facilities planning and construction. But part of it seemed to be the feeling that no matter how much an individual consumer learned, he or she would always know less than the provider.[13]

While it is certainly difficult to generalize to the rest of the country on the basis of this one report, conversations between a HRG staff member and members of other CHP's tends to confirm the prevalence of this deference to health professionals.

Areawide planning agencies have been dependent on hospitals, nursing homes, Blue Cross, and medical societies for much of their operating budgets. Hospitals, the largest private contributors, have used this dependency to influence agency decisions on construction projects.

> 25 percent of local budgets for health planning agencies have come from private pockets and hospital associations are the largest single contributor of these dollars.[14]
>
> A 1973 study by Interstudy, a midwest research group, established the strong positive relationship between the amount of time local agencies spent reviewing new building projects and the total hospital dollars that flowed into the coffers of the agency.[15]
>
> The General Accounting Office, after surveying Comprehensive Health Planning in California, Maryland, and Ohio, concluded that private contributors were using their dollars as a lever to control decisions. Dollar cut-offs, or threats to do so, were made when hospitals and other donors disliked the stands taken by the agencies.[16]

The picture which emerges seems clear. Comprehensive Health Planning Agencies, unwilling to interfere in the private fiefdom of administrators, trustees, and medical staffs have done little to check the national pattern of hospital overuse. Dominated by health professionals on their boards, dependent on hospitals for their funding, and relying on the health industry for their ideas, these agencies have failed to serve the public. Far from acting forcefully to "assure comprehensive health services of high quality for every person" they, like Blue Cross and Hill-Burton

Agencies, have become handmaidens for the nation's hospitals.

—Selections from "The $8-Billion Hospital Bed Overrun: A Consumer's Guide to Stopping Wasteful Construction," by Barry Ensminger, Public Citizen's Health Research Group, 2000 P Street, N.W., Washington, D.C. 20036 (1975).

THE MALPRACTICE BLOW-UP: Fighting Over the Carcass

Thomas Bodenheimer

On May 1, 1975, many northern California anesthesiologists packed up their nitrous oxide tanks and went home. All but the most urgent surgery stopped. Private hospital wards emptied out. Public hospital beds bulged with surgical and obstetric patients. Private hospitals—already financially overextended from their excess building—talked of enormous monetary losses, even of permanently closing. By May 10, over 3,000 lower-paid hospital workers, disproportionately minorities and women, had been laid off. Some of these workers, particularly the nonunionized, may never go back to work.

Argonaut Insurance Company, the nation's second largest malpractice insurer, had terminated its group coverage of 4,000 northern California doctors, offering individual malpractice insurance at a 384 percent rate increase. While many doctors swallowed hard and paid up, the anesthesiologists, their premiums zooming from $5,377 to $18,164, resoundingly said no, demanding government intervention to guarantee reasonable malpractice rates.

California doesn't stand alone. In December, 1974, the New York State Insurance Commissioner denied Argonaut a 197 percent rate incerase on its malpractice coverage of 20,000 New York State physicians. The company immediately announced cancellation of its insurance coverage as of June 30, 1975.

In Maryland, a judge ordered the St. Paul Fire and Marine Insurance Company to continue its coverage of 85 percent of the state's doctors. The company had planned to cancel its insurance by April 30 when a 48 percent rate increase was denied by the State Insurance Commission.

Doctors in Pennsylvania are suing Argonaut to prevent the company from reneging on its five-year contract with the state medical society.

In February, 1975, Argonaut notified Florida hospitals that malpractice premiums would increase by at least 500 percent over 1974.

Health providers in 21 states face crises of stupendous rate increases or cancellations of malpractice insurance. Thousands of doctors talk of walking out on their patients. It is a new manifestation of America's continuing and deepening health-care crisis.

HOW MALPRACTICE INSURANCE WORKS

Malpractice insurance is a subscriber of the health-care system with its own peculiar political economy. Last year about $500 million entered this subsector, with payments (premiums) from doctors, dentists and hospitals going principally to ten insurance companies. The money, of course, comes from health consumers as part of hospital daily charges and doctor fees. But a mere 16 percent of this money ever gets back to the consumer in awards for injuries caused by medical negligence.[1] The rest is siphoned off, mainly to insurance companies and lawyers.

The dynamics of malpractice insurance are rooted in the inherent conflicts among insurance companies, lawyers and health providers (doctors and hospitals) over who will pocket patients' money. Lawyers, who take a steep percentage of the award or settlement, want more suits with larger awards. Insurance companies want fewer suits and smaller awards, as do doctors. But doctors also want insurance companies to keep the premiums low, whereas the companies make their profits by keeping them high. Doctors, hospitals and insurers charge that lawyers cause the malpractice inflation because they are paid by contingent fees: between one-third and one-half of the settlement, with no payment if the injured person loses. Lawyers reply that the contingent-fee system allows the poor access to malpractice litigation and add that the insurance companies are raising rates to increase their already significant profits.

WHY THE CURRENT CRISIS?

The flurry of accusations back and forth obscures the fundamental issue: The malpractice situation exists because Americans are receiving poor quality health care. In the largest malpractice award to date, $4,025,000, a jury found San Francisco's Mt. Zion Hospital and one of its doctors liable in the case of an 11-

year-old boy who was not treated following a head injury and is now paralyzed and unable to speak. In another celebrated case, Albert Gonzales, a grocery clerk in constant pain from an unnecessary and bungled back operation, is sharing with his lawyer a $3.7 million award against Dr. John Nork and Mercy Hospital in Sacramento. The judge alluded to Dr. Nork as "an ogre, a monster feeding on human flesh" who "for nine years made a practice of performing unnecessary surgery and performing it badly, simply to line his pockets." Nork himself admitted to needlessly maiming at least 30 patients over the years; many of his colleagues knew but remained silent. The judge assailed the Sacramento County Medical Society, Mercy Hospital and the State Board of Medical Examiners for doing nothing about Nork.

These are the extremes. But poor quality care is not restricted to a tiny minority of incompetent doctors. Two million operations, about 15 percent of all surgery, are entirely unnecessary, performed to profit surgeons; these operations account for the deaths of at least 10,000 people annually.[2] A study of prescribing habits in Ohio revealed that 65.6 percent of antibiotics were unnecessary or incorrectly administered and that in 92 percent of cases with adverse drug reactions to antibiotics, the prescription was questionable or clearly faulty.[3] Ninety percent of antibiotic injections given to a group of patients in New Mexico were unnecessary.[4] Excessive use of antibiotics, pushed by the highly profitable drug industry, has been charged with causing roughly 100,000 deaths per year.[5]

But why have the number of malpractice cases increased 70 percent from 1973 to 1974?[6] Has the quality of care dropped precipitously in the past year?

Probably not, but mass consciousness has risen. The consumer movement, though new and unformed, is having its effect. Between 1966 and 1974, the percent of Americans who have "a great deal of confidence" in their doctors dropped from 72 to 50 percent.[7] Also, people are conscious of an expensive society that discards its ill and disabled; large malpractice awards are the only economic recourse.

In addition to the number of claims, the average claim size is going up—20 percent from 1973 to 1974. Though 89 percent of settlements are less than $10,000, California has seen 16 million-dollar verdicts since 1969. While the lawyer's fee system feeds the rise in claim size, a more basic factor is the economy and its rising prices.

In fact, malpractice claims themselves influence prices in the health arena since doctors now practice "defensive medicine," going overboard on diagnostic tests that serve only to protect themselves from suits without necessarily improving the quality of care. HEW Secretary Caspar Weinberger estimates that $3 to $5 billion is spent on such unnecessary procedures, including one-third of the $1.4 billion spent annually on X-rays. Thus the profit incentive that creates unnecessary and dangerous care leads to malpractice suits that in turn cause another kind of unnecessary care.

Inflation is only half the linkage between the general economic crisis and the malpractice insurance blow-up. Recession completes the chain. Part of the insurance industry's withdrawal from the malpractice field is related to that crucial determinant of insurance company behavior—investment of their multimillion-dollar premium income. 1974 was the worst year ever for casualty insurers, who were hit by a staggering $6-

billion drop in their investment portfolios.[8] The conglomerate Teledyne, Inc. ordered its subsidiary Argonaut out of the malpractice market when Argonaut's investments fell. Argonaut is continuing its less risky workmen's compensation business. Again, the profit basis of private insurance, disregarding any considerations of health care, determines whether a company will fulfill its needed function or will simply pull out, leaving behind massive disarray.

—From the Health/PAC *Bulletin*, May/June, 1975. (abridged)

THE MALPRACTICE CRISIS: Evasive Medicine

Louise Lander

Evading the root causes of a social problem is perhaps a natural reaction for those whose careers and mind-sets would be put at risk by facing up to them. When those same people are in a position to channel public discussion of the problem—even to determine the public's conception of what the problem is—the possibility that the larger society will effectively deal with the problem is sacrificed for the sake of particularistic interests. And ultimately the unaddressed problem will inevitably reassert itself in even more insidious forms.

Something like this process seems to be unfolding in relation to the medical malpractice issue. Long-developing signals of discontent from the patient population—aided and abetted by bench and bar—only became a "crisis" when an economic threat to professionals and institutions erupted. Then those with the power to define the crisis presented it almost entirely in terms of the insurance industry, the legal profession and the judicial system. Problems of the medical profession and the health-care system themselves have been acknowledged only glancingly, if at all. What follows will consider the profession's and the system's reactions to the crisis, surface and subterranean, and will attempt to glean those underlying causes that have been so elusive to public debate thus far.

THE TRIUMPH OF ECONOMICS

What gave the medical malpractice problem the status of a full-blown crisis in the eyes of the medical profession—and, through its reaction, in the public eye—had less to do with malpractice claims per se than with the price-hiking and withdrawal tactics of the malpractice insurance carriers. Those tactics were in turn as much a reaction to the plummeting of the stock market as to the escalation of malpractice litigation. (The 1974 bear market removed what for many insurers had been the incentive for entering the malpractice field: The so-called long tail—the long lapse of time between the paying in of a malpractice insurance premium and the paying out of a settlement or judgment—allows for a handsome profit on investment during a bullish market.)

The fact that economics more than medicine was the immediate catalyst of the crisis helped the medical profession initially to ignore the medical issues underlying malpractice claims; at the same time, however, the profession's outraged reaction to the carriers' conduct put it in the anomalous position of attacking economic behavior that simply reflected a set of free-market incentives that it had long found it in its interest staunchly to defend.

The physicians' strikes then saw large segments of the profession launching into the further circularity of exercising their own freedom to withdraw their services in an attempt to rectify the effects of the industry's unseemly withdrawal. That tactic created still another incongruity, namely the spectacle of a profession that had long argued that the least government is the best government demanding that state governments take an active role in the economics of medical practice.

THE INTERSECTION OF ECONOMICS AND MEDICINE

While the 1974 bear market wrought havoc with the reserves of all kinds of insurers, one characteristic of the economics of professional liability insurance made it a particularly unattractive business. Here the profession found it hard to avoid some consideration of problems of medical practice, for those economics made a direct connection between escalating premiums and disappearing insurers and the profession's traditional, if weakening, resistance to any limitation of its members' freedom to practice any and all forms of medicine, subject only to the laws of supply and demand. That stance became a problem for the insurers —and thus eventually for the physicians—because their risk-spreading base of physician-insureds, unlike the broad base provided by their life insurance or auto insurance customers, is dangerously narrow. Thus a relatively small number of malpractice settlements or judgments, unlike a small number of deaths or auto accidents, can throw a carrier's loss experience for an untenable loop.

That relatively small, though economically threatening, number of payments may represent an even smaller number of physicians: A study of malpractice suits filed in the tricounty Metropolitan Detroit area over the five-year period 1970 through 1974, for example, showed that 2.1 percent of the area's physicians—those sued more than once—accounted for 46.2 percent of the suits.[1] The single infamous case of Dr. John Nork in Sacramento, with its $3.7 million jury verdict, alone accounted for 12 percent of the California losses of American Mutual Liability Company, the unlucky carrier.[2]

Moreover, those physician-defendants threatening their insurers' economic security were not necessarily totally incompetent—as Dr. Nork apparently was—but might be unqualified to perform certain complex procedures and unwilling to admit their limitations. Thus a study by Empire Casualty Company of Denver of its 72 largest settlements and judgments over a 15-year period found that "some of the biggest payouts . . . were for physicians who overestimated their ability to do such things as treat compound fractures, read X-rays, handle difficult deliveries, or perform special surgery. In each case, prompt referral to, or consultation with, an appropriate specialist could have forestalled a malpractice claim."[3]

The inherent instability of medical malpractice insurance was not a problem for the industry (or, by extension, the profession) when malpractice suits were a relative rarity and their success even more rare and/or when a bullish stock market was inflating the carriers' reserves. The increasing willingness of the patient population and its allies at the bar to sue and the increasing willingness of the judiciary to ease the legal barriers to a successful suit, when combined with the decreasing viability of the stock market, left a traditionally important segment of the profession hoisted on its own petard. Those physicians, that is to say, who had stoutly defended the inviolability of the license to practice from limitation or reexamination found that the incompetence, absolute or relative, of some of their brothers was making that stance more expensive than they had ever foreseen.

Thus some elements of the profession, with much encouragement from the insurance industry,[4] have moved from economics to medical care to the extent of beginning to support legislative measures aimed at strengthening regulation of physicians. That development augurs for an increase in the intraprofessional split between primarily office-based generalists and primarily hospital-based subspecialists and for a boost to the already increasing power of the latter. The elite of the profession can well afford to recognize the economic and public-relations disadvantages of incompetents, absolute or relative, practicing medicine and in fact stand to reap economic benefit from a reduction in competition from generalists practicing their superspecialized skills.

THE TRIUMPH OF THE INSTITUTION

Shifting the scene from the office to the institution, however, presents the profession—here joined by the hospitals—with another problem that it would prefer not to confront. American medicine has always proudly exhibited a bias toward high-technology treatment, toward inpatient hospital care and toward surgery.

Given that an estimated 74 percent of incidents that become malpractice claims occur in hospitals and that about 57 percent of such incidents involve surgery,[5] the always questionable cost/benefit ratio of that bias is finally—in the short term at least—hurting physicians and hospitals as much as their patients. (While those statistics to some extent reflect the incompetence, absolute or relative, of surgeons,[6] they undoubtedly also reflect the environmental risks unique to hospitals, the potential defects of technology available only in hospitals and the potential for harm inherent in any surgical procedure.) Physicians' and hospitals' malpractice insurance premiums might be lower, that is, if they had heeded the charges made by critics of the system that it is fraught with unnecessary hospitalization and unnecessary surgery; their reason for evading that issue of course is that their incomes would be lower as well.

So while at least passing concern is expressed for the problem of medical incompetence, the problem of inherent systemic risks is not only ignored but flouted. For there appears to be a movement, inspired by various ramifications of the economics of malpractice insurance, toward increasing numbers of physicians relating to an institutional base in preference to a solo private practice. There are, for example, the repeatedly reported cases of academic physicians giving up their part-time private practices because their increased malpractice premiums (which fail to distinguish between full-time and part-time practice) make such practices hopelessly uneconomic to maintain. There is the ad placed by a medical employment agency in which the inducement "Free Malpractice" appears in type twice as large as the inducement "Med School Affiliations."[7] There is the report from the Defense Department that the incentive of malpractice insurance as a fringe benefit is bringing the armed forces record numbers of applications for medical commissions.[8] Or there is the announcement by a South Dakota insurance carrier that doctors coming to that state will only be insured by it if they join an established group practice.[9] A collection of incentives and disincentives, all ultimately related to the malpractice crunch, thus seem to be accelerating the movement of medical practice from office to group and institution.

As doctors increasingly move to an institutional base, that base is likely to exercise increasing control over their medical practice within it, again for reasons relating to the economics of malpractice. That control may itself take an economic form, as in an insistence that physicians not provided with insurance by the institution obtain it in adequate amounts on their own; thus a federal district court in New Orleans has upheld the right of a hospital to suspend the privileges of a member of its medical staff for failing to comply with its requirement that staff physicians maintain a minimum amount ($1 million) of malpractice insurance coverage.[10]

In terms of medical practice, the increased willingness of the judiciary to hold hospitals liable for the conduct of their medical staffs has given hospitals an economic incentive to increase their scrutiny of that conduct. According to one commentator, "This concern [about their potential liability] has been a tremendous impetus for hospitals to demand that their medical staffs undertake more effective auditing procedures of their members." [11] Here the hospitals are being forced to juggle the need to minimize their liability by instituting review and regulatory mechanisms affecting their medical staffs and the need not to jeopardize the good will of those same physicians, on which they depend for the maintenance of occupancy rates that alone guarantee an adequate cash flow. Thus the most advantageously situated institution is the one that is least dependent on private practitioners for its patient supply, a fact that may further reinforce the trend toward institutionally based medicine. Conversely, the most disadvantageously situated practitioner is the one lacking the preference or the talents for maneuvering in an increasingly bureaucratic setting.

A HEALING RELATIONSHIP OR A MARKET TRANSACTION?

While ignoring the increased risks of high-technology, institutionally based medical care, those with the power to define the content of the malpractice crisis have equally ignored a more fundamental problem: A perceived medical injury is a necessary but not sufficient ingredient of a malpractice claim, the essential catalyst being that quantum of resentment that can transform an unfortunate state into a hostile act.

If the patient perceives his physician as being primarily motivated by a concern for his well-being (a concern that would include an unwillingness to risk performance of a procedure beyond the scope of the physician's skills), the patient will have no reason to seek a pound of flesh when the results were not what he and his doctor had hoped for. But if the patient sees the physician as a highly paid entrepreneur (or employee) who in turn sees him as a defective commodity to be repaired for the sake of profit, his reaction to an untoward result will be the same as is his reaction when his auto mechanic charges a hefty price for failing to fix his car. (The probability of the latter perception is recognized by the insurance industry, which advises its physician-customers: "Keep your charges reasonable—the doctor who has the biggest fees can be the biggest target, too." [12])

The fact that American medical practice is based on a system of economic incentives (whether the fee-for-service system or the prepayment system) creates an inherent conflict of interest for the physician—an altruistic interest is his patients' maximum well-being frequently conflicts with his economic self-interest in maximizing his patients' profitability. The larger society, that is, has created an occupational group that it expects to exhibit an altruistic concern for the welfare of others but has simultaneously placed that group within a system of market incentives having no necessary relationship to the degree to which that welfare is furthered. (The profession itself of course has been an active participant in the creation of this dilemma.) Insofar as an injured patient perceives the economics as dominating the altruism, it is not surprising that he seeks an economic solution to a therapeutic problem.

In the context of a capitalist economy, the practice of scientific medicine can only heighten the patient's uncomfortable sense of himself as a damaged commodity, whatever it can offer him in terms of reduced morbidity and mortality. Scientific medicine is most markedly market medicine when its practice overlaps with the profit-based market for the products of a technological age. Thus the patient risks ceasing to be half of a social relationship and becoming instead an appendage of a machine whose use increases the income of the corporation that manufactured it, the hospital that bought or leased it and the physician who has prescribed its use. This result is not inherent in the machine per se but stems from an economic and social system in which the incentive for the development of new technology is to maximize profits rather than human potential.

Or the incentive for use of the mystique of scientific medicine on the practitioner's part may be to maximize his status, which thereby increases the psychic distance between him and his patient: In their classic study of Yale–New Haven Hospital, Duff and Hollingshead found that "Sometimes . . . 'scientific' medicine was used as 'insulating' medicine between patients and physicians. In that process the physician assumed superior knowledge and discounted or even ignored the report of the patient." [13] Thus science becomes identical with mystification instead of furthering human autonomy.

Financing mechanisms exacerbate the commodification phenomenon even further. The economic incentives of insurance-based payment mechanisms distort the choice of what care to provide in what setting from being a matter for doctor-patient agreement based on therapeutic and human considerations to being a matter of channeling care into those modalities that the insurance company has made an economic decision to cover. And the economic incentives usually coincide with that modality—inpatient hospital care—that is both most risky and most depersonalized.

Social policy in the form of Medicare and Medicaid, because based on the payment principle rather than the service principle, has extended the economic incentives of the market to new arenas. Thus Medicaid has brought us free enterprise with a vengeance, in the form of scandal-ridden Medicaid mills in New York, prepaid health plans in California and nursing-home chains all over. It has also extended to the poor the same risks of excessive hospitalization and excessive surgery to which the American medical system has long subjected the middle class. Medicare has abolished as superfluous the altruistic (albeit patronizing) medical tradition of treating the elderly poor at rates they could afford to pay. The loudly heralded rights to care these programs were said to have created were more accurately rights to call on government to pay for a bureaucratized commodity rather than rights to enter freely into a healing relationship.

Given that patients see medical care being furnished and financed as a product, whether dispensed by an individual entrepreneur or a large corporation, it is not surprising that they increasingly seek economic satisfaction when the product turns out to be defective. Here they receive reinforcement from the legal system, where the sanctity of property rights on which it is based reifies human existence and makes the ghoulish equation between pain and suffering and monetary damages.

But if the patients, who have few if any alternatives, are chasing an illusion, the profession, which is appreciably more powerful, is exacerbating the commodification of health care—and the "legalized and legitimated doctor-patient hostility"[14] that goes with it—even further. In part that exacerbation relates to the apparent trend already noted of increasingly providing health care in an institutional, and therefore further depersonalized, setting. More concretely, it relates to the physician's common reaction to the alienation and hostility of the patient turned plaintiff. (That reaction can be quite colorful, as in the statement of a physician-member of the HEW Commission on Medical Malpractice: "The doctor feels put upon. He feels nude on the corner of the Main Street of life. He often tries to cover himself with pride, and even occasionally arrogance, only to find himself being castrated. He really doesn't want to believe the hostility he feels."[15]) In terms of conduct, that reaction duplicates the patient's alienation and hostility in the form of what has come to be known as defensive medicine.

Of course one practitioner's defensive medicine may be another practitioner's standard practice. What distinguishes the phenomenon is not its content but its motivation: The patient is not an object of altruistic concern but a potential enemy against whom defensive measures must be taken, which must in turn be disguised as procedures undertaken for the patient's benefit. Thus outright deception joins economic motivation in insuring that what should be a healing relationship will have more of the character of a market transaction, and one between parties with opposing interests at that.

THE FOAM-RUBBER-PILLOW SYNDROME

Ultimately the evasiveness of the malpractice debate is destined to get its participants—and the American public—only a bad case of the foam-rubber-pillow syndrome (attack the problem here and it pops up there). The smorgasbord of purported solutions to the crisis that the medical profession and its allies in the insurance industry have been dishing out, aside from the admittedly short-term expedients for patching up the insurance market, address patient hostility as expressed in malpractice claims by seeking either to suppress it (e.g., by shortening the statute of limitations and abrogating various common-law doctrines of liability) or to channel it into hopefully less expensive outlets (e.g., arbitration or compensation systems modeled on workmen's compensation).

Perhaps it is to be expected that the medical profession will treat symptoms rather than causes, but for the sake of pursuing its short-term self-interest it is ignoring the importance of starting with a correct diagnosis. Thus patient hostility is obtusely blamed on the avariciousness of that other profession, whose members, however greedy, don't have a case until they have a client angry enough to undertake the ordeal of a lawsuit.

The doctors' dilemma of course is that the alternative to such short-sightedness is perhaps as painful as the hostility of the patient-litigant. The commodification of medical care, despite its inherent cycle of risk-alienation-injury-hostility-counter-hostility and so on, has brought ample economic rewards to the profession and to the delivery system within which it operates. When those rewards are threatened by the economics of patient hostility, the natural reaction is to seek to render that hostility less economically rewarding rather than to call into question the economic basis of one's own well-heeled livelihood. What threatens an onset of the foam-rubber-pillow syndrome is the fact that the hostility is not going to go away but is going to seek new channels for its expression with the help of a profession that thrives on hostility. Thus the malpractice crisis in one form or another is destined to be a permanent feature of the American scene unless and until social conditions make possible a solution based on social and ethical values rather than on the crudities of economic motivations.

—From the Health/PAC *Bulletin*, January/February, 1976.

11

National Health Insurance

This chapter begins with a cogent article written in 1970 and reprinted in *The American Health Empire*, in which Health/PAC staff members John Ehrenreich and Oliver Fein argued that the new political impetus for enactment of national health insurance legislation stemmed from health-care providers who had become financially overextended in the free-spending days of Medicare and Medicaid. The authors argued that any national health insurance program would fail economically because it would fuel health-care cost inflation through uncontrolled spending, just as Medicare and Medicaid did. At the same time, national health insurance would not address problems of health-care consumers, such as inaccessibility and unaccountability, precisely because it is an *insurance* program dealing primarily with finances. Thus national health insurance "is not clearly either a step towards or a step away from a national health care system . . . it's more of a shuffle sideways."

The second selection in this chapter is "Who Will Pay Your Bills?" This is a Health/PAC special report analyzing the major national health insurance proposals. It contrasts and compares these bills, understanding from the outset that even the best of the bills would result only in limited reforms of the health-care system.

NATIONAL HEALTH INSURANCE: The Great Leap Sideways

John Ehrenreich and Oliver Fein

There's a lot of commotion in the halls of Congress, among the leaders of labor, and within the Nixon Administration itself about National Health Insurance. A flood of bills proposing one or another form of National Health Insurance has already hit Congress. AFL-CIO President George Meany spent virtually his entire Labor Day speech pushing National Health Insurance as "labor's number one legislative goal" for the early Seventies. One Deputy Undersecretary in the Department of Health, Education, and Welfare, Robert Patricelli recently declared, "Next year will be 'health year' at the Department of Health, Education, and Welfare just as 1970 was 'welfare year.' " Even the American Medical Association, historically the leader of the anti-National Health Insurance forces, has chosen not to oppose National Health Insurance outright, but rather to toss its own plan into the legislative ring.

VESTED INTEREST

Proposals for National Health Insurance are nothing new in the nation's health history. What is new in the 1970 situation is the army of political forces forming to push for some form of National Health Insurance. On the one flank is the public, led on by the mass media to expect ever-greater miracles from the medical magicians, but increasingly frustrated in their ability to obtain even ordinary nostrums. On the other flank is labor, management, the hospitals, Blue Cross, the companies that manufacture and sell hospital supplies, and local and state governments, each faced with an increasingly serious set of problems growing out of the horse-and-buggy methods of financing medical services, each coming to one or another brand of National Health Insurance as a possible solution to its own special health care crisis.

"Labor's number one legislative goal . . . is National Health Insurance," declared AFL-CIO President George Meany, "and the AFL-CIO believes it can—and must—be enacted." Labor needs National Health Insurance to eliminate the hassle at the bargaining table over health fringe benefits, which have taken increasingly larger bites out of the wage package. In 1965, for example, in the steel industry, 19 cents an hour, or 4% of the average steel workers' total wages and benefits, went for health and life insurance. Today, because medical prices have gone up two to three times as fast as prices in general, as much as 8% to 10% of any new wage and benefit package must go to health and life insurance, just to maintain the existing health benefits. At a time when the real disposable income of American workers has stopped growing for the first time in 35 years (due largely to inflation and increased taxes because of the Vietnam war), labor is desperate to find ways to augment workers' wages. Relegating health insurance to the government leaves more dollars and cents for wage increases.

Increasingly, elements of management, particularly in big business, are also flirting with National Health Insurance. For these businessmen, health insurance premiums have become a significant and rapidly rising component of their overall labor costs. Businesses would like to stabilize the contribution they make for their employees' health care: predictability of costs permits planning for larger profits. In addition, National Health Insurance may shift part of management's labor costs (i.e., the health insurance component) onto government, leading to greater profits. This shift of labor costs from management to government would be limited to those large industrial employers whom labor has already compelled to make substantial contributions to health insurance. The marginal, small shop and agricultural employer who now makes little or no contribution to health insurance for his employees, may find National Health Insurance increases his labor costs. While management is not unified on the issue of National Health Insurance, those that count (big business and industry) are increasingly for one or another form of such insurance.

Of the medical-industrial complex—the hospital supply and equipment companies, the medical electronics and computer companies, and at least those drug companies who are diversified into hospital supplies—all would benefit from National Health Insurance. Their experience with Medicare and Medicaid has been profitable. National Health Insurance, like Medicare before it, would provide the dollars to guarantee the demand, and thereby still the lingering doubts that many companies have about the advisability of government involvement in health.

For the voluntary (private, nonprofit) hospitals, almost any program of National Health Insurance would be better than the present Medicaid program. Eligibility has become so restricted under Medicaid that many patients are no longer covered. That leaves the hospitals stuck with the bills of patients who are too rich for Medicaid but too poor to pay. A National Health Insurance program allows the possibility of universal coverage without eligibility restrictions. Equally important, National Health Insurance would stabilize hospital income by guaranteeing a certain level of reimbursement. Government will be reluctant to cut a program that affects a large cross-section of Americans. Of course, the voluntaries would prefer a National Health Insurance plan which merely subsidized their operations with minimal interference from government. But almost any form of National Health Insurance would be better than none.

Blue Cross/Blue Shield, the most important nongovernmental health financer, while certainly not wild about any government take-over of the health insurance business, would settle for a brand of National Health Insurance that would expand Blue Cross hegemony over the health insurance market. Although Blue Cross enrollment has flowered over the last decades, its percentage of the health insurance market has been declining. In 1945, Blue Cross insured 61% of the hospital insurance market compared to 33% by the commercial insurance companies. Today, that figure is reversed for the population under age 65, with Blue Cross garnering only 34% of the hospital insurance market compared to 60% by the commercial insurance companies. However, Medicare and Medicaid represented a big boost to Blue Cross since virtually every state turned over administration of their programs to Blue Cross. It is just such a relationship to National Health Insurance that Blue Cross wishes to foster. Parenthetically, even the commercial insurance companies are not total in their opposition to all varieties of National Health Insurance. For example, the president of Aetna has said, "A program of universal health insurance . . . could be structured to retain the advantages of competition and the profit incentive. . . . I have full confidence in our ability to work successfully in partnership with government."

Finally, local and state governments see rising costs for their health programs (state and city hospitals, Medicaid, etc.) as an unlimited drain on already scarce funds. Any program that shifts parts of the burden off their backs is welcome. As a result, even the most ardent states' righters voted enthusiastically to support New York Governor Nelson Rockefeller's National Health Insurance proposals at the 1969 National Governors' Conference.

Labor, big business, parts of the medical-industrial complex, the voluntary hospitals, Blue Cross, and local governments—all are attracted by some form of National Health Insurance. The growing consensus on the need for a National Health *Insurance* program will increase pressure on the Nixon Administration to respond with more than minor "reforms." In any event, it is certain that each "interest" group will try to shape National Health Insurance to its perception of THE crisis in health.

CONSUMER CRISIS VS. PROVIDER CRISIS

In fact, however, THE crisis in health is not just one crisis but two: the crisis felt by the consumers of health services, on the one hand, and the crisis experienced by the providers of health services, on the other. For the consumer, the crisis is the failure of the present system to deliver adequate health care at any price. Though not limited to poor people, black and Puerto Rican communities have been the most articulate in their criticisms. Medical care, they say, is fragmented and isolated from the social, economic, and environmental causes of pathology. People are experimented on and used as teaching material. The doctor's priorities come first. And the patient's needs run a poor second. Doctors and hospitals are totally unaccountable and unresponsive to the needs of the users of service. Increasingly, middle-class people are raising the same criticisms. They too experience long waits in overcrowded doctors' waiting rooms, constantly increasing bills, and the growing awareness that despite the wonders of heart transplants, it is increasingly difficult to find a doctor to treat ordinary ills.

Those who provide and pay for health care face a different crisis—the breakdown of the old systems of financing. The hospitals find themselves near collapse as costs skyrocket and financing fails to keep up. This threatens not only the institutions themselves, but also the multibillion-dollar drug and hospital supply companies who depend on the hospitals as a retail outlet for their products. At the same time that the hospitals weep because of "inadequate" funds, the providers of funds groan under the weight of the hospitals. Blue Cross is forced to raise its rates and face its enraged subscribers. The trade unions find themselves allocating an ever-increasing portion of wage hikes merely to maintain their present level of health benefits. Employee health plans cut an ever bigger bite out of corporate profits. Even the government feels the pinch as

Medicare and Medicaid costs knock the budget for a loop.

Since the providers and financiers of medical care feel only part of the crisis—the part concerning the financing of medical care—it is little wonder that their solution to the "crisis" concerns only that. The various plans for health insurance being discussed by such groups and figures as the AMA, Walter Reuther, the AFL-CIO, Nelson Rockefeller, Blue Cross President Walter McNerney, the American Hospital Association, and Senators Javits and Kennedy are all primarily programs to put the financing of medical care on a sounder basis. The issues which are debated—coverage, benefits, sources of financing, administrative mechanisms, etc.—all attempt to answer the question of how to finance existing health services. None of the proposals confronts other parts of the crisis—the basic issues of the organization of delivery systems, the relationship between the providers and recipients of care, power in the health delivery system or priorities in the system.

INSURANCE WON'T WORK

National Health *Insurance*, to be sure, may well be a useful reform for many Americans. It may help a few people pay for medical services which they otherwise would not get. It may shore up a few hospitals in low income areas whose total collapse would be a tragedy for the people of the community. It is hard to oppose a measure which, in however limited a way, may help a few people, at least, to have greater access to badly needed health services. But National Health *Insurance*, in the end, (1) won't work, and (2) will have regressive effects as well as progressive ones.

The problem is that National Health Insurance will be a mechanism to funnel money out of the pockets of workers and taxpayers into the hands of the people who now run (and mis-run) the health service delivery system—the doctors, the hospital administrators, and the medical-industrial complex which fattens off people's illness. It will thus strengthen those forces that insist that all health care must center on the doctor and the hospital, rather than the forces who wish to totally reorganize the delivery of health care.

At the same time, National Health Insurance will throw a cloud over what is really happening. To liberals, for whom National Health Insurance has long been a goal, it will appear that the problems of the medical system are being solved. Middle-class doubts as to the organization of care may quiet down temporarily if part of the bill is paid by someone else. The accelerating movement for more fundamental reorganization of the medical care system will be de-fused, at least for a while.

Meanwhile, National Health Insurance will solve nothing. First, it is unlikely that any of the proposed plans will be very effective in meeting people's health needs. For this we have the evidence of Medicaid and Medicare. Medicaid, for example, clearly showed that giving the poor an unlimited credit care for medical service did not end the two-class system of medicine. There are other stumbling blocks: institutional inaccessibility, the relationship between doctor and patient, the control by the doctors of priorities for allocating funds, time, and equipment among research, teaching, and patient care, and the unaccountability of the hospital to the medical needs of the community. Medical care is sold in a monopolistic, not a free, marketplace. The effect of National Health Insurance, as with Medicaid and Medicare, may well be a sizeable number of individuals who are enabled to pay for better care. But it will not create and make accessible high-quality medical services for the great majority of poor and middle-class people.

Second, the hopes of some of the insurance plan advocates that the medical-care system can be reorganized through incentives linked to the insurance scheme's repayment system will almost certainly be dashed. For example, there has been much talk of giving doctors and hospitals incentives to operate efficiently. This might save money, but at best, it would have no effect on the patterns of care in the institutions, on the relations of the institution to the community, on the quality of care, etc. In fact, unless very stringent controls by the consumer were introduced, the likely result would be that the hospital would cut down on service in order to save money and pick up its incentive reward. For another thing, economic incentives can at best only conquer economic obstacles to change. They have no power over the other pillars of the two-class medical system. For example, economic incentives may encourage a hospital to be more economical, but they are unlikely to persuade a hospital to accept community control, or to convince $50,000-a-year doctors to put care of the indigent ahead of prestigious research. Finally, incentives are slow. We can't wait 20 or 30 years just to get doctors into group practices.

The third way in which National Health Insurance will fail will be economically. We have seen in the past few years how Medicaid and Medicare fed galloping medical inflation. The mechanisms are clear: the medical establishment which commanded the use of the funds, used them for their own priorities—prestigious and expensive and "interesting" medical technology and high salaries for doctors and administrators. As a result, costs soared, while patient care improved only slightly, if at all. There is no reason to think the same thing would not be repeated under National Health Insurance. No workable cost-control law has yet been devised, and, in any case, the impulse of hospital administrators is to cut costs at the expense of patients and hospital workers. It is entirely conceivable that in 1975, under National Health Insurance, the nation will be spending $90 billion a year instead of the present $60 billion for health services, and $200 a day for a hospital bed without any significant improvement in the quality of care for the average citizen.

NHI EVADES BASIC QUESTIONS

National Health Insurance will fail because it fails to face the fundamental questions about our health system—control, accountability, accessibility, priorities, responsibility to the community. And it fails this test precisely because it is National Health *Insurance*. Under an *insurance* mechanism, no matter how liberal, the private delivery system performs a certain service and the public funding (insurance) system pays for it. The public insurers may try to persuade the controllers of the private delivery system to change the system, but no attempt is made to take the power to control away from them. The key issues about the health system are thus removed from the discussion, right from the start. To this dead end, we can only propose the fundamental alternative: The only way to fundamentally change the health system so that it provides adequate, dignified care for all is to take power over health care away from the people who now control it. Not merely the funding of the health system, but the system itself must be public. It then becomes possible to face such questions as how we decentralize the "National Health Care *System*" to make it responsible to the community and accountable to it, how we ensure that patient care is the primary priority of the system, how we ensure equal access to health institutions and to practitioners, and so on.

Many people have suggested that National Health Insurance might be a step toward such a national health system. Others argue it will be retrogressive: by providing financing, it will stave off the collapse of the present system for a few short years and will strengthen some of the enemies of such a system. At the same time, though, it will establish the necessity for the government to guarantee the right to health care for all, and it will arouse ever greater expectations of adequate health care. Thus National Health Insurance is not clearly either a step towards or a step away from a national health care system . . . it's more of a shuffle sideways.

—Adapted from an editorial in the Health/PAC *Bulletin*, January, 1970, and reprinted in Chapter XII of *The American Health Empire* (New York: Vintage Books, 1971).

WHO WILL PAY YOUR BILLS? A Health/PAC Special Report on National Health Insurance (1974)

The United States is the only industrial nation without a comprehensive program of government health insurance or a national health service. Most of us pay for our health care through private insurance. Only the elderly and some low-income people have government insurance.

But national statistics, added to the personal experiences of millions of people, show that our system fails to do the job. 20 million people have no private or government health insurance at all. Private insurance pays just over one-third of the average family's medical bills. This means that most families, who spend $400 a year for their health insurance, have to pay several hundred extra dollars when sickness strikes. Severe illness can leave a family with thousands of dollars in bills not covered by insurance. In fact, *medical bills are the number one cause of bankruptcy in the United States today.*

The most talked-about solution to this crisis is national health insurance. The American Medical Association (AMA) promises "to make sure that high quality medical and health care are available to every person" by passage of its national health insurance program. President Nixon announces his own national health insurance plan "to provide adequate health insurance for the American people." Senator Kennedy introduces yet a different national health insurance bill in Congress that is supposed to "end our current health crisis." All of us will be affected by the outcome of the current national health insurance debate.

For most of us, national health insurance is a thick and confusing stack of documents containing endless legal and financial terms. But behind the fine print lie concepts that are more important than the details of the bills themselves. To appreciate these concepts, it's worth taking a look at the history and present structure of health care finances.

The idea of national health insurance has been around for a long time. Almost 100 years ago European governments began to pay for the health care of their citizens. In the United States there were two early drives for national health insurance. [See "Origins of the Government Health Insurance Issue," by Theodore Marmor, in Chapter 8.] The first was begun by pro-labor professionals just before World War I and was defeated by the AMA and local medical societies, in concert with Samuel Gompers, president of the American Federation of Labor.[1] The second was begun during the New Deal in the 1930s and was finally defeated by a national AMA drive preceding the 1950 congressional elections. The issue remained relatively dormant during the 1950s.

In spite of inaction on national health insurance, the health care system as a whole changed markedly by 1960. Thorugh the '40s and '50s a giant private health insurance industry came into being, composed of Blue Cross, Blue Shield and commercial companies such as Aetna, Occidental and Connecticut General. These companies offer considerable hospital protection to working families who can afford to buy policies and are in a generally healthy age group. But the companies fail to pay most medical bills outside the hospital. And people who fall chronically ill or lose their jobs lose their insurance as well.

Low-income people, of course, couldn't afford insurance, and the companies didn't want to insure the elderly because of their high rate of illness. So a new drive for national health insurance began around 1960, concentrating on the poor and the elderly. In 1965 Congress passed Medicare for those over 65 and Medicaid for people unable to work.

MEDICARE AND MEDICAID: THE BEGINNINGS OF NATIONAL HEALTH INSURANCE

Medicare takes money from people's paychecks, under Social Security, and uses it to pay medical bills of the elderly. Medicare is limited, paying on the average only half of these bills. Though a step forward for people who pile up thousands of dollars in hospital costs, it ignores a sizeable portion of the bills charged in doctors' offices.

A woman in New Jersey used to pay $120 a year in doctor bills. After Medicare her doctor raised his fees, with the yearly bill coming to $228. Medicare left $133.60 for the woman to pay herself, so she pays more now than she did before Medicare. She is no exception. *People over 65 pay an average of $400–$500 each year in medical bills not covered by Medicare. Due to the rise in costs, that is more than the average senior citizen paid in total health costs before Medicare was passed.*

Medicaid has also failed to meet the needs of the 40 million poor people in the country (the government defines "poor" as a family of four earning less than $4,300.) More than 20 million of them are not covered at all. Those who are covered receive limited services. And Medicaid patients have a hard time finding doctors and dentists who will see them. In one Los Angeles county hospital, 23% of outpatients switched to private doctors right after Medicaid was passed, but twelve months later most of these patients chose to come back to the county hospital. Other studies confirm that private medicine has failed to care for many of the poor even when paid to do so.[2] Yet city and county hospitals, which used to treat people free, increasingly are charging for their services. Thus low-income people may actually have a harder time finding care than they did before Medicaid arrived.

The main thing about Medicare and Medicaid is that they caused medical costs to skyrocket. [For details, see Chapter 8.] Hospitals, doctors and nursing homes were allowed to decide how much to charge, and they were paid through private insurance intermediaries, usually Blue Cross and Blue Shield, who made no attempt to control these charges. The first year after Medicare and Medicaid started, hospital costs were up 19% and doctor fees 7%.[3] In the first six years of the programs, medical prices increased by over 40% compared to an increase of 20% in the six years before the programs started. And the fees didn't go up just for Medicare and Medicaid patients: they rose for all of us.

Medicare and Medicaid were a financial shot in the arm for the health industry. Doctors' average incomes now top $40,000 with many specialists earning over $100,000. The insurance intermediaries expanded their business by $10 billion a year, including several hundred million for "administrative expenses." This means high executive salaries (Blue Cross President Walter McNerney earns $80,000), new buildings, newspaper and radio ads and Congressional lobbying. Medical equipment and drug companies increased their sales and profits. Nursing home stocks boomed. Hospitals added on new beds at a rate three times greater than the population increase. As a result, 25% of hospital beds are now empty, upping the rates to all patients. So Medicare and Medicaid—our country's first taste of national health insurance—though designed to help the patient, have largely profited doctors, hospitals and medical businesses.

THE CONGRESSIONAL PROPOSALS

The experience of Medicare and Medicaid tells us a lot about national health insurance. It tells us that health costs could zoom up even faster, that large medical bills could remain uncovered, and that payment for a doctor doesn't guarantee being able to find one. National health insurance won't be a carbon copy of Medicare and Medicaid, but its basic principle—government-assisted financing of private health providers —is the same.

The idea of national health insurance came in with a bang in the early '70's. By 1971 no fewer than 13 bills, representing every major interest in the health system and ranging from the all-encompassing Kennedy-labor bill to the very minimal AMA Medicredit bill, were facing Congress. Many predicted that national health insurance would be a reality within a year or two, and certainly it would be a major issue in the 1972 presidential campaign.

Yet prophecy is a risky vocation and suddenly it seemed like the fires under national health insurance had died out. It was hardly mentioned in the 1972 campaign. Only in 1974 did it begin once more to gain momentum. By this time the processes of political compromise were well at work. Three bills emerged as front runners, clearly defining the boundaries of what is likely to be passed.

Early in 1974 both President Nixon and Senator Russell Long submitted considerably liberalized versions of the national health insurance proposals they had previously sponsored. Senator Long's catastrophic illness proposal was expanded to include health-care benefits for the poor, and President Nixon's new proposal included both more comprehensive benefits and equal benefits for all groups. Shortly thereafter, Senator Kennedy abandoned his all-public, cradle-to-grave Health Security Act for a more limited and conservative measure, which includes a system of benefits with deductibles and coinsurance similar to the Nixon proposals and which allows a substantial role for the insurance companies.

Once serious debate begins on national health insurance, the outcome will not be the passage of one or another of these particular bills. Ideas from various bills will get mixed up into a national health insurance law. Also, national health insurance won't come in one big leap. It's likely to come step by step over the next ten years or more.

WHAT TO LOOK FOR IN NATIONAL HEALTH INSURANCE

The tangle of national health insurance plans before Congress is so confusing that most people give up before trying to sort it out. But there is an easy way to judge the various proposals by asking a few simple questions:

Who is covered? National health insurance could pay the medical bills of everyone in the country, or it could restrict itself to some groups of people and leave others out.

Which services are paid for? National health insurance could pay for all health services (doctor, dentist, hospital, eyeglasses, mental health, drugs, extended care and nursing homes) or it could cover, for example, only doctor, hospital and extended care costs, making people themselves pay for the other services.

Do large out-of-pocket expenses remain? National health insurance could pay the entire cost of health services, or it could leave deductibles, coinsurance and limitations for people to pay themselves. A deductible means that you pay the first $50 or $100 of a hospital or doctor bill and the health insurance pays the rest. A 25% coinsurance on a $400 hospital bill means that you pay 25% of the bill, $100, and the insurance pays the rest. A limitation means, for example, that the insurance pays for only 30 days of hospital care or only six doctor visits a year. Studies show that coinsurance tends to keep low-income people away from seeking health care more than middle-income people, and that it particularly reduces people's use of preventive health services.

Who pays? A national health insurance plan could be financed by regressive or progressive payments. A "regressive" payment means that lower-income people pay a greater portion of their income than wealthier people pay. Economists agree that social security taxes are extremely regressive.[8] Insurance premiums (for example, $400 per family regardless of family income) are also regressive. A "progressive" payment means that higher income people pay a greater percent of their income than lower-income people, for example, a graduated income tax without loopholes.

Will costs be controlled? If national health insurance, like Medicare and Medicaid, allowed doctors and hospitals to set their own fees, it would produce an enormous rise in the costs of health care. Strict controls are required to keep costs from rising. There are two ways to control costs. One is to keep patients away by making them pay a substantial part of the costs (large coinsurance and deductibles); this discriminates against people with less money and discourages preventive care. The other method of cost control is to limit fees and profits.

Is access to service guaranteed? Providing money to pay for health care does not guarantee finding health care. We have a shortage of doctors and other health personnel especially in rural areas and inner cities. In addition, health care is fragmented among different specialists so that at least one-third of Americans have no personal physician who feels true responsibility for their total care. A national health insurance plan could ignore these problems or could provide improvements in the overall supply, geographic distribution and organization of services.

Who profits? National health insurance means government-assisted financing of private health practitioners and institutions. Since money is the fuel that runs private enterprise, national health insurance always brings profit to private providers of care.

Let's look closely at three proposals and briefly at four others. Remember, more important than the details are the principles underlying the plans.

THE LONG-RIBICOFF CATASTROPHIC HEALTH INSURANCE AND MEDICAL ASSISTANCE REFORM ACT

The Catastrophic Health Insurance and Medical Assistance Reform Act is sponsored by Senator Russell Long, chairman of the key Senate Finance Committee, and Abraham Ribicoff, long-standing Senate liberal who hails from Hartford, Connecticut, the insurance capital of the world. Senator Long's previous bill provided only catastrophic health insurance, whereas the new bill adds a new health insurance program for the poor.

The Long-Ribicoff bill assumes that most health needs can be handled adequately by the present health insurance industry and that for persons who cannot be covered profitably, the government should step in to provide protection. Consequently the bill would leave Medicare for the elderly intact and would extend benefits similar to those of Medicare to the poor and those suffering from catastrophic illness.

The Long-Ribicoff bill has three parts: Title I, providing insurance against catastrophic illness; Title II, providing a federalized health insurance program for the poor; and Title III, establishing voluntary guidelines for the sale of private health insurance covering the remaining health needs.

Title I will cover Social Security beneficiaries (95% of the population). Its most important features are its deductibles and coinsurance. *It is not intended to pay most medical bills, and, in fact, it will assist only the 2% of the population that suffers devastating illness.*

The plan has a 60-day hospital deductible. This means that the federal government covers hospital costs only after a person has been hospitalized for 60 days. People would have to rely on private insurance, Medicare and Medical Assistance to pay for the first 60 days. Those without such insurance or with inadequate insurance might spend several thousand dollars before getting help from catastrophic health insurance. And even after the 60th hospital day, Title I makes patients pay $21.00 coinsurance each day.

For nonhospital services, every family has a yearly deductible of $2,000. *A family must spend $2,000 for doctor bills, X-rays and laboratory tests before receiving aid from Title I.* Even then, the plan pays only 80% of costs, leaving each family with 20% coinsurance. Only after total coinsurance payments reach $1,000 does Title I pay the whole cost. And even then dental care, eyeglasses and drugs are left out. Title I is financed by the regressive Social Security system (0.3% tax on wages up to $9,000 paid by both employers and employees).

Title II would replace Medicaid, providing medical coverage for individuals with annual incomes up to $2,400 and families of four with incomes up to $4,800. The low-income ceilings mean that many poor people who presently receive Medicaid will be ineligible for Medical Assistance. For those who do qualify there would be no deductibles, and coinsurance would be only $3 per doctor visit for the first ten visits per year. The Medical Assistance Plan is financed 75% by the federal government through general revenues and 25% by the states. Both Titles I and II would be administered through the Social Security Administration, with private health insurance companies acting as financial intermediaries as they do presently under Medicare.

Title III of the Long-Ribicoff bill would establish

guidelines that would presumably guarantee that all persons who are not included in the above programs could buy an insurance policy covering a particular set of services for a reasonable price. Companies that do not comply would be disqualified as fiscal intermediaries for the other programs. Other than this, the Long-Ribicoff bill provides no cost or quality controls and no provision for improving the supply, distribution or organization of services.

NIXON'S COMPREHENSIVE HEALTH INSURANCE PLAN

The President's 1971 measure was a hastily thrown together johnny-come-lately to the national health insurance scene. Although the influential Committee for Economic Development, representing the nation's largest corporations, and the Health Insurance Association of America supported plans similar to it, the President's proposal failed to gain substantial congressional support and even received criticism from within the Administration.

Consequently in early 1974, just as the fires of Watergate were heating up, President Nixon submitted a new national health insurance proposal. The Comprehensive Health Insurance Plan (CHIP) maintains the basic structure of the President's earlier measure, but its benefits are broader and are supposedly uniform for all groups. *CHIP does not guarantee anyone health insurance. Rather CHIP makes it possible for everyone to buy a standardized private health insurance policy.*

It does this in three ways: Full-time employees may purchase health insurance by paying 35% of the annual premium cost (later to become 25%); employers will be required to pay the rest. The annual premium cost is presently estimated to be $600, so a family could expect to pay $210 a year. The poor, unemployed, part-time employed and those considered high medical risks will receive a government subsidy based on income to purchase premiums. Their share can range from zero to 150% of the premium cost. The elderly will continue on Medicare, but will also have to pay a share of premium cost based on income. The plan is voluntary.

CHIP offers greatly expanded benefits compared with the 1971 Nixon proposal. Also, CHIP ostensibly offers the same benefits to everyone, unlike the earlier proposal, which would have given much less to the poor. Benefits include unlimited hospital and physician services, prescription and other life-saving drugs; laboratory tests, X-rays, medical devices and ambulance service; limited treatment for mental illness, alcoholism and drug addiction; certain nursing home, convalescent and home health services; and services to children, including preventive care, eye and ear examinations, and dental care to the age of 13.

However, these benefits are limited by a system of deductibles and coinsurance that will mean that families will seldom benefit from their health insurance. The individual must pay the first $150 in medical costs each year, with a limit of $450 per year per family (the deductible). After that he must make coinsurance payments of 25% of succeeding costs up to a maximum of $250 per person or $1,500 per family per year. (For the poor, deductibles and coinsurance are graduated according to income.) This means that most ordinary family health needs will not be met by CHIP. *Including the $210 they pay for the premium, a family could pay $660 before getting any help from*

CHIP whatsoever. Basically CHIP would provide catastrophic illness insurance, and it would positively discourage preventive care or early treatment.

More than this, although CHIP purports to be universal, many people would be left out. Because it is voluntary and the individual expenses can be considerable, many economically marginal people will risk not being insured. *For instance, part-time and temporary workers are not covered by the employee plan, and to be insured under the plan for the poor and unemployed, they would have to pay most of the $600 premium cost themselves.* And the elderly may be worse off under CHIP than they are presently under Medicare. Medicare provides many services automatically and free of charge, whereas CHIP would require the elderly to pay their share of premium cost, coinsurance and deductibles for all of their benefits.

Furthermore, health care costs would be enormously regressive under CHIP, particularly for the lower-income worker. The estimated $210 employee share of premium cost would be the same for the $7,000-a-year worker and the $70,000-a-year executive, even though it comprises 3% of the worker's salary and 0.3% of the executive's salary. Likewise, the maximum out-of-pocket expense of $1,500 will be 21% of this worker's income—easily enough to throw a family into bankruptcy—while it will be only 2% of the executive's income. Only for the poor (families under $7,000 and individuals under $5,000) would the costs be graduated.

Finally, CHIP would perpetuate the two-class health care system. It would allow some health care providers, particularly doctors, to charge out-of-pocket fees to patients covered under the employee plan, above and beyond what CHIP will pay. For those people, this will destroy the notion of a maximum liability for medical expenses. For the poor and elderly, it would mean discrimination as usual, since they would continue to be less profitable patients to treat.

The Medicare portion of CHIP would be run by the federal government, which can contract out administration to private health insurers, as it does presently under Medicare. The employee plan and the plan for the poor would be administered according to 50 different state plans (presuming all 50 states choose to participate). The federal government's role would be limited to approving state plans and establishing benefits and eligibility standards. Left to the states would be such crucial functions as reviewing rates charged by doctors and hospitals, regulating insurance company profits, monitoring employer contributions and administering cost and quality controls.

Nixon's plan favors the creation of health maintenance organizations (HMO's). HMO's are heralded as a better way to deliver health care. They bring doctors, hospitals, nursing homes, labs and pharmacies together under one management. We would sign up with an HMO, and our insurance company would pay that HMO a fixed sum each year. We would seek care from the HMO's affiliated doctors and hospitals, but would have to pay extra for getting care elsewhere.

Some of us have been receiving care from HMO's for years: from Kaiser on the West Coast, HIP in New York City, Group Health in Seattle, and others. *It's important to realize that HMO's get the same amount of money regardless of how many services we use, which gives them a financial interest in providing less rather than more services.* This has the advantage of discouraging the HMO's doctors from performing excessive surgery or putting people in the hospital unnecessarily. But HMO's have a tendency to go overboard in limiting services, often making it hard for us even to get needed doctors' appointments.

In its overall strategy, Nixon's plan opens new doors for large companies to receive a larger share of the $83 billion health care pie at the expense of individual private doctors and smaller nonprofit hospitals. Particularly the health insurance industry stands to gain. According to *Business Week,* an additional $3 billion would be channeled to health insurers each year.[4] The AFL-CIO points out that "The partnership proposed by the Nixon Administration is a partnership between the federal government and the private insurance industry—a most profitable arrangement for the industry but very costly for the American people." This is no surprise, since rich insurance executives contributed heavily to Nixon's political campaigns. W. Clement Stone, for example, chairman of the large Combined Insurance Company, gave Nixon $2.8 million in 1968 and another $2 million in 1972.[5]

Why are private insurance companies needed at all under national health insurance? Money could be collected by the government and paid directly to doctors and hospitals. Government financing would save a great deal of the $3 billion used each year by the insurance industry for advertising, high executive salaries, other largely unnecessary administrative costs and profits. The $3 billion could be put to other uses —it is enough to operate well-staffed health centers in 3000 communities.

By controlling the use of billions of dollars of health care money the insurance industry is more and more in the position of deciding who gets health care, what kind of care it is, and how much it costs. Nixon's plan, and its current counterpart, the Health Insurance Association of America's 1973 bill, would increase this power of insurance companies, placing our care even more in the hands of people who are not primarily concerned with health.

THE NATIONAL HEALTH INSURANCE PROGRAM (KENNEDY-MILLS)

Shortly after President Nixon and Senator Long introduced their new bills in Congress, Senator Kennedy, working with Representative Wilbur Mills, came forth with a compromise measure, the National Health Insurance Program (NHIP). In it Kennedy attempted to preserve some of the merits of his earlier, cradle-to-grave, entirely public, comprehensive national health insurance proposal while incorporating measures designed to gain support from both of his chief contenders. Consequently NHIP is a major retreat from his first bill.

NHIP will cover everyone except those receiving Medicare and will be compulsory, unlike the other two bills. Its benefits are virtually the same as those of the Nixon bill, including unlimited physician's services and hospitalization, limited inpatient and outpatient psychiatric care, post-hospital extended care and home health services, outpatient prescription drugs, X-rays, lab tests, medical devices and other services presently provided by Medicare, prenatal, well-child and family planning services, and ear, eye and dental care for children under 13.

Like the Nixon bill, NHIP will include deductibles and coinsurance. *With the exception of preventive and children's services, a patient would receive no benefits from NHIP until he had spent $150 a year* *(or a maximum of $300 per family) in medical expenses. Then he would have to pay 25% of succeeding costs until he had paid a maximum out-of-pocket cost of $1,000 per year.* Then NHIP would take over. The maximum liability is graduated according to income. Not only are these out-of-pocket costs a disincentive for early treatment, but as health care costs go up, these will be an increasing financial burden on the consumer.

Also like the Nixon bill, consumers will receive a credit card through which providers will be paid in full for their services. If deductibles or coinsurance are involved, they will be paid by the consumer to the insurance company or Social Security Administration, whichever is administering the program.

The Kennedy-Mills bill will be financed primarily by a 4% payroll tax—1% to be paid by employees on wages up to $20,000 and 3% to be paid by employers. Self-employment income will be taxed at 2.5% and unearned income will be taxed at 1%. Health care for the poor will be partially financed by general revenues and state contributions.

NHIP will be administered by a new, independent Social Security Administration. Administration of the program can be contracted out to private health insurance carriers as Medicare is now—a significant concession to the health insurance industry. For controlling cost and quality of services, the Kennedy-Mills bill incorporates PSRO review, incentives for delivery of health care through HMO's, prospective reimbursement for hospitals, reimbursement of physicians on the basis of a fee schedule and planning agency approval of character and quantity of services. No mention is made of consumers in the administration of the bill. NHIP will create a Health Resources

Development Board, which will eventually be funded at 2% of NHIP revenues.

SOME OTHER PROPOSALS

Other national health insurance proposals are similar to the Nixon plan in basic concepts: private insurance for working people and government-supported private insurance for the poor.[6] One of these bills is "Medicredit," written by the AMA. The AMA plan has two parts, catastrophic insurance similar to CHIP and basic health insurance. Like Nixon's plan, Medicredit relies completely on the private insurance industry, supplying government assistance for people unable to buy insurance. Coinsurances, deductibles and uncovered services abound. The plan minimizes the government's role in health care and gives, in the AMA's words, "free choice by every physician as to how he will conduct his practice." This means that doctors can decide when and where to set up an office, regardless of need; to choose which patients to see and which to reject; and to remain the highest paid occupation in the country. Medicredit guarantees insurance companies an additional $5 billion in private insurance payments and $6 billion in federal tax money, causing the AFL-CIO to call the provisions of the plan "thinly disguised efforts to protect vested interests and insurance company profits."

Not surprisingly, the National Healthcare Act of 1973, sponsored by the Health Insurance Association of America, provides incentives for all working people to buy more private insurance. Poor and "uninsurable" people receive private insurance at government expense. Coinsurance payments are higher for hospital care than for doctors' services, supposedly to discourage expensive hospitalization. But since most hospital care is decided on by the doctor, not the patient, the coinsurance would be costly for many people. The government-supported portion of the bill is administered by the states, reflecting the usual friendly relations between insurance companies and state insurance commissioners.

The American Hospital Association's bill seeks to convert the health system from reliance on private doctors to a network of "health care corporations." These corporations differ from Nixon's HMO's mainly in being centered around nonprofit hospitals rather than for-profit companies. As in Nixon's plan, employers and employees buy private insurance and low-income people receive federal assistance for their insurance. Payments might go to insurance companies or directly to health care corporations. Patients face a complicated array of coinsurance and service limitations.

Under discussion by some Nixon Administration officials is the proposal of Harvard economist Martin Feldstein. Feldstein thinks that all national health insurance plans will worsen the Medicare-Medicaid inflation. His solution? Provide as little insurance as you can get away with.

Feldstein proposes a plan similar to catastrophic insurance. The government, through private insurance intermediaries, would pay for all health care expenses above 10% of family income (for example, above $500 for a family earning $5000). Families above $8000 would pay no more than $800 a year. People who run up medical bills of several hundred dollars could get government-guaranteed low-interest loans to pay the bills over time. Feldstein believes that people would stop buying private insurance (since the insurance costs almost as much as their maximum health bill) and would pay doctor and hospital bills directly. The effect is supposed to be cost consciousness by the patient and therefore less inflation. The Feldstein plan is the most extreme form of controlling costs by discouraging patients from seeking care. Everyone, especially low-income people, will think twice before getting a Pap smear. No attempt is made to control costs by limiting fees or profits.

THE KENNEDY BILL

The national health insurance plan originally introduced by Senator Kennedy expresses many ideals about good health care for all Americans.[7] (In 1974 Senator Kennedy abandoned this bill for the Kennedy-Mills bill but reintroduced it in the 1975 session of Congress.) Supported by the country's labor leaders, the bill virtually eliminates private insurance companies from the health system. But it does not guarantee that health care will be available when and where people are sick.

Under Kennedy's bill we pay a larger amount of money to the federal government through income taxes and social security payments. In return, everyone in the country can visit doctors, receive hospital care and obtain laboratory tests, X-rays and some drugs free of charge. We are not burdened with deductibles and coinsurance payments. Some types of care such as dentists, treatment for mental illness and nursing homes are not free and could be a considerable burden to many families. But of all the national health insurance bills, Kennedy's coverage is the broadest.

No more health insurance premiums or hospital bills plague us under Kennedy's plan. Instead, money to pay doctors and hospitals comes from social security and income taxes.[8] But these payments are a burden also, especially to working people. Social security is unfair because families with low-paying jobs have to contribute as much as those with higher incomes. A bus driver with income of $9000 might pay $400 to social security while an engineer earning $19,000 also pays $400. And while workers pay social security out of their hard-earned wages, big investors pay nothing on the large dividends that fall into their laps.

Income taxes, the other source of money for Kennedy's plan, are more fair but still allow many rich businessmen to pay little or nothing. In 1969, 56 millionaires paid no income tax at all. And other millionaires pay fewer taxes than the average factory worker. So the Kennedy plan makes working Americans pay for the country's health bills and doesn't force top corporation executives to pay their share.

Kennedy's plan does not allow doctors and hospitals to set their own fees. It attempts to slow rising health costs by limiting these fees. Unnecessary surgery and excessive building and equipping of hospitals is discouraged. However, literature printed by the bill's supporters promises doctors that their high incomes will not suffer, so the commitment to cost control is unclear.

The plan calls for HMO's to take over a large share of health care delivery. Yet Senator Kennedy affirmed in 1973 that his plan will "not remove the freedom of every physician to choose where and how he provides health care." Like other national health insurance plans, the Kennedy bill fails to provide a family doctor for everyone in each neighborhood and town. Even though much of the care is free, we could get sick and be unable to find a doctor to take care of us.

The profit motive remains under the Kennedy bill. In fact, Senator Kennedy recently said, "I believe in maintaining the free enterprise system in this country and in American medicine." His HMO's, technically nonprofit, can accumulate millions of dollars of patients' money for growth, advertising, lobbying and high salaries. Drug companies, among the most profitable businesses in America, remain unchanged. The bill does reduce profit making by phasing out private insurance companies. But it leaves most other health-related profits untouched.

Even with the Kennedy bill, decisions about our health care will be made by businessmen and doctors, and by high government officials who listen mainly to businessmen and doctors. Of course doctors should be making medical decisions and skilled administrators should do the day-to-day running of hospitals. But it doesn't take a doctor or a businessman to decide how much doctors are paid, how a hospital spends it money, or during what hours care should be available.

All of us who work in or receive service at a hospital could be in on decisions about spending half a million dollars for a new research laboratory versus using that money for programs of preventive medicine in the community. Employees and patients of a hospital or clinic have a right to decide whether ten doctors are hired at $40,000 each or whether it is better to have twenty doctors at $20,000. If the entire health system were run by all of us rather than by doctors, it's likely that doctors couldn't get away with the incomes they now demand.

The Kennedy bill is the only national health insurance plan that could significantly relieve our health-care crisis. But it would be so expensive that taxpayers might be unwilling to support the plan. If Kennedy and the labor unions wanted real changes in health care, they might have demanded new governing bodies for hospitals and clinics. It seems pretty certain that if all people who use and who work in a hospital or clinic decided how health care money is used, more would go for needed services and less for high salaries and profits. Then we could really get more health care for less cost.

NATIONAL HEALTH INSURANCE AND PROFITS

Of the $83 billion that Americans spent for health in 1972 at least 10% went directly for profits.[9] Drug companies earn over $600 million in profits each year and spend $1.5 billion more in advertising. The health insurance industry collected $20 billion in premiums in 1970 and paid out only $17 billion in health care benefits. The companies kept $3 billion for administration, advertising and profits. The income of doctors is excessive as compared to the income of other highly trained professionals (professors or lawyers) in the amount of $2 billion per year. Nursing homes, proprietary hospitals and medical supply companies together earn $600 million in profits. So each year $8 billion in people's money leaves the health-care system as profits and profit-creating advertising and administration.

And that's only part of the picture. How about the 2 million needless operations performed each year that serve only to bring more income to surgeons? How about the 30% of days spent in the hospital that are unnecessary, costing $100 per patient per day and leading to the expensive overbuilding and overequipping of hospitals? How about the 60% of drug prescriptions that have no therapeutic value at all, prescribed because doctors receive most of their post-graduate education from drug company representatives and advertisements? According to testimony by Melvin Glasser of the United Auto Workers before the Senate Finance Committee in 1971, "*Approximately 20% of the total national expenditures for health, personal health services, is wasted, down the drain of unnecessary hospitalization, needless surgery, duplication of facilities, fragmentation and duplication of administrative costs." 20% means $16.6 billion dollars in 1972.*

Not only are these profit distortions expensive, they actually cause many people to die. At least 10,000 people die each year from operations that should never have been done. Additional thousands die from the side effects of drugs that should never have been prescribed. Both of these excesses are closely linked to the profits of surgeons and drug companies. Profit-making in health care is an extremely risky activity, and those of us who take the risks don't reap the benefits.

National health insurance is no cure for harmful profits. In fact, most of the plans are designed to increase profits. Under national health insurance, Americans will pay more for health care in private insurance payments, social security and taxes. This means a constant stream of money for doctors, hospitals, insurance companies, construction firms, equipment, supply and drug companies. Medicare and Medicaid showed the health industry that government insurance is good business.

National health insurance, then, is not a massive popular movement for better health care. 1970's-style national health insurance is mainly the creation of large health businesses to insure their economic well-being. So profits can be expected to have a clear edge over service in deciding health care priorities.

PUBLIC OR PRIVATE HEALTH CARE?

Any of the national health insurance plans would help those of us who become seriously ill and run up thousands of dollars in medical bills. The Kennedy bill would also help us pay most other health care costs. But further inflation caused by rising fees and profits could wipe out the gains made by a national health insurance law. And though national health insurance may help pay for health care, it doesn't promise that the care will be available.

The alternative to national health insurance—which is government-assisted financing of private health providers—is a public system of health care. Such a system would really have a chance to eliminate all financial worry about health care, make available family doctors when and where they are needed, and work toward eliminating the causes of ill health in our society.

According to Dr. George Silver, public health professor at Yale Medical School, "those insured under a national health insurance act will be physicians and hospitals, not patients. . . . The guarantee will be of payment to the providers, not of service to the patient." National health insurance provides money for private individuals and institutions to take care of our illnesses if, when and where they choose to do so. In contrast, under a public system the government feels responsible for our health. The public has control over the country's health resources and the government has the obligation to make an adequate supply of these resources available to everyone.

Many of us have had some experience with publicly run health care, whether county hospitals, Veterans Administration hospitals, or state mental institutions. The experience is usually a dismal one. Public facilities are shortstaffed, poorly administered, and grossly underfinanced.

There's a reason why public health institutions are so poorly financed. It has to do with their relation to the dominant private health sector. Private hospitals have overwhelming advantages over public hospitals in attracting money and manpower. The privates began with ample capital and with private doctors to admit paying patients to them. With the ability to get paying patients, private hospitals had a source of income that public hospitals, which derived from poorhouses, were denied. Medicare then provided large sums of tax money that private hospitals, with their superior resources, could also pull away from public hospitals. It is the usual up-or-down spiral characteristic of an economic system based on private capital: institutions and individuals that start out with money can always attract more money whereas those without money remain impoverished.

Public financing of private providers channels more money away from public institutions. Local taxpayers, predominantly working families, are forced to pay in three different ways: for their own health insurance allowing them to use private doctors and hospitals, for the billions in public money that pays through Medicare and Medicaid over 50% of private hospital budgets, and for the local public hospital to care for the cast-offs from the privates. Small wonder that the public sector can't get the money it needs to provide adequate services.

Private hospitals have always misused their public counterparts. Even with their massive public financing, privates take paying patients and send non-paying and "undesirable" patients to public hospitals. This "patient-dumping" reaches enormous proportions; *in Chicago, 18,000 emergency patients were refused admission to private hospitals in 1970.* The most fortunate ended up at Cook County Hospital; the unlucky —at least 50 people—died in the course of transfer.[10]

As long as a small, underfinanced public system coexists with a large wealthy private one, the private system will successfully compete for paying patients, doctors, money and power. If a health system is to be built that gets away from the distortions and high costs of the profit motive, it must eventually be entirely controlled by the public.

References

THE HEALTH STATUS OF AMERICANS (Ch. 1)

1. Nancy Worthington, "National Health Expenditures, 1929–74," *Social Security Bulletin* (February, 1975) p. 3.
2. *The Budget of the United States Government, Fiscal Year 1975*, U.S. Government Printing Office (Washington, 1975) p. 51.
3. U.S. National Center for Health Statistics, *Monthly Vital Statistics Report*, Vol. 23, No. 13 (May 30, 1975) p. 5.
4. Ibid., p. 15.
5. U.S. National Center for Health Statistics, *Infant Mortality Rates: Socioeconomic Factors*, Series 22, No. 14 (Rockville, Md., 1972).
6. David Kessner et al., *Infant Death: An Analysis by Maternal Risk and Health Care*, Institute of Medicine, National Academy of Sciences (Washington, D.C., 1973).
7. U.S. National Center for Health Statistics, *Vital Statistics of the United States, 1973*, Vol. 2, Section 5 (Rockville, Md., 1975) pp. 5-15.

8. U.S. National Center for Health Statistics, *Facts of Life and Death* (Rockville, Md., 1974) p. 7.
9. United Nations, *Demographic Yearbook 1973*, 25th Issue (New York, 1974) pp. 94–100.
10. United Nations, *Demographic Yearbook 1957*, 9th Issue (New York, 1957) pp. 558–588.
11. *The New York Times*, February 1, 1973.
12. Charles A. Hill, Jr., and Mozart I. Spector, "Natality and Mortality of American Indians Compared with U.S. Whites and Nonwhites," *HSMHA Health Reports*, Vol. 86, No. 3 (March, 1971) p. 229.
13. Robert E. Roberts and Cornelius Askew, Jr., "A Consideration of Mortality of Three Subcultures," *HSMHA Health Reports*, Vol. 87, No. 3 (March, 1972) p. 262.
14. U.S. National Center for Health Statistics, *Limitation of Activity and Mobility Due to Chronic Conditions, United States—1972*, Series 10, No. 96 (Rockville, Md., 1974) p. 3.
15. Ibid., p. 15.
16. Ibid., p. 7.
17. U.S. National Center for Health Statistics, *Health Characteristics of Low-Income Persons*, Series 10, No. 74 (Rockville, Md., 1972) p. 12.
18. U.S. National Center for Health Statistics, *Limitation of Activity*, op. cit., pp. 76–77.
19. U.S. House of Representatives, Committee on Ways and Means, *Basic Facts on the Health Industry*, U.S. Government Printing Office (Washington, D.C., 1971) p. 128.
20. Ibid., pp. 77–79.
21. U.S. National Center for Health Statistics, *Health Resources Statistics: Health Manpower and Health Facilities, 1974* (Rockville, Md., 1974) p. 202.
22. A. Donabedian et al. (eds.), *Medical Care Chartbook*, 5th edition, University of Michigan School of Public Health (Ann Arbor, 1972) p. 135.
23. Ibid., p. 181.

24. U.S. Bureau of the Census, *The Social and Economic Status of the Black Population in the United States, 1972,* U.S. Department of Commerce (Washington, D.C., 1973) p. 92.
25. U.S. House of Representatives, Committee on Ways and Means, op. cit., p. 132.
26. H. G. Mather et al., "Acute Myocardial Infarction: Home and Hospital Treatment," *British Medicine,* Vol. 3 (1971) p. 334.
27. Suzanne Arms, *Immaculate Deception,* Houghton Mifflin (Boston, 1975).
28. Doris Hair, *The Cultural Warping of Childbirth,* International Childbirth Education Association (Seattle, 1972).
29. U.S. Bureau of the Census, *Statistical Abstract of the United States: 1974,* 95th edition, U.S. Government Printing Office (Washington, D.C., 1974), p. 825.
30. Nancy Worthington, op. cit., p. 5.
31. A. Donabedian et al., op. cit., pp. 96–97.
32. U.S. House of Representatives, Committee on Ways and Means, op. cit., p. 18.
33. Ibid., p. 16.
34. U.S. House of Representatives, Committee on Ways and Means, op. cit., pp. 52–53.
35. Marjorie Smith Mueller, "Private Health Insurance in 1973: A Review of Coverage, Enrollment, and Financial Experience," *Social Security Bulletin* (February, 1975) p. 28.
36. Ibid., p. 37.
37. Howard West, "Five Years of Medicare—A Statistical Review," *Social Security Bulletin* (December, 1971), p. 17.
38. U.S. Office of Management and Budget, *Social Indicators, 1973,* U.S. Government Printing Office (Washington, D.C., 1973), p. 41.
39. Health Care Message from the President of the United States (February 6, 1974).

WHAT PEOPLE GET FROM HEALTH INSURANCE (Ch. 3)

1. Mueller, M. S. Private health insurance in 1971: Health care services, enrollment, and finances. *Social Security Bulletin* 36(2): 3–22, 1973.
2. Of paying and queuing. *Notes on Health Politics* 1: 1–2, September 1, 1973.
3. Hoyt, E. *Your Health Insurance: A Story of Failure.* The John Day Company, New York, 1970.

BLUE CROSS: WHAT WENT WRONG? (Chapter 3) *

1. See Herman M. and Anne R. Somers, "Private Health Insurance: Problems, Pressures and Prospects," 46 *Calif. L. Rev.* 508, 555–57 (1958). See also L. Barrett, "Retreat from Idealism: Blue Cross," *The Nation*, Jan. 9, 1960, pp. 26–32; E. T. Chase, "Can Blue Cross Survive Its Own Success?" 21 *The Reporter*, 18–19 (Oct. 29, 1959).
2. *Basic Facts on the Health Industry*, Report by the Staff of the House Committee on Ways and Means, 92nd Cong., 1st Sess., pp. 8 and 42 (1971).
3. Figures for Medicare and other federal programs are from SSA, BHI, *Quarterly Report to Providers* (1970). Medicaid figures are from internal data, Research and Development Dept., Blue Cross Association.
4. Dr. Odin W. Anderson, quoted in F. R. Hedinger, *The Social Role of Blue Cross as a Device for Financing the Costs of Hospital Care*, Health Care Research Series, No. 2, Iowa, p. 3 (1966). Hereinafter cited as Hedinger.
5. For a description of pre-Blue Cross hospital insurance,

* Comments are not included in the footnotes. They are designated here as "Footnote"; the reader may consult the original publication for the full text.

see T. J. Richardson, "*The Origin and Development of Group Hospitalization in the United States, 1890–1940*," 20 *University of Missouri Studies*, No. 3, pp. 15–18 (1945). See also Hedinger, Ref. 4, pp. 6–9; and Robert Eilers, *Regulation of Blue Cross and Blue Shield Plans*, Huebner Foundation Studies (Homewood, Ill.: Irwin, 1963), pp. 8–9. Hereinafter cited as Eilers.

6. R. G. Brodrick, M.D., Presidential Address, *Bulletin of the American Hospital Association*, October, 1927, pp. 25–27.
7. See Asa S. Bacon, "Hospital Budget-Savings Plan for Prospective Mothers," *Bulletin of the American Hospital Association*, January 1928, p. 68.
8. "A Statistical Analysis of 2,717 Hospitals," *Bulletin of the American Hospital Association*, July 1931, p. 68.
9. Louis S. Reed, *Health Insurance: the Next Step in Social Security* (N.Y.: Harper, 1937), p. 189.
10. See Hedinger, Ref. 4, pp. 4–13.
11. Justin Ford Kimball, "Prepayment and Hospital," *Bulletin of the American Hospital Association*, July 1934, p. 44. On the early history of Blue Cross, see also Duncan M. MacIntyre, *Voluntary Health Insurance and Rate Making* (Ithaca, N.Y.: Cornell University Press, 1962), pp. 166 et seq.; HEW, SSA, *Private Health Insurance and Medical Care* (1968); O. W. Anderson, *State Enabling Legislation for Non-Profit Hospital and Medical Plans*, Public Health Economics, Research Series, No. 1 (Ann Arbor, Mich.: University of Michigan, 1944).
12. Approval Program for Blue Cross Plans, AHA, 2M–12/70–1575, 1964, Standard No. 5.
13. Footnote. See also *Illinois Hospital Service, Inc. v. Gerber*, 18 Ill.2d 531, 165 N.E.2d 279 (1960).
14. Hedinger, Ref. 4, p. 24; MacIntyre, Ref. 11, p. 155.
15. Harry Becker, ed., *Financing Hospital Care in the United States* (N.Y.: McGraw-Hill, 1955), pp. 8–11.
16. *Research and Statistic Note*, No. 17 (Washington, D.C.: HEW, SSA, Oct. 13, 1965), p. 6; M. S. Mueller,

"Enrollment, Coverage and Financial Experience of Blue Cross and Blue Shield Plans, 1969," *Research and Statistic Note*, No. 4 (Washington, D.C.: HEW, SSA, April 21, 1971), p. 1; *National Health Insurance Proposals*, Hearings before the House Committee on Ways and Means, 92nd Cong., 1st Sess., p. 342 (1971).

17. R. Rorem, *Non-Profit Hospital Service Plans*, (Chicago: Commission on Hospital Service, 1940), p. 24.
18. Herman M. and Anne R. Somers, *Doctors, Patients, and Health Insurance* (Washington, D.C.: The Brookings Institution, 1961), p. 304.
19. Eilers, Ref. 5, p. 89; MacIntyre, Ref. 11, p. 154. Footnote. See also J. Stuart, "Blue Cross and Insurance: The Difference;" 33 *Hospitals* 51 (Feb. 16, 1959).
20. See O. D. Dickerson, *Health Insurance*, 3d ed. (Homewood, Ill.: Irwin, 1968), ch. 18, pp. 568–601; Frank Joseph Angell, *Health Insurance* (N.Y.: Ronald Press, 1963), pp. 363–66 and 478–90; and Edwin J. Faulkner, *Health Insurance* (N.Y.: McGraw-Hill, 1960), ch. 11, pp. 364–405, for an explanation of rate setting by commercial insurers. Moral, racist, and sexist factors not based on actuarial experience have played a role in selection of risks and determination of rates. See generally Edwin J. Faulkner, *Accident-and-Health Insurance* (N.Y.: McGraw-Hill, 1940), pp. 115–19 and 126–27. Footnote.
21. The number of persons hospitalized per 1,000 population per year broken down by family income and age. Footnote from HEW, Public Health Service, National Center for Health Statistics, *Persons Hospitalized by Number of Hospital Episodes and Days in a Year, United States—1968*, National Health Survey, Series 10, Number 64, DHEW Publication No. (HSM) 72–1029, p. 4 (1971).
22. On pressure by organized labor for experience rating see MacIntyre, Ref. 11, p. 155 et seq.; Hedinger, Ref. 4, pp. 65 et seq. Footnote from MacIntyre, Ref. 11, p. 161.
23. Unpublished data provided by the Public Relations

Department of the Blue Cross Association, 840 N. Lake Shore Drive, Chicago, Ill. 60611. The Vermont-New Hampshire plan has remained committed to community rating.

24. U.S. Service Mark Registration Number 554,448, registered Feb. 5, 1952; No. 554,817, registered Feb. 12, 1952; and 554,818, registered Feb. 12, 1952.
25. "The name 'Commission on Hospital Service' was subsequently changed to 'Hospital Service Plan Commission' and, finally, to 'Blue Cross Commission' in 1946. Legally, the Blue Cross Commission was a subordinate trust of the American Hospital Association. The Board of Trustees of the AHA could disapprove any course of action of the commission. Thus, the Blue Cross Commission was in a literal sense an arm or 'commission' of the American Hospital Asociation." Eilers, Ref. 5, p. 58.
26. "AHA and Blue Cross Split but Still a Twosome," *Medical World News*, Sept. 10, 1971, p. 20.
27. Telephone interview with Robert L. Mickelsen, Senior Director, Approval and Licensure, Blue Cross Association, June 28, 1973. (Prior to the transfer Mr. Mickelsen was an employee of the AHA, with the title Blue Cross Specialist.)
28. Bylaws, AHA and BCA. The 1971 organizational changes are reported in *AHA Convention Daily*, Aug. 25, 1971; *Modern Hospital*, September 1971, p. 37.
29. *Modern Hospital*, ibid. In June 1972 the AHA committee searching for a new president of that organization recommended Walter J. McNerney, President of BCA, *Washington Report on Medicine and Health*, No. 1305, July 3, 1972. The committee's recommendation was not accepted.
30. Footnote. Hearings before the Subcommittee on Antitrust and Monopoly of the Senate Committee of the Judiciary, 91st Cong., 2nd Sess., Pt. 2, p. 51 (January 1971). Herinafter cited as Hart Committee Hearings.
31. Id. at pp. 31, 54.
32. Ibid.

33. Id. at pp. 32–33, 61.
34. Id. at pp. 36–37, 48.
35. Id. at pp. 188–89.
36. Id. at p. 55. Footnote. Id. at p. 51.
37. *Blue Cross-Blue Shield Fact Book 1972*, (Chicago, BCA), p. 12.
38. Hart Committee Hearings, Ref. 30, p. 26.
39. For example, the Evaluation of Part A Intermediary Performance, SSA, March 19, 1971, based on the 18 months ending December 1970, indicated that the Richmond plan was one of the three Blue Cross plans in the nation that had an "unsatisfactory" composite of unit cost per bill processed. Footnote.
40. The Washington Blue Cross is called Group Health Association Inc. See *Administration of Federal Health Benefit Programs*, Hearings before a Subcommittee of the House Committee on Government Operations, 91st Cong., 2nd Sess., pp. 274–75 (1970).
41. Id. at pp. 274–75. Footnote. Id. at pp. 228, 255 and 261.
42. Footnote. A. Bajonski, "The Blue Cross Double Cross," 5 *Chi Journalism Rev.*, No. 2, p. 4 (February 1972), and A. Bajonski, "Further Notes on the Blue Cross Double Cross," 5 *Chi. Journalism Rev.*, no. 6, p. 19 (June 1972).
43. Hart Committee Hearings, Ref. 30, pp. 40–41.
44. Footnote on Congressional testimony by Walter McNerney regarding membership of Blue Cross boards.
45. For example, *N.J. Stat. Ann.* §17:48–5 (Supp. 1973); *Calif. Stat. Ann. Insurance* §11498 (1972); *Wisc. Stat. Ann.* §182.032(3)(a) (1957); *N.Y. Ins. Law* §250.1-a (Supp. 1973).
46. Hart Committee Hearings, Ref. 30, Pt. 2, p. 184. Footnote.
47. Id. at p. 131.
48. Footnote. Hart Committee Hearings, Ref. 30, p. 131.
49. See Sen. Edward Kennedy, *In Critical Condition* (N.Y.: Simon and Schuster, 1972), pp. 209–10.
50. According to BCA data, the board of directors or cor-

porate membership selects the public board members in 44 plans. Hart Committee Hearings, Ref. 30, pp. 177–82. Footnote.

51. Hart Committee Hearings, Ref. 30, at pp. 178 et seq. Footnote.
52. Ibid. Footnote.
53. See *Philadelphia Inquirer*, Jan. 30, 1972, p. 26; Feb. 14, 1971, p. F17, col. 1; Feb. 23, 1972, p. 17; *Philadelphia Bulletin*, Jan. 26, 1972, p. 9; Feb. 23, 1972, p. 38, col. 4. Footnote.
54. Footnote from Minutes, Associated Hospital Service, Nov. 22, 1972.
55. Footnote. Detailed data on each member of the Philadelphia plan board is compiled in an unpublished paper, "Conflicts of Interest on the 1970 Blue Cross of Greater Philadelphia Board," on file at the Health Law Project, 133 So. 36th Street, Philadelphia, Penn. 19174.
56. Footnote. Ibid.
57. The information upon which this tabulation is based was presented in *Physician Training Facilities and Health Maintenance Organization*, Hearings before the Subcommittee on Health of the Senate Committee on Labor and Public Welfare, 92nd Cong., 1st. Sess., Pt. 3, pp. 1043 ff. (Nov. 2, 1971). Footnote.
58. Footnote. See also *Administration of Federal Health Benefit Programs*, Ref. 40, p. 228
59. Footnote from Hart Committee Hearings, Ref. 30, p. 220. Dr. Harry Becker, a health economist long associated with Blue Cross and organized labor, estimates that the single most important objective of Blue Cross plan subscriber relations is to keep the blue chip accounts happy. Interview, May 6, 1971, New York, N.Y.
60. C. Silberstein, "Non-Group and Small Group Coverage: What's Available and How Much Does it Cost?" (Unpublished ms, Nov. 11, 1971). Se also *The American Health Empire*, A Report from the Health Policy Advisory Center (N.Y.: Random House, 1970), pp. 151–54.

61. The New York Insurance Department recently proposed regulations that would require insurance companies to maintain experience data for determining rates. Proposed Amendments to 11 N.Y.C.R.R. 52, issued Dec. 20, 1972.
62. Dr. Harry Becker explains that labor representatives impressed by the opportunity to meet, work, and socialize with financial and professional leaders take an accommodating and unquestioning role in exchange for amiable relationships on the board. Ref. 59.

COMMERCIAL INSURANCE COMPANIES: CAPITALIZING ON ILLNESS (Ch. 3)

1. *Source Book of Health Insurance Data*, pp. 36, 43. Health Insurance Institute, New York, 1973–1974.
2. *Best's Insurance Reports, Life-Health, 1971*. A. M. Best Company, Morristown, N.J., 1971.
3. Menshikov, S. *Millionaires and Managers*. Progress Publishers, Moscow, 1959.
4. Perlo, V. *The Empire of High Finance*. International Publishers, New York, 1957.
5. Rich Nixon contributor: Price favoritism denied. *San Francisco Chronicle*, p. 6, October 6, 1972.
6. *Basic Facts on the Health Industry*. Committee on Ways and Means, June 1971.

GETTING A FIX: THE U.S. DRUG MONOPOLY (Ch. 4)

1. Harvard Business School, *A Note on the U.S. Prescription Drug Industry*, Part 1, p. 6.
2. Hearings before the Subcommittee on Monopoly, Select Committee on Small Business, U.S. Senate, p. 5067 (Nelson Hearings).
3. *Up Against the Lab Bench II*, 1968.

4. Richard Goodman, "The Law and Monopoly, The Case of Tetracycline," *New University Thought*, Vol. 3, No. 4, p. 48, 1963.
5. Harvard Business School, exhibit 2.
6. H.E.W., *Task Force on Prescription Drugs*, U.S. Government Printing Office, 1968, pp. 12–13.
7. *Task Force on Prescription Drugs*, p. 19.
8. Nelson Hearings, p. 1903.
9. Harvard Business School, Part I, p. 18.
10. Harvard Business School, Part II, p. 42.
11. *Standard & Poor, Trade & Securities*, "Drugs, Cosmetics, Basic Analysis," May 2, 1968.
12. Nelson Hearings, p. 4299.
13. Harvard Business School, Part I, pp. 20–21.
14. Nelson Hearings, pp. 4487–4488.
15. Nelson Hearings, pp. 3216–3218.
16. Nelson Hearings, p. 3506.
17. Ibid.
18. Nelson Hearings, p. 3508.
19. Harvard Business School, Part II, p. 24.
20. Nelson Hearings, p. 4351.
21. Harvard Business School, Part II, p. 27.
22. *New Republic*, March 6, 1971.
23. FDA Commissioner Ley, Quoted in *Science*, Aug. 29, 1969, p. 877.
24. Borda, *J.A.M.A.*, 205:645, 1968.

THE HEALTH WORKFORCE: BIGGER PIE, SMALLER PIECES (Ch. 5)

1. *Statistical Abstract of the United States* (1973).
2. U.S. Department of Health, Education and Welfare, *Health Manpower Source Book: Allied Health Manpower, 1950–1980* (1970).
3. American Hospital Association, *Hospital Statistics: 1974 Edition* (Chicago, 1974).
4. William L. Kissick, "Health Manpower in Transition,"

Millbank Memorial Fund Quarterly, XLVI (January, 1968), 53–90.

5. National Center for Health Statistics, *Health Resources Statistics: Health Manpower and Health Facilities 1972–73.*
6. National Center for Health Statistics, *Health Resources Statistics: Health Manpower and Health Resources 1968.*
7. HEW Manpower Administration, *Technology and Manpower in the Health Service Industry 1965–75* (May, 1967).

DIVISION OF LABORERS (Ch. 6)

Government Publications*

1. Report on Licensure and Related Health Personnel Credentialling, DHEW Pub. No. (HSM) 72–11, June 1971.
2. Report of the National Advisory Commission on Health Manpower, Vols. I and II, U.S. Government Printing Office, Nov., 1967.
3. Equivalency and Proficiency Testing. Division of Allied Health Manpower, PHS, NIH, DHEW.
4. Health Manpower Source Books, PHS Pub. No. 263, 1970.
5. Health Manpower in Hospitals, Bureau of Health Manpower Education, PHS, DHEW, 1970.
6. Selected Training Programs for Physician Support Personnel, DHEW Pub. No. (NIH) 72–83, May 1972.
7. Hospitals: Industry Wage Survey, U.S. Dept. of Labor, BLS, Bulletin No. 1688, March, 1969.
8. Health Manpower, A County and Metropolitan Area Data Book, PHS Pub. No. 2044, June, 1971.
9. State Licensing of Health Occupations, PHS Pub. No. 1758, DHEW, 1968.

* DHEW is the U.S. Department of Health, Education and Welfare. PHS is the Public Health Service, a branch of DHEW. NIH is the National Institutes of Health.

10. Accreditation and Certification . . . in Relation to Allied Health Manpower, DHEW, PHS-NIH, (NIH) Pub. No. 71–192, Bureau of Health Manpower Education, 1971.

Other References

1. Study of Accreditation of Selected Health Educational Programs, Final Report and Staff Working Papers, Parts I and II, SASHEP, 1 Dupont Circle, Washington NW, D.C.
2. Physician Associate. Journal of the American Academy of Physician Associates, 6900 Grove Road, Thorofare, N.J.
3. The Physician Assistant: Today and Tomorrow, Alfred M. Sadler, Blair L. Sadler and Ann A. Bliss, New Haven: Yale University Press, 1972.
4. Allied Health Trends, Newsletter of the Association of Schools of Allied Health Professions, 1 Dupont Circle NW, Washington, D.C.
5. Medical Licensure and Discipline in the U.S., Robert C. Derbyshire, Baltimore: Johns Hopkins Press, 1969.
6. Allied Health Manpower: Trends and Prospects, Harry Greenfield and Carol A. Brown, New York: Columbia University Press, 1969.
7. Health Manpower Development and Utilization. A Framework for Advocacy Focusing on Physician Assistant Development, William Plumb, Berkeley, California. Available at Health/PAC.
8. Witches, Midwives and Nurses, A History of Women Healers, Barbara Ehrenreich and Deirdre English. (Oyster Bay, N.Y.: Glass Mountain Pamphlets).
9. Hospital Workers: A Case Study in the "New Working Class," John and Barbara Ehrenreich, *Monthly Review*, Jan., 1973. See Chapter 5.

ORIGINS OF THE GOVERNMENT HEALTH INSURANCE ISSUE (Ch. 8)

1. Odin W. Anderson, "Compulsory Medical Care Insurance, 1910–1950," *The Annals of the American Academy of Political and Social Science*, CCLXXIII (January, 1951), 106–113. Reprinted in Eugene Feingold (ed.), *Medicare: Policy and Politics* (San Francisco: Chandler Publishing, 1966), p. 89.
2. Ibid., Feingold, p. 90.
3. *Congress and the Nation, 1945–1964* (Washington, D.C.: Congressional Quarterly Service, 1965), pp. 4, 7.

CORPORATE MEDICINE: THE KAISER HEALTH PLAN (Ch. 9)

1. *The Big Foundations*, Waldemar Nielsen, 20th Century Fund Study, Columbia University, 1973, pages 245–46.
2. *Kaiser Wakes the Doctors*, Paul de Kruiff, 1948.
3. *Chicago Sun*, June 20, 1945.
4. *The Kaiser-Permanente Medical Care Program*, A Symposium, Anne R. Somers, editor, The Commonwealth Fund, New York, 1971, page 13.
5. Nielsen, op. cit., page 247.
6. Ibid., page 248.
7. See section 37.59 Kaiser Hospital General Specifications, City Hall, Redwood City, California, February 15, 1966.
8. *The Case for American Medicine*, Harry Schwartz, 1972, page 174.
9. Somers, op. cit., page 42.
10. Ibid., page 42.
11. *Health Insurance Effects*, Roemer, Hetherington, Hopkins, Gerst, Parson and Long, School of Public Health, The University of Michigan, 1972.

12. "Social Class Differences in Utilization of Pediatric Services in a Prepaid Direct Service Medical Care Program," Nolan, Schwartz, Simonian, *American Journal of Public Health*, January, 1967.
13. *Feelings About the Kaiser Foundation Health Plan on the Part of Northern California Carpenters and Their Families*, April 5, 1973, CCHPA, 1870 Ogden Drive, Burlingame, Cal., 94010.
14. Somers, op cit., page 16.
15. *Kaiser-Permanente Health Plan, Why It Works*, Greer Williams, The Henry J. Kaiser Foundation, Oakland, Cal., 1971, page 38.
16. Nolan, et al., op. cit., page 48.
17. Roemer, et al., op cit., page 45.
18. Ibid., page 32.
19. Nolan, et al. op cit., pages 38–40.
20. Ibid., page 45.
21. Williams, op cit., page 48.
22. "An Evaluation of Prepaid Group Practice," Avedis Donabedian, *Inquiry*, Vol. VI, Number 3, pages 1–15.
23. Nolan, et al., op cit., page 42.
24. Hearings Before the Subcommittee on Health of the Committee on Labor and Public Welfare, United States Senate, Part 4, page 1484.
25. Somers, op cit., page 91.
26. Personal Communication.
27. Roemer, et al., op cit.
28. *The Federal Employees Health Benefits Program*, 1971, studies utilization from 1961–68 in four different types of health insurance plans which were offered Federal employees and their families across the nation. The four types are group practice (seven plans, four of them are Kaiser), the Blues, commercial plans, and what they call individual-practice plans, such as the San Joaquin Foundation for Medical Care.
29. *The Report of the Medical and Hospital Advisory Council to the Board of Administration of the California State Employees' Retirement System* (The Sacramento Study) presents data gathered for 1962–63

from California state employees who were members of the same four different types of health insurance plans as in the Federal study.

30. *Family Medical Care Under Three Types of Health Insurance*, Columbia University, 1962, compares the 1958 experiences of members of Kaiser in northern California, New Jersey Blue Cross-Blue Shield and a commercial plan, General Electric, in the Midwest. A major drawback of this study is that the data are now 15 years old.
31. Footnotes 27, 28, 29.
32. The Columbia study found a similarly low rate for tonsillectomies at Kaiser, but found no differences in adult surgery rates.
33. Roemer, et al., op cit., pages 27–34.
34. Footnotes 27, 28, 29.
35. Roemer, et al., op cit., page 45.
36. *Financial Study of the Kaiser Medical Care Program*, Working Paper Number 12, Robert A. Vradiu, David B. Starkweather, and Alfred W. Childs. University of California, Berkeley, Unpublished manuscript.
37. Personal Communication.

THE $8-BILLION HOSPITAL BED OVERRUN

1. P.L. 89–749, §2, Comprehensive Health Planning and Public Health Services Amendments of 1966, codified as 42 U.S.C. 246 et. seq.
2. Hearings before the Committee on Interstate and Foreign Commerce on H.R. 6418, The Partnership for Health Amendments of 1967, pp. 15–16 (1967).
3. The newly created local Comprehensive Health Planning Agencies were, by and large, updated versions of already existing agencies in the voluntary health planning structure—former hospital planning or health and welfare councils—groups that traditionally had spent much of their time on hospital construction

proposals. See Ardell, D. R., "Public Regional Councils and Comprehensive Health Planning: A Partnership?" *Journal of the American Institute of Planners*, p. 397 (1970); *The American Health Empire: Power, Profits, and Politics* (Random House, 1970), pp. 199–213; "A Descriptive Analysis of CHP "B" Agencies," p. 78.

4. See note 1.
5. *Comprehensive Health Planning as Carried Out by State and Areawide Agencies in Three States*, General Accounting Office, April, 1974.
6. D. Donoghue, P., Bryant, A., and Shaughnessy, P., "A Descriptive Analysis of CHP 'B' Agencies," Interstudy (1973) p. 9.
7. "Health Agency Faulted to Hospital Bed Oversupply," *The Daily Oklahoman*, November 15, 1974.
8. Interview with Ms. Julia Borbely-Brown, Citizens Concerned about Durham Health Care, Durham, North Carolina.
9. Letter to the Honorable Francis B. Burch from Mr. Frank M. Kratovil, March 27, 1974.
10. "A Descriptive Analysis of CHP "B" Agencies," p. 20.
11. Id.
12. Anderson, D., and Anderson, N. N., "Comprehensive Health Planning in the States: A Current Status Report," p. 3, Health Services Research Center, American Rehabilitation Foundation, Minneapolis, Minnesota (1969).
13. Danaceau, P., "The Puget Sound Health Planning Council, A Case Study of Consumer Participation in Seattle, Washington." An unpublished paper prepared for the Health Services Institute for Children and Families, Inc., Rosslyn, Virginia.
14. "A Descriptive Analysis of CHP 'B' Agencies," pp. 15, 78.
15. Id. p. 79.
16. *Comprehensive Health Planning As Carried Out by State and Areawide Agencies in 3 States*, by the Comptroller of the United States, April 13, 1974.

THE MALPRACTICE BLOW-UP: FIGHTING OVER THE CARCASS

1. *San Francisco Chronicle*, February 13, 1975.
2. *Washington Post*, July 18, 1972.
3. Silverman, M. and Lee, P. R., *Pills, Profits and Politics* (Berkeley: University of California Press, 1974), p. 290.
4. *San Francisco Chronicle*, April 9, 1975.
5. Silverman and Lee, op. cit., p. 290.
6. Thomas, D. L., "Malpractice Epidemic," *Barron's*, March 31, 1975.
7. David, L., "A Physician Answers His Critics," *Physicians' World*, December, 1974.
8. Thomas, *op. cit.*

THE MALPRACTICE CRISIS: EVASIVE MEDICINE

1. Physicians Crisis Committee, *Court Docket Survey* (Detroit: The Committee, 1975), calculated from data at pp. 42–43.
2. "Argonuat and Malpractice: A Tangled Web," *Medical World News* 16:23–25 at p. 25 (July 14, 1975).
3. Howard Eisenberg, "New Light on the Costliest Malpractice Mistakes," *Medical Economics* 50:146–163 at p. 147 (August 20, 1973).
4. One insurance official is quoted as telling the AMA Board of Trustees that "this is not an insurance problem but a medical-insurance problem. We need the medical profession's help in weeding out those physicians who are contributing to the problem." "AMA Trustees Seek a Solution," *American Medical News*, June 23–30, 1975.
5. U.S. DHEW, *Report of the Secretary's Commission on Medical Malpractice* (Washington, D.C.: The Department, 1973), p. 9.
6. That hospital-linked malpractice statistics need to be

analyzed in terms of the types of practitioners involved is suggested by the Detroit-area study, which examined the number of patient admissions per malpractice case for 55 hospitals and found that of the 17 university-affiliated teaching hospitals that sample included, 12 had better-than-average malpractice case ratios. Physicians Crisis Committee, *op. cit.*, p. 39.

7. Advertisement for Saffer Medical Consultants, *New York Times*, Sunday, August 24, 1975, Section 4.
8. Everett R. Holles, "Doctors Are Joining Services to Avoid Malpractice Insurance Costs," *New York Times*, March 22, 1975.
9. Lawrence K. Altman, "Malpractice Rates Drive Up Doctor Fees," *New York Times*, July 27, 1975.
10. "Court Upholds Hospital Rule on Malpractice Coverage," *Hospitals* 49:171 (March 16, 1975).
11 Don Harper Mills, "Malpractice Litigation: Are Solutions in Sight?," *JAMA* 232:369–373 at p. 373 (April 28, 1975).
12. Eisenberg, *op. cit.*, p. 163.
13. Raymond S. Duff and August B. Hollingshead, *Sickness and Society* (New York: Harper & Row, 1968), p. 380.
14. From "We have been concerned to show the connections between the growth of commercial practices in certain sectors of medical care and the increasing application of the laws of the marketplace—of legalized and legitimated doctor-patient hostility. The second is a logical consequence of the first." Richard M. Titmuss, *The Gift Relationship* (New York: Pantheon Books, 1971), p. 170.
15. George W. Northrup, D.O., quoted in "How the Commission Arrived at a Report," *Medical World News* 14:44–48 at p. 48 (October 5, 1973).

WHO WILL PAY YOUR BILLS?

1. Feingold, E. *Medicare: Policy and Politics* (San Francisco, Chandler Publishing Co., 1966), 86–101.

2. Kisch, A. and Gartside, F. "Use of a county hospital outpatient department by MediCal recipients" *Medical Care*, Nov.-Dec. 1968.; Blake, E. "Medicaid: the fading of a dream," *Health PAC Bulletin*, April, 1973 (see references at end of the article); *Heal Yourself* (available from American Public Health Association, 1015 18th St., N.W. Washington, D.C. 20036), p. 35.
3. *Medical Care Costs and Prices: Background Book* (Department of Health, Education and Welfare, January, 1972), pp. 23, 41.
4. *Business Week*, February 27, 1971.
5. *San Francisco Chronicle*, July 13, 1973.
6. Congressional bills are available from your Senator or Congressperson. The "Medicredit" bill is S. 444 (in the Senate) and H.R. 2222 (in the House). An explanation of the bill, "Medical and Health Care for All" can be obtained from the American Medical Association, 535 N. Dearborn St., Chicago, Ill. 60610.

   The Health Insurance Association of America's bill is S. 1100/H.R. 5200 and the American Hospital Association bill is H.R. 1. For Feldstein's proposal, see Feldstein, M. "A new approach to national health insurance," *The Public Interest*, Spring, 1971.
7. The Kennedy plan is S. 3/H.R. 22. For more information from the supporters of the proposal, write to the Committee for National Health Insurance, 806 15th St., N.W. Washington, D.C. 20005. A detailed analysis of the Kennedy bill and the 1971 Nixon plan was prepared by the National Health Law Program, School of Law, University of California, Los Angeles, Calif. 90024 on January 1, 1972.
8. For further discussion of social security and taxation, see Pechman, J. et al., *Social Security: Perspectives for Reform* (Washington: The Brookings Institution, 1968); Pechman, J. *Federal Tax Policy* (Washington: The Brookings Institution, 1971); and Stern, P. *The Rape of the Taxpayer* (New York: Random House, 1973).
9. Documentation for these three paragraphs:

Profits in general: "The medical-industrial complex" *Health PAC Bulletin*, November, 1969.

Drug advertising: Burack, R. *The New Handbook of Prescription Drugs* (Ballantine Books, 1970), p. 20.

Deaths from prescription drugs: Testimony by Dr. Henry Simmons of the FDA, December 7, 1972.

Doctors' incomes: If each of the 200,000 practicing doctors earns an average of $10,000 in excess income, the total comes to $2 billion each year.

Insurance industry administrative costs: Data compiled by the Health Professionals for Political Action (Box 386, Kenmore Station, Boston, Mass. 02215, August 1, 1973) shows that government-administered insurance is substantially cheaper to run than private insurance.

Unnecessary hospitalization: Testimony of Dr. Amos Johnson, past president of the American Association of General Practice, before the Senate Antitrust and Monopoly Subcommittee, February 24, 1970.

For information on unnecessary surgery, see: Bunker, J. "Surgical manpower. A comparison of operations and surgeons in the United States and in England and Wales" *New England Journal of Medicine*, Jan. 15, 1960; Denenberg, H. "A shopper's guide to surgery: 14 rules on how to avoid unnecessary surgery" available from the State of Pennsylvania Insurance Commissioner; the figure of 10,000 deaths from unnecessary surgery comes from Ralph Nader's Health Research Group (*San Francisco Chronicle*, December 17, 1971); another estimate is that unneeded operations kill 24,000 people each year (*Washington Post*, July 18, 1972).

20% of health expenditures are wasted: Melvin Glasser, in Hearings before the Senate Finance Committee, "National health insurance" April, 1971, p. 130.

15. Roemer, M. and Mera, J. "'Patient-dumping' and other voluntary agency contributions to public agency problems" *Medical Care*, Jan.-Feb. 1973.

Index

THE HEALTH POLICY ADVISORY CENTER is an independent, nonprofit research and educational organization engaging in analysis on issues of health policy, for an audience that includes health-care workers, community groups and students. Established in New York City in 1968, Health/PAC opened a West Coast office in 1971 in San Francisco. It publishes a bi-monthly journal, the Health/PAC *Bulletin* and issued its first book-length report, *The American Health Empire*, in 1970.

DAVID KOTELCHUCK, who received his Ph.D. in physics from Cornell University, served on the faculty of Vanderbilt University and Mt. Sinai School of Medicine before joining Health/PAC in 1972. His area of expertise is occupational health, and he serves as a consultant to the United Electrical Workers Union and other union and community groups.

8—76

VINTAGE HISTORY—WORLD

V-286 ARIES, PHILIPPE *Centuries of Childhood*
V-59 BEAUFRE, GEN. ANDRÉ *NATO and Europe*
V-44 BRINTON, CRANE *The Anatomy of Revolution*
V-250 BURCKHARDT, C. J. *Richelieu: His Rise to Power*
V-393 BURCKHARDT, JACOB *The Age of Constantine the Great*
V-391 CARR, E. H. *What Is History?*
V-67 CURTIUS, ERNST R. *The Civilization of France*
V-746 DEUTSCHER, ISAAC *The Prophet Armed*
V-747 DEUTSCHER, ISAAC *The Prophet Unarmed*
V-748 DEUTSCHER, ISAAC *The Prophet Outcast*
V-471 DUVEAU, GEORGES *1848: The Making of a Revolution*
V-707 FISCHER, LOUIS *Soviets in World Affairs*
V-475 GAY, PETER *The Enlightenment: The Rise of Modern Paganism*
V-277 GAY, PETER *Voltaire's Politics*
V-114 HAUSER, ARNOLD *The Social History of Art* through V-117 (Four Volumes)
V-201 HUGHES, H. STUART *Consciousness and Society*
V-50 KELLY, AMY *Eleanor of Aquitaine and the Four Kings*
V-728 KLYUCHEVSKY, V. *Peter the Great*
V-246 KNOWLES, DAVID *Evolution of Medieval Thought*
V-83 KRONENBERGER, LOUIS *Kings and Desperate Men*
V-287 LA SOUCHÈRE, ÉLÉNA DE *An Explanation of Spain*
V-43 LEFEBVRE, GEORGES *The Coming of the French Revolution*
V-364 LEFEBVRE, GEORGES *The Directory*
V-343 LEFEBVRE, GEORGES *The Thermidorians*
V-474 LIFTON, ROBERT J. *Revolutionary Immortality: Mao Tse-Tung and the Chinese Cultural Revolution*
V-92 MATTINGLY, GARRETT *Catherine of Aragon*
V-703 MOSELY, PHILIP E. *The Kremlin and World Politics:* Studies in Soviet Policy and Action
V-733 PARES, SIR BERNARD *The Fall of the Russian Monarchy*
V-285 PARKES, HENRY B. *Gods and Men*
V-719 REED, JOHN *Ten Days That Shook the World*
V-176 SCHAPIRO, LEONARD *Government and Politics of the Soviet Union* (Revised Edition)
V-375 SCHURMANN & SCHELL (eds.) *The China Reader: Imperial China,* I
V-376 SCHURMANN & SCHELL (eds.) *The China Reader: Republican China,* II
V-377 SCHURMANN & SCHELL (eds.) *The China Reader: Communist China,* III
V-312 TANNENBAUM, FRANK *Ten Keys to Latin America*
V-322 THOMPSON, E. P. *The Making of the English Working Class*
V-749 TROTSKY, LEON *Basic Writings of Trotsky*
V-724 WALLACE, SIR D. M. *Russia:* On the Eve of War and Revolution
V-206 WALLERSTEIN, IMMANUEL *Africa: The Politics of Independence*
V-729 WEIDLÉ, W. *Russia:* Absent and Present
V-122 WILENSKI, R. H. *Modern French Painters,* Volume I (1863-1903)

V-123 WILENSKI, R. H. *Modern French Painters,* Volume II (1904-193[illegible])

V-106 WINSTON, RICHARD *Charlemagne:* From the Hammer to the Cross

VINTAGE HISTORY—AMERICAN

V-365 ALPEROVITZ, GAR *Atomic Diplomacy*
V-334 BALTZELL, E. DIGBY *The Protestant Establishment*
V-198 BARDOLPH, RICHARD *The Negro Vanguard*
V-42 BEARD, CHARLES A. *The Economic Basis of Politics* and Related Writings
V-60 BECKER, CARL L. *Declaration of Independence*
V-17 BECKER, CARL L. *Freedom and Responsibility in the American Way of Life*
V-191 BEER, THOMAS *The Mauve Decade:* American Life at the End of the 19th Century
V-199 BERMAN, H. J. (ed.) *Talks on American Law*
V-211 BINKLEY, WILFRED E. *President and Congress*
V-513 BOORSTIN, DANIEL J. *The Americans: The Colonial Experience*
V-358 BOORSTIN, DANIEL J. *The Americans: The National Experience*
V-44 BRINTON, CRANE *The Anatomy of Revolution*
V-37 BROGAN, D. W. *The American Character*
V-72 BUCK, PAUL H. *The Road to Reunion, 1865-1900*
V-98 CASH, W. J. *The Mind of the South*
V-311 CREMIN, LAWRENCE A. *The Genius of American Education*
V-190 DONALD, DAVID *Lincoln Reconsidered*
V-379 EMERSON, THOMAS I. *Toward A General Theory of the First Amendment*
V-424 FOREIGN POLICY ASSOCIATION, EDITORS OF *A Cartoon History of United States Foreign Policy—Since World War I*
V-368 FRIEDENBERG, EDGAR Z. *Coming of Age in America*
V-264 FULBRIGHT, J. WILLIAM *Old Myths and New Realities* and Other Commentaries
V-463 GAY, PETER *A Loss of Mastery: Puritan Historians in Colonial America*
V-31 GOLDMAN, ERIC F. *Rendezvous with Destiny*
V-183 GOLDMAN, ERIC F. *The Crucial Decade—and After:* America, 1945-1960
V-95 HOFSTADTER, RICHARD *The Age of Reform*
V-9 HOFSTADTER, RICHARD *American Political Tradition*
V-317 HOFSTADTER, RICHARD *Anti-Intellectualism in American Life*
V-120 HOFSTADTER, RICHARD *Great Issues in American History,* Volume I (1765-1865)
V-121 HOFSTADTER, RICHARD *Great Issues in American History,* Volume II (1864-1957)
V-385 HOFSTADTER, RICHARD *The Paranoid Style in American Politics and Other Essays*
V-242 JAMES, C. L. R. *The Black Jacobins*
V-367 LASCH, CHRISTOPHER *The New Radicalism in America*
V-386 MCPHERSON, JAMES *The Negro's Civil War*
V-318 MERK, FREDERICK *Manifest Destiny in American History*
V-84 PARKES, HENRY B. *The American Experience*
V-371 ROSE, WILLIE LEE *Rehearsal for Reconstruction*
V-212 ROSSITER, CLINTON *Conservatism in America*
V-285 RUDOLPH, FREDERICK *The American College and University:* A History
V-394 SEABURY, PAUL *Power, Freedom and Diplomacy*

V-530 SCHLESINGER, ARTHUR M. *Prelude to Independence*
V-52 SMITH, HENRY NASH *Virgin Land*
V-345 SMITH, PAGE *The Historian and History*
V-432 SPARROW, JOHN *After the Assassination: A Positive Appraisal of the Warren Report*
V-388 STAMPP, KENNETH *The Era of Reconstruction 1865-1877*
V-253 STAMPP, KENNETH *The Peculiar Institution*
V-244 STEBBINS, RICHARD P. *U. S. in World Affairs, 1962*
V-110 TOCQUEVILLE, ALEXIS DE *Democracy in America, Vol. I*
V-111 TOCQUEVILLE, ALEXIS DE *Democracy in America, Vol. II*
V-103 TROLLOPE, MRS. FRANCES *Domestic Manners of the Americans*
V-265 WARREN, ROBERT PENN *Legacy of the Civil War*
V-368 WILLIAMS, T. HARRY *Lincoln and His Generals*
V-208 WOODWARD, C. VANN *Burden of Southern History*